Clinical Neurogenetics

Editor

BRENT L. FOGEL

NEUROLOGIC CLINICS

www.neurologic.theclinics.com

Consulting Editor
RANDOLPH W. EVANS

November 2013 • Volume 31 • Number 4

ELSEVIER

1600 John F. Kennedy Boulevard • Suite 1800 • Philadelphia, Pennsylvania, 19103-2899

http://www.theclinics.com

NEUROLOGIC CLINICS Volume 31, Number 4
November 2013 ISSN 0733-8619, ISBN-13: 978-0-323-26108-1

Editor: Donald Mumford

Photocopying

Single photocopies of single articles may be made for personal use as allowed by national copyright laws. Permission of the Publisher and payment of a fee is required for all other photocopying, including multiple or systematic copying, copying for advertising or promotional purposes, resale, and all forms of document delivery. Special rates are available for educational institutions that wish to make photocopies for non-profit educational classroom use. For information on how to seek permission visit www.elsevier.com/permissions or call: (+44) 1865 843830 (UK)/(+1) 215 239 3804 (USA).

Derivative Works

Subscribers may reproduce tables of contents or prepare lists of articles including abstracts for internal circulation within their institutions. Permission of the Publisher is required for resale or distribution outside the institution. Permission of the Publisher is required for all other derivative works, including compilations and translations (please consult www.elsevier.com/permissions).

Electronic Storage or Usage

Permission of the Publisher is required to store or use electronically any material contained in this periodical, including any article or part of an article (please consult www.elsevier.com/permissions). Except as outlined above, no part of this publication may be reproduced, stored in a retrieval system or transmitted in any form or by any means, electronic, mechanical, photocopying, recording or otherwise, without prior written permission of the Publisher.

Notice

No responsibility is assumed by the Publisher for any injury and/or damage to persons or property as a matter of products liability, negligence or otherwise, or from any use or operation of any methods, products, instructions or ideas contained in the material herein. Because of rapid advances in the medical sciences, in particular, independent verification of diagnoses and drug dosages should be made.

Although all advertising material is expected to conform to ethical (medical) standards, inclusion in this publication does not constitute a guarantee or endorsement of the quality or value of such product or of the claims made of it by its manufacturer.

Neurologic Clinics (ISSN 0733-8619) is published quarterly by Elsevier Inc., 360 Park Avenue South, New York, NY 10010–1710. Months of issue are February, May, August, and November. Periodicals postage paid at New York, NY, and additional mailing offices. Subscription prices are $285.00 per year for US individuals, $489.00 per year for US institutions, $140.00 per year for US students, $359.00 per year for Canadian individuals, $586.00 per year for Canadian institutions, $397.00 per year for international individuals, $586.00 per year for international institutions, and $199.00 for Canadian and foreign students/residents. To receive student/resident rate, orders must be accompanied by name of affiliated institution, date of term, and the *signature* of program/residency coordinator on institution letterhead. Orders will be billed at individual rate until proof of status is received. Foreign air speed delivery is included in all *Clinics* subscription prices. All prices are subject to change without notice. **POSTMASTER:** Send address changes to *Neurologic Clinics*, Elsevier Health Sciences Division, Subscription Customer Service, 3251 Riverport Lane, Maryland Heights, MO 63043. **Customer Service: Telephone: 1-800-654-2452 (U.S. and Canada); 314-447-8871 (outside U.S. and Canada). Fax: 314-447-8029. E-mail: journalscustomerservice-usa@elsevier.com (for print support); journalsonlinesupport-usa@elsevier.com (for online support).**

Reprints. For copies of 100 or more of articles in this publication, please contact the Commercial Reprints Department, Elsevier Inc., 360 Park Avenue South, New York, New York, 10010-1710; Tel.: +1-212-633-3874; Fax: +1-212-633-3820, and E-mail: reprints@elsevier.com.

Neurologic Clinics is also published in Spanish by Nueva Editorial Interamericana S.A., Mexico City, Mexico.

Neurologic Clinics is covered in *Current Contents/Clinical Medicine, MEDLINE/PubMed (Index Medicus), EMBASE/Excerpta Medica,* and *PsycINFO,* and *ISI/BIOMED.*

Printed and bound by CPI Group (UK) Ltd, Croydon, CR0 4YY

Transferred to digital print 2012

Contributors

CONSULTING EDITOR

RANDOLPH W. EVANS, MD
Clinical Professor, Department of Neurology, Baylor College of Medicine, Houston, Texas

EDITOR

BRENT L. FOGEL, MD, PhD
Program in Neurogenetics, Department of Neurology, David Geffen School of Medicine, University of California Los Angeles, Los Angeles, California

AUTHORS

ROBERT H. BALOH, MD, PhD
Associate Professor of Neurology, Director of Neuromuscular Medicine, ALS Program; Director, Department of Neurology, Regenerative Medicine Institute, Cedars-Sinai Medical Center; Associate Professor-in-Residence, Department of Neurology, University of California, Los Angeles, California

YVETTE M. BORDELON, MD, PhD
Associate Clinical Professor, Department of Neurology, David Geffen School of Medicine at UCLA, Los Angeles, California

ABIGAIL COLLINS, MD
Assistant Professor, Pediatrics and Neurology, School of Medicine, Children's Hospital Colorado, University of Colorado Denver, Aurora, Colorado

ROHINI COORG, MD
Pediatric Epilepsy Fellow, Department of Neurology, Washington University School of Medicine, St Louis, Missouri

KRISTIN E. D'ACO, MD
Assistant Professor, Division of Medical Genetics, Department of Pediatrics, Golisano Children's Hospital, University of Rochester Medical Center, Rochester, New York

BRENT L. FOGEL, MD, PhD
Program in Neurogenetics, Department of Neurology, David Geffen School of Medicine, University of California Los Angeles, Los Angeles, California

PEYMAN GOLSHANI, MD, PhD
Assistant Professor, Department of Neurology, David Geffen School of Medicine, University of California, Los Angeles, California

DEBORAH A. HALL, MD, PhD
Associate Professor, Department of Neurological Sciences, Rush University, Chicago, Illinois

MATTHEW B. HARMS, MD
Assistant Professor of Neurology, Neuromuscular Division, Department of Neurology, Hope Center for Neurological Disorders, Washington University School of Medicine, St Louis, Missouri

JENNIFER M. KWON, MD
Associate Professor, Division of Child Neurology, Departments of Neurology and Pediatrics, University of Rochester Medical Center, Rochester, New York

GUSTAVO H.B. MAEGAWA, MD, PhD, FACMG
Assistant Professor, Department of Pediatrics, McKusick-Nathans Institute of Genetic Medicine, The Johns Hopkins University School of Medicine, Baltimore, Maryland

SUNIL Q. MEHTA, MD, PhD
Health Sciences Clinical Instructor, Department of Psychiatry and Biobehavioral Sciences, David Geffen School of Medicine, University of California, Los Angeles, California

JOAN A. O'KEEFE, PT, PhD
Assistant Professor, Department of Anatomy and Cell Biology, Rush University, Chicago, Illinois

GREGORY M. PASTORES, MD
Associate Professor, Departments of Neurology and Pediatrics; Neurogenetics Laboratory, New York University School of Medicine, NYU at Rivergate, New York, New York

NATALIA S. ROST, MD, MPH
Associate Professor, Department of Neurology, JP Kistler Stroke Research Center, Massachusetts General Hospital, Boston, Massachusetts

VIKRAM G. SHAKKOTTAI, MD, PhD
Department of Neurology, University of Michigan, Ann Arbor, Michigan

NUTAN SHARMA, MD, PhD
Department of Neurology, Massachusetts General Hospital, Harvard Medical School, Boston, Massachusetts

PERRY B. SHIEH, MD, PhD
Associate Professor, Director of Neuromuscular Program, Department of Neurology, UCLA School of Medicine, Los Angeles, California

JEFFREY L. WAUGH, MD, PhD
Department of Neurology, Massachusetts General Hospital, Harvard Medical School; Department of Neurology, Boston Children's Hospital, Boston, Massachusetts

JUDITH L.Z. WEISENBERG, MD
Assistant Professor, Department of Neurology, Washington University School of Medicine, St Louis, Missouri

ERIC WEXLER, MD, PhD
Department of Psychiatry, Center for Neurobehavioral Genetics, Semel Institute, University of California Los Angeles School of Medicine, Los Angeles, California

MICHAEL WONG, MD, PhD
Associate Professor, Department of Neurology, Washington University School of Medicine, St Louis, Missouri

Contents

Preface   xi

Brent L. Fogel

Clinical Neurogenetics: Recent Advances in the Genetics of Epilepsy   891

Rohini Coorg, Judith L.Z. Weisenberg, and Michael Wong

Epilepsy represents a diverse group of disorders with primary and second-ary genetic etiologies, as well as non-genetic causes. As more causative genes are identified, genetic testing is becoming increasingly important in the evaluation and management of epilepsy. This article outlines the clinical approach to epilepsy patients, with emphasis on genetic testing. Specific targeted tests are available for numerous individual genetic causes of epilepsy. Broader screening tests, such as chromosome micro-array analysis and whole exome sequencing, have also been developed. As a standardized protocol for genetic testing has not been established, individualized diagnostic approaches to epilepsy patients should be used.

Clinical Neurogenetics: Stroke   915

Natalia S. Rost

Understanding the genetic architecture of cerebrovascular disease holds promise of novel stroke prevention strategies and therapeutics that are both safe and effective. Apart from a few single-gene disorders associated with cerebral ischemia or intracerebral hemorrhage, stroke is a complex genetic phenotype that requires careful ascertainment and robust associ-ation testing for discovery and validation analyses. The recently uncovered shared genetic contribution between clinically manifest stroke syndromes and closely related intermediate cerebrovascular phenotypes offers effec-tive and efficient approaches to complex trait analysis.

Clinical Neurogenetics: Amyotrophic Lateral Sclerosis   929

Matthew B. Harms and Robert H. Baloh

Our understanding of amyotrophic lateral sclerosis (ALS), a fatal neuro-degenerative disease, is expanding rapidly as its genetic causes are uncovered. The pace of new gene discovery over the last 5 years has accelerated, providing new insights into the pathogenesis of disease and highlighting biological pathways as targets for therapeutic develop-ment. This article reviews our current understanding of the heritability of ALS and provides an overview of each of the major ALS genes, highlighting their phenotypic characteristics and frequencies as a guide for clinicians evaluating patients with ALS.

Clinical Neurogenetics: Autism Spectrum Disorders   951

Sunil Q. Mehta and Peyman Golshani

Autism spectrum disorders are neurodevelopmental disorders character-ized by deficits in social interactions, communication, and repetitive or restricted interests. There is strong evidence that de novo or inherited genetic alterations play a critical role in causing Autism Spectrum Disorders, but non-genetic causes, such as in utero infections, may also play a role. Magnetic resonance imaging based and autopsy studies indicate that early rapid increase in brain size during infancy could underlie the deficits in a large subset of subjects. Clinical studies show benefits for both behavioral and pharmacological treatment strategies. Genotype-specific treatments have the potential for improving outcome in the future.

Clinical Neurogenetics: Dystonia From Phenotype to Genotype   969

Jeffrey L. Waugh and Nutan Sharma

Dystonia can arise from genetic syndromes or can be secondary to nongenetic injuries; both causes can produce pure dystonia, dystonia plus other movement disorders, or paroxysmal mixed movement disorders. Genetic causes of dystonia are inherited through dominant, recessive, X-linked, and mitochondrial mechanisms, may show anticipation, are variably penetrant, and may be limited to small ethnic populations or single families. In this article, the genetic causes of dystonia, an algorithm for their diagnosis and management, information on common medications and surgical treatments, and resources for affected families and those interested in advancing research are presented.

Clinical Neurogenetics: Autosomal Dominant Spinocerebellar Ataxia   987

Vikram G. Shakkottai and Brent L. Fogel

The autosomal dominant spinocerebellar ataxias are a diverse and clinically heterogeneous group of disorders characterized by degeneration and dysfunction of the cerebellum and its associated pathways. Clinical and diagnostic evaluation can be challenging because of phenotypic overlap among causes, and a stratified and systematic approach is essential. Recent advances include the identification of additional genes causing dominant genetic ataxia, a better understanding of cellular pathogenesis in several disorders, the generation of new disease models that may stimulate development of new therapies, and the use of new DNA sequencing technologies, including whole-exome sequencing, to improve diagnosis.

Clinical Neurogenetics: Muscular Dystrophies and Other Genetic Myopathies   1009

Perry B. Shieh

With advances in the genetics of muscle disease, the term, *muscular dystrophy*, has expanded to include mutations in an increasing large list of genes. This review discusses the genetics, pathophysiology, and potential treatments of the most common forms of muscular dystrophy: Duchenne muscular dystrophy, Becker muscular dystrophy, facioscapulohumeral muscular dystrophy, and myotonic dystrophy. Other forms of muscular dystrophy and other genetic muscle disorders are also discussed to provide an overview of this complex clinical problem.

Clinical Neurogenetics: Neurologic Presentations of Metabolic Disorders   1031

Jennifer M. Kwon and Kristin E. D'Aco

This article reviews aspects of the neurologic presentations of selected treatable inborn errors of metabolism within the category of small molecule disorders caused by defects in pathways of intermediary metabolism. Disorders that are particularly likely to be seen by neurologists include those associated with defects in amino acid metabolism (organic acidemias, aminoacidopathies, urea cycle defects). Other disorders of small molecule metabolism are discussed as additional examples in which early treatments have the potential for better outcomes.

Clinical Neurogenetics: Neuropathic Lysosomal Storage Disorders   1051

Gregory M. Pastores and Gustavo H.B. Maegawa

The lysosomal storage disorders are a clinically heterogeneous group of inborn errors of metabolism, associated with the accumulation of incompletely degraded macromolecules within several cellular sites. Affected individuals present with a broad range of clinical problems, including hepatosplenomegaly and skeletal dysplasia. Onset of symptoms may range from birth to adulthood. Most are associated with neurologic features. Later-onset forms are often misdiagnosed as symptoms, which might include psychiatric manifestations, are slowly progressive, and may precede other neurologic or systemic features. Symptomatic care, which remains the mainstay for most subtypes, can lead to significant improvement in quality of life.

Clinical Neurogenetics: Fragile X–Associated Tremor/Ataxia Syndrome   1073

Deborah A. Hall and Joan A. O'Keefe

This article summarizes the clinical findings, genetics, pathophysiology, and treatment of fragile X–associated tremor ataxia syndrome. The disorder occurs from a CGG repeat (55–200) expansion in the *fragile X mental retardation 1* gene. It manifests clinically in kinetic tremor, gait ataxia, and executive dysfunction, usually in older men who carry the genetic abnormality. The disorder has distinct radiographic and pathologic findings. Symptomatic treatment is beneficial in some patients. The inheritance is X-linked and family members may be at risk for other fragile X–associated disorders. This information is useful to neurologists, general practitioners, and geneticists.

Clinical Neurogenetics: Huntington Disease   1085

Yvette M. Bordelon

Huntington disease (HD) is an autosomal dominant, adult-onset, progressive neurodegenerative disease characterized by the triad of abnormal movements (typically chorea), cognitive impairment, and psychiatric problems. It is caused by an expanded CAG repeat in the gene encoding the protein huntingtin on chromosome 4 and causes progressive atrophy of the striatum as well as cortical and other extrastriatal structures. Genetic testing has been available since 1993 to confirm diagnosis in affected adults and for presymptomatic testing in at-risk individuals. This review covers HD signs, symptoms, and pathophysiology; current genetic testing issues; and current and future treatment strategies.

Clinical Neurogenetics: Friedreich Ataxia   1095

Abigail Collins

Friedreich ataxia is the most common autosomal recessive ataxia. It is a progressive neurodegenerative disorder, typically with onset before

20 years of age. Signs and symptoms include progressive ataxia, ascending weakness and ascending loss of vibration and joint position senses, pes cavus, scoliosis, cardiomyopathy, and arrhythmias. There are no disease-modifying medications to either slow or halt the progression of the disease, but research investigating therapies to increase endogenous frataxin production and decrease the downstream consequences of disrupted iron homeostasis is ongoing. Clinical trials of promising medications are underway, and the treatment era of Friedreich ataxia is beginning.

Clinical Neurogenetics: Behavioral Management of Inherited Neurodegenerative Disease   **1121**

Eric Wexler

Psychiatric symptoms often manifest years before overt neurologic signs in patients with inherited neurodegenerative disease. The most frequently cited example of this phenomenon is the early onset of personality changes in "presymptomatic" Huntington patients. In some cases the changes in mood and cognition are even more debilitating than their neurologic symptoms. The goal of this article is to provide the neurologist with a concise primer that can be applied in a busy clinic or private practice.

Index   **1145**

NEUROLOGIC CLINICS

FORTHCOMING ISSUES

February 2014
Neuroimaging
Lazslo Mechtler, MD, *Editor*

May 2014
Secondary Headache
Randolph W. Evans, MD, *Editor*

August 2014
Myopathies
Mazen M. Dimachkie, MD, and
Richard J. Barohn, MD, *Editors*

RECENT ISSUES

August 2013
Advances in Neurologic Therapy
José Biller, MD, FACP, FAAN, FANA, FAHA,
Editor

May 2013
Peripheral Neuropathies
Richard J. Barohn, MD, and
Mazen M. Dimachie, MD, FAAN, *Editors*

February 2013
Spinal Cord Diseases
Alireza Minagar, MD, FAAN, and
Alejandro A. Rabinstein, MD, FAAN,
Editors

RELATED INTEREST

Psychiatric Clinics of North America, March 2010
Psychiatric Genetics
James B. Potash, *Editor*

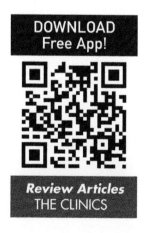

DOWNLOAD
Free App!

Review Articles
THE CLINICS

NOW AVAILABLE FOR YOUR iPhone and iPad

Preface

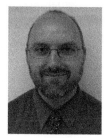

Brent L. Fogel, MD, PhD
Editor

We are presently in the midst of a rapid acceleration in the discovery of novel genetic etiologies for neurologic disorders, the development of greater insights into molecular pathogenesis, and the emergence of new technologies to facilitate efficient diagnosis of diseases spanning the breadth of Neurology. Consequently, the role of human genetic variation in neurologic disease has never been more at the clinical forefront than it is today. In this issue of *Neurologic Clinics*, this rapidly burgeoning relationship is elegantly presented through a collection of articles covering a broad cross—section of neurologic disease, illustrating how such recent genetic advances have impacted the clinical practice of neurology.

In this issue, we are treated to a broad perspective across the neurologic landscape demonstrating how neurogenetic discoveries have modified the clinical approach to common neurologic diseases and symptoms, as well as improved our understanding of known genetic diseases. Genetic contributions will be highlighted across a variety of diverse neurologic conditions, including epilepsy, stroke, amyotrophic lateral sclerosis, and autism spectrum disorders. Additional articles discuss the genetic etiologies to be considered in patients presenting with dystonia or spinocerebellar ataxia. Of many, one theme that stands out among these various topics is the impact of next—generation sequencing on gene discovery and the important clinical role for genomic medical techniques, such as diagnostic whole exome sequencing, moving forward.

For clinicians who currently treat or may encounter patients with known genetic disorders, relevant updates in the muscular dystrophies and genetic myopathies, metabolic disorders, and lysosomal storage disorders are presented. Focused articles describe current clinical knowledge in the specific genetic diseases Fragile X—associated tremor/ataxia syndrome, Huntington disease, and Friedreich ataxia. Finally, a comprehensive discussion of the treatment of comorbid behavioral manifestations in patients with inherited neurodegenerative disease reminds us that although underlying molecular etiologies may differ, in the absence of disease-specific treatments, symptomatic approaches benefit a wide variety of neurogenetic patients, irrespective of etiology.

It is becoming clear that as the numbers of disease genes and related mutations rise, primary care and community physicians will be presented more and more often

Neurol Clin 31 (2013) xi–xii
http://dx.doi.org/10.1016/j.ncl.2013.06.001
0733-8619/13/$ – see front matter © 2013 Published by Elsevier Inc.

with patients affected by (or at risk for) neurogenetic disease. Therefore, comprehensive clinical reviews, providing focused discussions for a genetically targeted approach to a patient with a distinct presentation or disease, or, alternatively, for the management of patients with specific neurogenetic conditions, will become essential for day—to—day practice. In the development of this series of articles, I thank the dedicated clinicians and neuroscientists who have enthusiastically contributed their expertise to this issue, as well as Donald Mumford, for his editorial experience and guidance. To you, the readers, those both well versed in genetics and those newly acquainted to the field, I present this issue as an illustration of the current state of clinical neurogenetics and the bright future which lies ahead.

Brent L. Fogel, MD, PhD
Department of Neurology, Program in Neurogenetics
David Geffen School of Medicine at the University of California, Los Angeles
695 Charles E. Young Drive South
Gonda 1206
Los Angeles, CA 90095, USA

E-mail address:
bfogel@ucla.edu

Clinical Neurogenetics
Recent Advances in the Genetics of Epilepsy

Rohini Coorg, MD, Judith L.Z. Weisenberg, MD,
Michael Wong, MD, PhD*

KEYWORDS

- Epilepsy • Seizure • Genetics

KEY POINTS

- Epilepsy is not a single disease. It can result from many diseases, and may be classified into primary genetic, structural/metabolic, or unknown causes.
- Electroclinical syndromes are specific types of epilepsy that have characteristic ages of onset, seizure types, electroencephalographic abnormalities, and other features. Many of these electroclinical syndromes are currently of unknown cause, but most are presumed to be genetic in origin and some have been found to have primary genetic causes.
- Other epilepsies are secondary to other well-defined structural or metabolic diseases or entities, which may also have genetic causes.
- Genetic testing is an increasingly useful way to establish a diagnosis and aid in treatment of epilepsy. An individualized approach to genetic testing should be adapted for each patient.
- Although at present there are limitations and challenges to genetic testing, ongoing and future research may expand the utility and applications of genetics in epilepsy.

INTRODUCTION
Definitions

A seizure is a transient, stereotyped change in behavior caused by abnormal neuronal activity in the brain.[1] Epilepsy is traditionally defined by the occurrence of 2 or more unprovoked seizures. An updated definition of epilepsy includes the occurrence of a single seizure in the context of a brain disorder predisposing to future seizures.[1] Epilepsy has a prevalence of 0.5% to 1% in the general population.[2] Epilepsy may itself be a primary disorder, often with a known genetic origin, or may be part of a group of symptoms comprising another disease. It may also exist secondary to a metabolic cause, structural brain malformation, or acquired injury.

Funding Sources: None (R. Coorg); NINDS (J.L.Z. Weisenberg, M. Wong); DOD (M. Wong).
Conflicts of Interest: None.
Department of Neurology, Washington University School of Medicine, Box 8111, 660 South Euclid Avenue, St Louis, MO 63110, USA
* Corresponding author.
E-mail address: wong_m@wustl.edu

Classification

The International League Against Epilepsy (ILAE) has recently revised the terminology and classification system for seizure types and epilepsy.[3] This system describes seizures as involving networks within the brain, rather than single areas. Seizures can have a wide range of clinical manifestations, and may be classified as focal or generalized. Focal seizures originate within networks localized to one hemisphere, whereas generalized seizures involve initiation and rapid propagation within distributed networks involving both hemispheres (**Box 1**).

From an etiologic standpoint, ILAE reorganized epilepsy into having a "genetic," "structural/metabolic," or "unknown" cause.[3] Electroclinical syndromes are specific types of epilepsy that share characteristic clinical features, seizure types, and patterns on an electroencephalogram (EEG). Electroclinical syndromes resulting from a known primary genetic abnormality are classified as epilepsies with a "genetic" cause (formerly known as "idiopathic" epilepsy). Most of the remaining electroclinical syndromes do not have an identified cause but are still presumed to have an underlying genetic cause, often polygenic in nature. In addition, epilepsy may be secondary to well-defined structural or metabolic abnormalities or diseases (formerly known as "symptomatic" epilepsy), some of which also have genetic causes. Finally, the remaining types of epilepsy without a known or presumed etiology are grouped as having an "unknown cause" (formerly known as "cryptogenic"). This article provides a brief overview of the different clinical presentations of epilepsy related to primary and secondary genetic etiology, and outlines the clinical approach to evaluation of patients with epilepsy, focusing on the role of genetic testing. Epilepsies attributable to nongenetic causes are outside the scope of this review.

Box 1
2010 ILAE classification of seizure types

Generalized seizures

    Tonic-clonic

    Absence

        Typical

        Atypical

        With special features: myoclonic, eyelid myoclonia

    Myoclonic

        Myoclonic

        Myoclonic atonic

        Myoclonic tonic

    Clonic

    Tonic

    Atonic

Focal seizures

Unknown

    Epileptic spasms

CLINICAL FINDINGS, GENETICS, AND ETIOLOGY
Primary Genetic Causes/Electroclinical Syndromes

Electroclinical syndromes with known genetic causes are summarized in **Table 1**. A few selected syndromes are discussed here, and are organized by age of onset: the neonatal period and infancy (the first 2 years of life), childhood (ages 2–11 years), and adolescence (ages 12–17 years).

Syndromes with onset in the neonatal period and infancy

Benign familial neonatal epilepsy is an autosomal dominant electroclinical syndrome with an 85% penetrance linked to a mutation in a voltage-gated potassium channel.[4,5] This syndrome may occur in otherwise developmentally normal infants, with age of onset during the first 3 months of life. These seizures may be of multiple types but are usually characterized as tonic, and may occur up to 30 times daily.[6] Resolution occurs 1 to 6 months after onset, but as many as 14% of neonates develop other seizure types later.[6] Benign familial neonatal-infantile epilepsy is an autosomal dominant sodium channelopathy with onset in the first 7 months, usually resolving by 12 months.[7] The seizures are brief, usually with focal features such as eye and head deviation, occur in clusters of 5 to 10 per day, and occur in the setting of normal development.[8]

Benign infantile epilepsy presents similarly with an onset between 3 and 20 months of age and is characterized by focal, brief seizures occurring in clusters during the day. These seizures may consist of behavioral arrest, head or eye deviation, or unilateral clonic activity.[8] It has been linked to regions in chromosome 19.[9] Of note, benign infantile epilepsy may occur with familial hemiplegic migraine owing to missense mutations in the *ATP1A2* transporter gene,[10] or with choreoathetosis caused by a mutation in *PRRT2* in chromosome 16.[11,12] In all 3 of these epilepsy syndromes, an interictal EEG obtained between seizures is normal and the long-term prognosis is relatively good.

Early infantile epileptic encephalopathy with suppression-burst (EIEE or Ohtahara syndrome), on the other hand, is a severe epilepsy occurring during the first 3 months of life characterized by tonic spasms occurring during wakefulness and sleep. Affected infants have abnormal neurologic examinations and a high risk of mortality, and a corresponding EEG showing a suppression-burst pattern.[6] This electroclinical syndrome has been linked to mutations in *ARX*,[13,14] *CDKL5*,[15] *STXBP1*,[16–18] *PLB1*,[19] and *KCNQ2*,[20] and affected infants who survive may have seizures that evolve into infantile spasms.[6]

Just as different genotypes may produce a shared epilepsy phenotype, mutations affecting a single gene may result in different phenotypes. *SCN1A* sodium channel–related disorders include generalized epilepsy with febrile seizures plus (GEFS+), severe myoclonic epilepsy of infancy (Dravet syndrome), and myoclonic-astatic epilepsy (myoclonic epilepsy of Doose). These syndromes may show incomplete penetrance or variable expressivity, and may also occur de novo.[21–23]

GEFS+ is a syndrome typically affecting multiple family members with different generalized seizure phenotypes, ranging from simple febrile seizures to Dravet syndrome. The EEG may be normal in up to 50% of children with GEFS+, or may demonstrate generalized polyspike-wave in the remainder, depending on the phenotype.[23] In addition to *SCN1A* other genes have been identified, which are listed in **Table 1**. In children with GEFS+, genotype does not predict phenotype or prognosis.[22]

Children with Dravet syndrome comprise the most severe phenotype caused by mutations in *SCN1A* (**Box 2**). Dravet syndrome is a rare and progressive epilepsy with onset within the first year of life, usually affecting previously developmentally

Table 1
Electroclinical syndromes with known genetic causes

Electroclinical Syndromes	Genes (or Locus, if Gene Unavailable)	Mode of Inheritance (if Known)	Available Testing	References
Generalized Epilepsies of Neonates and Infancy				
Benign familial neonatal epilepsy	KCNQ2, KCNQ3	Autosomal dominant	Sequence and deletion/ duplication analysis	4,5,54
Benign familial neonatal-infantile epilepsy	SCN2A	Autosomal dominant	Sequence analysis	5,7,54-56
Benign familial infantile epilepsy	(19q), PRRT2 (with choreoathetosis) ATP1A2 (with hemiplegic migraine)	Autosomal dominant	PRRT2: Sequence analysis ATP1A2: Sequence analysis	5,9-12,54,56
Early infantile epileptic encephalopathy with suppression-burst	ARX, CDKL5, STXBP1, PLB1, KCNQ2	ARX, CDKL5: X-linked dominant STXBP1: Autosomal dominant PLB1: Autosomal recessive KCNQ2: Autosomal dominant	All: Sequence and deletion/ duplication analysis	13-20,54,56
Familial infantile myoclonic epilepsy	TBC1D24	Autosomal recessive	Sequence analysis (not commercially available in USA)	54,56,57
Genetic/generalized epilepsy with febrile seizures plus (GEFS+)	Type 1: SCN1B Type 2: SCN1A Type 3: GABRG2 Other: SCN2A GABRD	SCN1A, SCN1B, SCN2A: Autosomal dominant	SCN1B, GABRG2, GABRD, SCN2A: Sequence analysis SCN1A: Sequence and deletion/ duplication analysis PCDH19: Sequence and deletion/ duplication analysis	21,22,45,54-56
Severe myoclonic epilepsy of infancy (Dravet syndrome)	SCN1A, SCN2A, GABRG2	SCN1A, SCN2A: Autosomal dominant	SCN1A: Sequence and deletion/ duplication analysis SCN2A: Sequence analysis GABRG2: Sequence analysis	21,22,45,54-56

Myoclonic-astatic epilepsy (myoclonic epilepsy of Doose)	SCN1A, SCN1B, GABRG2, SLC2A1 (5%)	SCN1A, SCN2A: Autosomal dominant; SLC2A: Autosomal dominant or recessive	SCN1A: Sequence and deletion/duplication analysis; SCN1B: Sequence analysis; SLC2A1: Sequence and deletion/duplication analysis; GABRG2: Sequence analysis	21,22,25,54-56
Epilepsy and mental retardation limited to females (EFMR)	PCDH19	PCDH19: X-linked	PCDH19: Sequence and deletion/duplication analysis	21,56,58,59
Generalized Epilepsies of Childhood and Adolescence				
Childhood absence epilepsy	GABRG2, GABRA1 (CAE with JME), SLC2A1 (early onset), GABRB3 (Austrian), CACNA1H (Chinese), CACNG3, LGI4	SLC2A: Autosomal dominant or Recessive; LGI4: Autosomal recessive, GABRA1: Autosomal dominant	All: Sequence analysis	27,28,30,43,54,56,60
Childhood absence epilepsy with febrile seizures	GABRG2		Sequence analysis	54,60
Childhood absence epilepsy with ataxia	CACNA1A		Sequence analysis	54,60
Juvenile absence epilepsy	ME2, INHA (Turkish)	ME2: Autosomal recessive	Testing not commercially available	54,56,60
Juvenile myoclonic epilepsy	GABRA1, EFHC1, BRD2, CACNB4	GABRA1: Autosomal dominant	All: Sequence analysis	54,61-65
Epilepsy and paroxysmal exercise-induced dyskinesia	SLC2A1	SLC2A1: Autosomal dominant	Sequence and deletion/duplication analysis	45,54,56,66

(continued on next page)

Table 1
(continued)

Electroclinical Syndromes	Genes (or Locus, if Gene Unavailable)	Mode of Inheritance (if Known)	Available Testing	References
Focal epilepsies				
Autosomal dominant nocturnal frontal lobe epilepsy	*CHRNA4, CHRNB2, CHRNA2*	Autosomal dominant	All: Sequence analysis	31–34,45,54
Autosomal dominant lateral temporal lobe epilepsy/ autosomal dominant partial epilepsy with auditory features	*LGI1*	Autosomal dominant	Sequence analysis	36,37,45,54
Benign epilepsy with centrotemporal spikes (BECTS)/benign childhood epilepsy with centrotemporal spikes (BCECTS)/benign Rolandic epilepsy/Rolandic epilepsy	*ELP4, KCNQ2* (1 report)	*KCNQ2:* One case, de novo post-benign neonatal seizures BECTS (heterozygous mutation)	Testing not commercially available	39,40,61
Autosomal dominant partial epilepsy with variable foci	(22q11–q12)	Autosomal dominant	Causative gene not identified	54,56,67–70
Familial mesial temporal lobe epilepsy	(4q13.2–q21.3), (7p21.3), (1q25 and 18q, digenic), (12q22–q23.3)	Complex Inheritance	Causative genes not identified	54,56,67,71–74

> **Box 2**
> **Case summary 1**
>
> A 2-year-old boy presented with seizures since 6 months of age. These seizures occurred multiple times a year with high fevers, and were characterized by generalized stiffening and rhythmic jerking of both arms and legs for up to 30 minutes. Seizures often resulted in hospital admissions for status epilepticus. His neurologic examination and development were initially normal but he began experiencing generalized tonic-clonic seizures, as well as myoclonic and focal seizures, without fever. These multiple seizures were poorly responsive to antiseizure medication and he started to develop signs of developmental delay. An electroencephalogram (EEG) performed during his most recent admission showed generalized slowing, and magnetic resonance imaging (MRI) of the brain was normal. Fragile X testing was performed and showed normal results. SCN1A gene sequencing was negative. A chromosomal microarray showed a loss in copy number of the long arm of chromosome 2 spanning a minimum of 0.015 Mb and maximum of 0.028 Mb. The deleted segment included part of the SCN1A gene. This case illustrates a typical presentation of a child with Dravet syndrome.

normal children.[23] For unknown reasons, twice as many boys as girls are affected.[23] A typical disease course may begin with a deceivingly mild period up to 6 months with febrile seizures, often generalized clonic or hemiclonic in nature. Afterward, multiple seizures types may ensue, including myoclonic, atypical absence, and focal seizures. Multiple episodes of status epilepticus and a severe encephalopathy may occur between the second and sixth year, followed by a relatively stable period. Ataxia and pyramidal signs may be seen.[23] The EEG may initially be normal, but often develops generalized or multifocal spikes later. Similar to GEFS+, Dravet syndrome may occur as a result of alterations in other genes in voltage-gated sodium or γ-aminobutyric acid channels (see **Table 1**).

Myoclonic epilepsy of Doose has also been linked to *SCN1A*, and is characterized by frequent head drops followed by myoclonic and astatic (atonic) seizures. Other seizure types include myoclonic-astatic, absence, and tonic-clonic seizures. The onset is usually between 2 and 5 years, and its clinical course and prognosis are variable.[22–24] Of note, 5% of children with myoclonic-astatic seizures were reported in one study to have glucose-1 transporter deficiency owing to a mutation in the *SCL2A1* gene. These children also had intellectual disability.[25]

Syndromes with onset in childhood and adolescence
Well-characterized generalized epilepsies with onset in childhood and adolescence include childhood absence epilepsy (CAE) and juvenile myoclonic epilepsy (JME). These electroclinical syndromes remain a primarily clinical diagnosis, and genetic testing is not routinely done. CAE is characterized by absence seizures beginning between 2 and 10 years of age corresponding with a 3-Hz generalized spike and wave pattern on EEG, activated by hyperventilation.[26] Absence seizures appear as sudden onset of activity arrest, lip-smacking, eye-blinking, and alteration of consciousness usually lasting between 4 and 20 seconds followed by immediate return to normal consciousness. Prognosis for epilepsy remission and developmental outcome with this syndrome is usually excellent.[26] Genes associated with rare familial cases of CAE are described in **Table 1**. Ten percent of children with absence epilepsy and early onset before 4 years of age may have a mutation in *SLC2A1*, making glucose-1 transporter deficiency an important diagnosis to consider in the differential.[27–30]

JME, a well-known and often life-long syndrome with a complex inheritance, has an onset between 5 and 20 years of age and consists of myoclonic seizures on awakening, generalized tonic-clonic seizures (in more than 90%), and absence seizures

---

Box 3
Case summary 2

A 6-month-old, former term infant was brought to clinic with seizures since 3 months of age. These seizures were first described as right-arm shaking. Now her parents described brief episodes of eye rolling and bilateral upper extremity extension occurring in clusters lasting 5 to 30 seconds long. Occasionally the family noticed she would have head drops with these episodes. Her neurologic examination was significant for mild axial hypotonia and multiple hypopigmented macules on her trunk and extremities. She also had a shagreen patch on her right elbow. An EEG was performed, which revealed hypsarrhythmia. An MRI scan of the brain showed a dominant left frontal tuber with extensive cortical tubers in both hemispheres **(Fig. 1)**. In addition, a 9 × 5-mm enhancing subependymal nodule was seen near the right foramen of Monroe. Her spasms responded to vigabatrin; however, the seizures consisting of right-hand shaking continued. By 2 years of age, she was using her left hand more than her right hand. She was referred for surgical evaluation. A complete tuberous sclerosis gene panel revealed a deletion of exon 15 in the TSC2 gene. This case demonstrates an infant diagnosed with tuberous sclerosis complex presenting with infantile spasms. It also highlights the importance of the physical examination, as her dermatologic findings aided in diagnosis.

(in more than one-third of patients).[26] Generalized tonic-clonic seizures can be provoked by sleep deprivation, stress, and fatigue.[26] An EEG typically shows fast (3–6 Hz) generalized spike and wave discharges and photoparoxysmal response in up to one-third of patients. **Table 1** displays a list of genes involved to date, including both channel and nonchannel proteins.

Focal epilepsy syndromes with an onset in late childhood or adolescence include autosomal dominant nocturnal frontal lobe epilepsy, autosomal dominant lateral temporal lobe epilepsy, and benign epilepsy with centrotemporal spikes (BECTS). Autosomal dominant nocturnal frontal lobe epilepsy is characterized by onset between 7 and 12 years (ranging from infancy to adulthood), and involves genes coding for nicotinic acetylcholine receptors.[31–34] Individuals with this syndrome experience brief, stereotyped nocturnal seizures, which may often be of bizarre semiology. Examples include thrashing, posturing, pedaling, or crawling behavior. These seizures tend to occur just before awakening and may secondarily generalize.[35] Electrographic changes during seizures may be seen on EEG in more than 80% of patients, and 20% to 30% of patients with this clinical syndrome may have positive genetic testing.[35]

Autosomal dominant lateral temporal lobe epilepsy, also known as autosomal dominant partial epilepsy with auditory features, has an onset in adolescence or adulthood. This syndrome is characterized by auditory hallucinations and rare nocturnal generalized tonic-clonic seizures. Visual changes, such as simple lights, colors, and shapes, can also occur. An interictal EEG is typically normal.[35,36] Mutations in *LGI1* have been linked to this electroclinical syndrome.[37]

BECTS, otherwise known as benign Rolandic epilepsy, is a common focal epilepsy syndrome presenting between 1 and 14 years of age. It is characterized by nocturnal focal motor seizures, primarily involving the face, and secondary generalized seizures with bilateral centrotemporal spikes on EEG with a horizontal dipole.[38] Although this syndrome remains a clinical diagnosis, it has been linked to mutations in *ELP4*.[39] A recent case report also suggests a relationship to *KCNQ2*, a gene associated with benign familial neonatal epilepsy[40] and EIEE.[20] Remission usually occurs 2 to 4 years after onset, with emerging evidence of potential cognitive long-term effects.[38]

Structural/Metabolic Causes

Epilepsy may be secondary to other structural, metabolic, and genetic syndromes. Many genetic disorders causing intellectual or other neurologic disability include an

Table 2
Malformations of cortical development with known genetic causes and commonly involving epilepsy

Structural/Metabolic Cause of Epilepsy: Malformations of Cortical Development	Genes	Mode of Inheritance (if Known)	Available Testing	References
Holoprosencephaly	SHH, PTCH1, ZIC2, SIX3, TGIF	Autosomal dominant (all)	Chromosome analysis, aCGH, All genes listed: Sequence analysis	56,75,76
Schizencephaly	EMX2		Sequence analysis (not commercially available in USA)	56,75
Lissencephaly	LIS1, ARX, DCX	ARX, DCX: X-linked LIS1: de novo	All: Sequence analysis	56,75,77
Double-cortex syndrome	DCX	X-Linked	Sequence analysis	75,77
Periventricular heterotopia, X-linked	FLN1 (FLNA)	X-Linked	Sequence analysis	75,78
Neurocutaneous syndromes				
Tuberous sclerosis	TSC1, TSC2	Autosomal dominant	Sequence analysis of both TSC1 and TSC2, Deletion/duplication of both TSC1 and TSC2	75,79
Neurofibromatosis type I	NF1	Autosomal dominant	Sequence analysis	75,80

Table 3
Inborn errors of metabolism commonly involving epilepsy

Structural/Metabolic Cause of Epilepsy: (Selected) Inborn Errors of Metabolism	Genes	Mode of Inheritance (if Known)	Available Testing	References
Pyridoxine (vitamin B6) deficiency	ALDH7A1	Autosomal recessive	Sequence analysis	81
Nonketotic hyperglycinemia (glycine encephalopathy)	GLDC, AMT	Autosomal recessive (all)	All: Sequence analysis	82
Biotinidase deficiency	BTD	Autosomal recessive	Targeted mutation analysis or sequence analysis	83,84
Peroxisomal disorders Zellweger syndrome Infantile Refsum disease Neonatal adrenoleukodystrophy	PEX1, PXMP3 (PEX2), PEX3, PEX5, PEX6, PEX10, PEX12, PEX13, PEX14, PEX16, PEX19, PEX26	Autosomal recessive (all)	Sequence analysis	85
Lysosomal storage disorders Metachromatic leukodystrophy (arylsulfatase A deficiency) Krabbe disease	ARSA, PSAP GALC	Autosomal recessive (all)	ARSA: Sequence analysis; PSAP: Sequence analysis; GALC: Targeted mutation analysis, sequence analysis	86,87
Congenital disorders of glycosylation: PMM2 deficiency (CDG1a) Fukuyama muscular dystrophy Walker-Warburg syndrome Muscle-eye-brain disease	PMM2 FCMD POMT1, POMT2 MEB	Autosomal recessive (all)	PMM2: Sequence analysis; FCMD: Targeted mutation analysis, sequence analysis; POMT1: Sequence analysis All others: Sequence analysis	75,88–90
Glucose transporter disorder (GLUT 1 deficiency)	SLC2A1	Autosomal dominant or recessive	Sequence and deletion/duplication analysis	27–30,45
Neuronal ceroid lipofuscinosis	PPT1, TPP1, CLN3, CLN5, CLN6, CLN7/ MFSD8, CLN8, CTSD	Onset before adulthood: autosomal recessive Onset during adulthood: autosomal dominant (suspected)	PPT1, TPP1, CLN3, CLN8: Targeted mutation and sequence analysis CLN5: Targeted mutation analysis, sequence and deletion/ duplication analysis; CLN6, CLN7/ MFSD8, CTSD: Sequence analysis	75,91

Table 4
Progressive myoclonic epilepsies

Structural/Metabolic Cause of Epilepsy: (Selected) Progressive Myoclonic Epilepsies	Genes	Mode of Inheritance	Available Testing	References
Unverricht-Lundborg disease	CSTB	Autosomal recessive	Targeted mutation analysis, sequence analysis	67,75,92,93
Lafora body disease	EPM2A, EPM2B (NHLRC1)	Autosomal recessive	All: Sequence analysis	67,75,94,95
Dentatorubro-pallidoluysian atrophy	DRPLA (ATN1)	Autosomal dominant, (trinucleotide expansion)	Targeted mutation analysis	75,96,97
Mitochondrial disorders				
Myoclonic epilepsy with ragged red fibers (MELAS)	tRNAlys (MT-TL1)	Mitochondrial inheritance	MT-TL1: Targeted mutation analysis	75,98,99
POLG-related disorders (includes: Alpers-Huttenlocher syndrome, progressive external ophthalmoplegia, myoclonic epilepsy myopathy sensory ataxia, POLG-related ataxia neuropathy spectrum disorders)	POLG1 (nuclear encoded gene that codes for a mitochondrial protein)	Autosomal recessive, except for progressive external ophthalmoplegia phenotype, which may be autosomal recessive or autosomal dominant	POLG1: Direct sequencing, targeted mutation, sequence and deletion/duplication analysis	

Table 5
Other genetic syndromes commonly involving epilepsy

Structural/Metabolic Cause of Epilepsy: Other Genetic Syndromes	Genes	Mode of Inheritance	Available Testing	References
Angelman syndrome	UBE3A	Maternal deletion, uniparental disomy (paternal contribution of both copies of chromosome 15), imprinting defect	DNA methylation analysis, sequence analysis	100
Fragile X syndrome	FMR1	X-Linked dominant (trinucleotide expansion, with anticipation)	PCR/Southern blot analysis	101
Rett syndrome	MECP2	X-Linked dominant	Sequence analysis	75,102
Trisomy 21 (Down syndrome)	N/A		Karyotype	75
William syndrome	ELN, LIMK1, GTF2I, STX1A, BAZ1B, CYLN2, GTF2IRD1, NCF1	All: Autosomal dominant	FISH, chromosomal microarray	75,103
Wolf-Hirschhorn syndrome	WHSCR, LETM1	Most de novo, others inherited from a parent with a balanced translocation	Conventional cytogenetic studies, FISH, genome-wide CMA	75,104

Abbreviations: CMA, chromosomal microarray analysis; FISH, fluorescence in situ hybridization; PCR, polymerase chain reaction.

increased risk of epilepsy, such as trisomy 21, Rett syndrome, and Angelman syndrome. Other epilepsies with distinct structural brain abnormalities, such as a spectrum of malformations of cortical development,[41] also have genetic etiology (**Box 3**). Owing to space limitations, these various disorders are not discussed in detail here. Rather, the reader is referred to **Tables 2–5** for a partial list of structural/metabolic conditions resulting in seizures, with associated genetic causes and the current testing availability. A careful history and physical examination, as well as imaging and other laboratory testing, should first raise high suspicion for particular diseases before individualized genetic testing for these disorders is performed.

EVALUATION AND MANAGEMENT
Strategies for Diagnosis

A history of the seizures is the most important tool for diagnosing epilepsy. The first step in the evaluation is deciding whether an event was a seizure. The second step is correctly classifying the seizure type (see Classification section and **Box 1**). The third step involves recognizing other clinical features (eg, developmental and family history), examination findings, and results of diagnostic studies, to clarify a cause or specific epilepsy syndrome (see Clinical Findings section). Initial diagnostic studies may include basic laboratory tests (complete blood count, chemistries, and cerebrospinal fluid [CSF]), an EEG, and imaging of the brain (in most cases magnetic resonance imaging [MRI]).[42] In many clinical settings, genetic testing can be a useful tool to establish a specific genetic cause, improve treatment, and aid in anticipatory care. As this article is focused on genetics, genetic testing is discussed in more detail.

With the growing number of clinically available genetic tests, a rational approach to testing will become increasingly important. Tests may be expensive and not covered by health insurance companies, although whole-exome sequencing may be significantly reduced in cost in comparison with previous years.[43,44] Testing for recently discovered genes may not be commercially available. Moreover, certain types of testing may require further testing of family members to fully interpret a result.

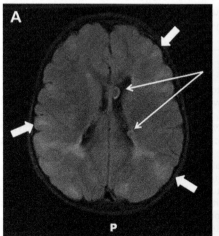
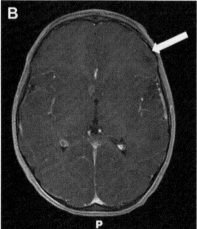

Fig. 1. (A) T2-weighted fluid-attenuated inversion recovery image showing subependymal nodules (*thin arrows*) and bilateral hemispheric tubers (examples, *thick arrows*) in a patient with tuberous sclerosis complex. (B) T1-weighted image showing subependymal nodules and a prominent left frontal cortical tuber (*thick arrow*).

The current diagnostic approach to genetic testing should be individualized to the patient, depending on the specific clinical features and suspected causes (as overviewed in the previous sections and accompanying tables), and whether the results would affect further diagnostic testing or management. **Tables 1–5** describe available genetic testing in primary genetic and structural/metabolic causes of epilepsy. Disease-causing copy number variations in a patient's genetic sequence may be revealed by studies such as specific gene testing, fluorescence in situ hybridization (FISH), a chromosomal microarray, or whole-exome sequencing. In general for specific gene tests, a sequence analysis is performed first, followed by deletion/duplication testing (if applicable). If commercial testing for a newly discovered gene is unavailable, whole-exome sequencing may be especially beneficial.

Further information on available testing for specific diseases mentioned in this article and others may be obtained from the Gene Tests Web site: http://www.ncbi.nlm.-nih.gov/sites/GeneTests.[56] At present, indiscriminately screening all patients with epilepsy using a single test or group of tests is not recommended.[28,45] On the other hand, in children with nonsyndromic intellectual disability, a recent evidence report recommended to consider obtaining genetic testing in this population, including karyotyping (4% diagnostic yield) and chromosomal microarray (8% yield).[46] This recommendation may similarly apply to screening children with epilepsy and comorbid developmental delay. Whole-exome sequencing is also increasingly used as a diagnostic approach in children with intellectual disability and autism.[44] One recent study produced a yield of 16% in individuals with severe intellectual disability, mostly de novo mutations.[47] Whole-exome sequencing may likewise prove a useful tool in epilepsy in the near future, but concerns remain about appropriate usage of these powerful methods, including problems with data interpretation and ethical issues of coincidentally found abnormalities.[28]

Although a universal, standardized approach to genetic testing for epilepsy is not currently recommended, some common principles can be used to guide an individualized testing strategy. First, genetic testing for patients with a high suspicion for treatable conditions should be a priority. For example, children with glucose transporter (*GLUT1*) mutations are optimally treated with the ketogenic diet and may require genetic testing because of high clinical suspicion despite normal CSF studies (see **Table 3**).[27–30] Of further complexity with *GLUT1* disorders, it has recently become

---

Box 4
Case summary 3

A 5-year-old boy presented to clinic with a history of epilepsy, ataxia, and developmental delay. His seizures began at 10 months of age and were characterized by brief 10-second periods of "blanking out" with occasional lip-smacking. These features increased in frequency to more than 40 times daily, which improved somewhat with antiepileptic medication. His history included delays in both language and motor areas. He began speaking his first words at 18 months, and by 2 years he began walking. His parents reported a tremor, with fine motor and gross motor difficulties since birth. Physical examination was notable for normal cognition, dysarthria, mildly decreased muscle bulk and tone, and a fine-action tremor of all extremities. MRI of the brain was normal. An EEG-video study captured absence seizures, characterized by subtle activity arrest, which corresponded with 3-Hz generalized spike and wave discharges (**Fig. 2**). Frequent interictal 2.5- to 4-Hz generalized epileptiform discharges were also present. A lumbar puncture revealed a cerebrospinal fluid (CSF) glucose level of 34 mg/dL, and a simultaneously drawn serum glucose level of 78 mg/dL. The CSF/serum glucose ratio was 0.44. SLC2A1 sequence analysis showed a heterozygous unclassified variant of unknown significance. Despite this, a diagnosis of GLUT1 transporter deficiency was established based on clinical and laboratory findings, and his seizure control improved after initiation of a ketogenic diet.

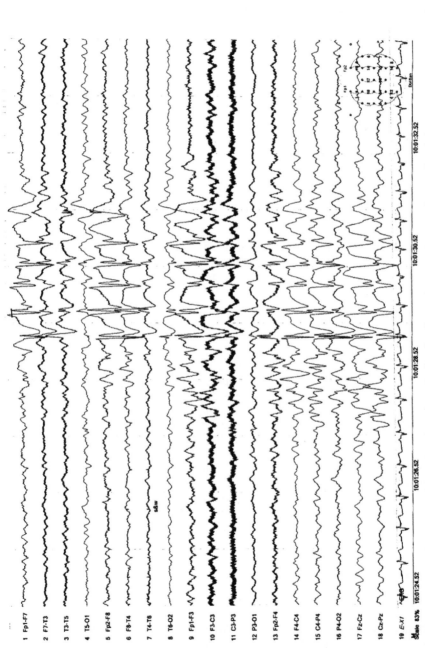

Fig. 2. Electroencephalogram showing ictal pattern of 3-Hz generalized spike and wave corresponding with subtle activity arrest in a patient with GLUT1 transporter deficiency.

apparent that some individuals with a glucose transporter defect may manifest in a similar fashion to more benign generalized epilepsy syndromes (**Box 4**).[48] Similarly, targeted genetic testing may be helpful in other severe epileptic encephalopathies where early diagnosis and treatment might influence prognosis, such as with *SCN1A* mutations and Dravet syndrome.[28] Other reasons to pursue genetic testing include future family planning or prevention of further unnecessary diagnostic testing. On the other hand, genetic testing may frequently not be needed if a clinical diagnosis is clear or if genetic testing is unlikely to change patient management. For example, it may not be necessary to obtain genetic confirmation of an infant with benign familial neonatal seizures, as this is usually a self-resolving condition with a relatively straight-forward clinical diagnosis.[45]

The presence of variable expressivity, reduced penetrance, and genetic heterogeneity in phenotype-genotype relationships with epilepsy syndromes complicate the application and interpretation of genetic testing.[45] Another common challenge involves the interpretation of a "variant of unknown significance." With chromosomal microarray and whole-genome sequencing, sequence variants (such as single-nucleotide polymorphisms) often occur in the normal genome. To clarify whether a variant is benign or causes disease, testing from both parents is necessary. If either parent carries the genetic change, the variant is usually benign. However, in some such cases the variant may actually be pathogenic but have variable penetrance, with the affected parent having a very mild phenotype. Furthermore, interpretation may prove impossible if one or both parents are unavailable or diseased. On the other hand, if a variant of unknown significance is found in a region previously described as associated with an epilepsy syndrome, a high level of suspicion may be concluded and steps taken in reporting this genetic variant.[49] As a further level of complexity, it is clear that in some cases interactions between multiple mutations may result in epilepsy.[50]

Current Management and Therapeutic Options

There are 4 types of proven treatment for epilepsy: medication, epilepsy surgery, ketogenic diet, and electrical stimulation. More than 20 antiseizure medications are available. Although overall most drugs are relatively equivalent in efficacy, some medications are more appropriate for specific seizure types (eg, focal vs generalized) or epilepsy syndromes. About one-third of all patients are intractable to medication.[51] For appropriate candidates, epilepsy surgery is sometimes the next best option, with a relatively high rate of freedom from seizure. Ketogenic diet and vagal nerve stimulation are additional nonmedical options for medically intractable epilepsy patients. As the focus of this article is on genetics, a detailed review of the different antiseizure medications and nonmedical treatments for epilepsy is beyond its scope. At present, there are no specific treatments (eg, gene therapy) that target underlying genetic defects directly causing epilepsy.

SUMMARY AND FUTURE DIRECTIONS

Genetic testing in epilepsy has improved our understanding of epilepsy and has inspired new questions pertaining to the selection of antiepileptic medication and anticipation of adverse drug reactions. Many studies have examined the relationship of genotype with the presence of medical intractability, drug selection, and dosage administration, but none have obtained conclusive results to date.[52] On the other hand, the identification of HLA-B*1502, an HLA-B allelic variation, was shown to be 100% sensitive and 97% specific in predicting the onset of Stevens-Johnson syndrome (a severe dermatologic hypersensitivity reaction) in Asian individuals with epilepsy treated with carbamazepine and, to a lesser extent, lamotrigine, phenytoin, and oxcarbazepine, demonstrating the clinical utility of this test.[52,53] Testing for this risk factor is now considered a standard of care in populations of Asian descent before starting these medications. Despite this encouraging application of pharmacogenomics in epilepsy, limited study sizes, a lack of standardization between centers, and a lack of prospective studies remain barriers to obtaining clinically relevant testing in other settings.[52]

Nevertheless, genetics is exploding with the potential to increase our understanding and management of epilepsy. In patients with epilepsy it should be determined by the treating physician, in careful discussion with the patients or their family, whether testing is necessary for establishing a diagnosis or affecting treatment. In potentially untreatable conditions, genetic testing should be pursued if the results are likely to affect future pregnancies or family planning. In such cases a careful review of the patient's history, suspected disease, and characteristics of available testing should help in selecting a test with the highest diagnostic probability for the individual. In all cases, informed consent should be obtained, with genetic counseling available to the patient and family before and after testing occurs. In the future, whole-genome sequencing and pharmacogenomics may have an even greater impact on the treatment of epilepsy.

REFERENCES

1. Fisher RS, van Emde Boas W, Blume W, et al. Epileptic seizures and epilepsy: definitions proposed by the International League Against Epilepsy (ILAE) and the International Bureau for Epilepsy (IBE). Epilepsia 2005;46(4):470–2.
2. Banerjee PN, Filippi D, Hauser A. The descriptive epidemiology of epilepsy—a review. Epilepsy Res 2009;85(1):31–45.
3. Berg AT, Berkovic SF, Brodie MJ, et al. Revised terminology and concepts for organization of seizures and epilepsies: report of the ILAE Commission on Classification and Terminology, 2005-2009. Epilepsia 2010;51(4):676–85.
4. Singh NA, Westenskow P, Charlier C, et al, BFNC Physician Consortium. KCNQ2 and KCNQ3 potassium channel genes in benign familial neonatal convulsions: expansion of the functional and mutation spectrum. Brain 2003;126(12): 2726–37.
5. Bellini G, Miceli F, Soldovieri MV, et al. Benign familial neonatal seizures (Last updated August 4, 2011). In: GeneReviews at GeneTests: medical genetics information resource (database online). Seattle (WA): University of Washington; 1997–2011. Available at: http://www.genetests.org. Accessed November 6, 2012.
6. Panayiotopoulos CP. Neonatal epileptic seizures and neonatal epileptic syndromes. In: A clinical guide to the epileptic syndromes and their treatment. 2nd edition. London: Springer-Verlag; 2007. p. 185–206.
7. Heron SE, Crossland KM, Andermann E, et al. Sodium-channel defects in benign familial neonatal-infantile seizures. Lancet 2002;360(9336):851–2.
8. Panayiotopoulos CP. Idiopathic epileptic seizures and syndromes in infancy. In: A clinical guide to the epileptic syndromes and their treatment. 2nd edition. London: Springer-Verlag; 2007. p. 207–22.
9. Guipponi M, River F, Vigevano F, et al. Linkage mapping of benign familial infantile convulsions (BFIC) to chromosome 19q. Hum Mol Genet 1997;6(3):473–7.
10. Vanmolkot KR, Kors EE, Hottenga JJ, et al. Novel mutations in the Na^+, K^+-ATPase pump gene ATP1A2 associated with familial hemiplegic migraine and benign familial infantile convulsions. Ann Neurol 2003;54(3):360–6.

11. Swoboda KJ, Soong B, McKenna C, et al. Paroxysmal kinesiogenic dyskinesia and infantile convulsions: clinical and linkage studies. Neurology 2000;55(2): 224–30.

12. Heron SE, Bronwyn GE, Kivity A, et al. PRRT2 mutations cause benign familial infantile epilepsy and infantile convulsions with choreoathetosis syndrome. Am J Hum Genet 2012;90:152–60.

13. Shoubridge C, Fullston T, Gécz J. ARX spectrum disorders: making inroads into the molecular pathology. Hum Mutat 2010;31(8):889–900.

14. Kato M, Saitoh S, Kamei A, et al. A longer polyalanine expansion mutation in the ARX gene causes early infantile epileptic encephalopathy with suppression-burst pattern (Ohtahara syndrome). Am J Hum Genet 2007;81(2):361–6.

15. Castrén M, Gaily E, Tengström C, et al. Epilepsy caused by CDKL5 mutations. Eur J Paediatr Neurol 2011;15(1):65–9.

16. Saitsu H, Kato M, Mizuguchi T, et al. De novo mutations in the gene encoding STXBP1 (MUNC18-1) cause early infantile epileptic encephalopathy. Nat Genet 2008;40(6):782–8.

17. Mignot C, Moutard ML, Trouillard O, et al. STXBP1-related encephalopathy presenting as infantile spasms and generalized tremor in three patients. Epilepsia 2011;52(10):1820–7.

18. Saitsu H, Kato M, Okada I, et al. STXBP1 mutations in early infantile epileptic encephalopathy with suppression-burst pattern. Epilepsia 2010;51(12):2397–405.

19. Kurian MA, Meyer E, Vassallo G, et al. Phospholipase C beta 1 deficiency is associated with early onset epileptic encephalopathy. Brain 2010;133(10):2964–70.

20. Weckhuysen S, Mandelstam S, Suls A. KCNQ2 encephalopathy: emerging phenotype of a neonatal epileptic encephalopathy. Ann Neurol 2012;71:15–25.

21. Miller IO, Sotero MA. SCN1A-Related seizure disorders (Last updated November 10, 2011). In: GeneReviews at GeneTests: medical genetics information resource (database online). Seattle (WA): University of Washington; 1997–2011. Available at: http://www.genetests.org. Accessed November 6, 2012.

22. Scheffer IE, Berkovic SF. Generalized epilepsy with febrile seizures plus: a genetic disorder with heterogeneous clinical phenotypes. Brain 1997;120:479–90.

23. Panayiotopoulos CP. Epileptic encephalopathies in infancy and early childhood. In: A clinical guide to the epileptic syndromes and their treatment. 2nd edition. London: Springer-Verlag; 2007. p. 223–71.

24. Stephani U. The natural history of myoclonic astatic epilepsy (Doose syndrome) and Lennox-Gastaut syndrome. Epilepsia 2006;47(2):53–5.

25. Mullen SA, Marini C, Suls A, et al. Glucose transporter 1 deficiency as a treatable cause of myoclonic astatic epilepsy. Arch Neurol 2011;68(9):1152–5.

26. Panayiotopoulos CP. Idiopathic generalised epilepsies. In: A clinical guide to the epileptic syndromes and their treatment. 2nd edition. London: Springer-Verlag; 2007. p. 319–62.

27. Suls A, Mullen SA, Weber YG, et al. Early-onset absence epilepsy caused by mutations in the glucose transporter GLUT1. Ann Neurol 2009;66:415–9.

28. Scheffer IE. Genetic testing in epilepsy: what should you be doing? Epilepsy Curr 2011;11(4):107–11.

29. Wang D, Pascual JM, De Vivo D. Glucose transporter type 1 deficiency syndrome (Last updated August 9, 2012). In: GeneReviews at GeneTests: medical genetics information resource (database online). Seattle (WA): University of Washington; 1997–2011. Available at: http://www.genetests.org. Accessed November 6, 2012.

30. Arsov T, Mullen SA, Damiano JA, et al. Early onset absence epilepsy: 1 in 10 cases is caused by GLUT1 deficiency. Epilepsia 2012;53(12):e204–7.

31. Kurahashi H, Hisose S. Autosomal dominant nocturnal frontal lobe epilepsy (Last updated September 20, 2012). In: GeneReviews at GeneTests: medical genetics information resource (database online). Seattle (WA): University of Washington; 1997–2011. Available at: http://www.genetests.org. Accessed November 6, 2012.

32. Steinlein OK, Mulley JC, Propping P, et al. A missense mutation in the neuronal nicotinic acetylcholine receptor alpha 4 subunit is associated with autosomal dominant nocturnal frontal lobe epilepsy. Nat Genet 1995;11(2):201–3.

33. Aridon P, Marini C, Di resta C, et al. Increased sensitivity of the neuronal nicotinic receptor alpha 2 subunit causes familial epilepsy with nocturnal wandering and ictal fear. Am J Hum Genet 2006;79(2):342–50.

34. De Fusco M, Becchetti A, Patrignani A, et al. The nicotinic receptor beta 2 subunit is mutant in nocturnal frontal lobe epilepsy. Nat Genet 2000;26(3):275–6.

35. Panayiotopoulos CP. Familial (autosomal dominant) focal epilepsies. In: A clinical guide to the epileptic syndromes and their treatment. 2nd edition. London: Springer-Verlag; 2007. p. 363–72.

36. Ottman R. Autosomal dominant partial epilepsy with auditory features (Last updated July 13, 2010). In: GeneReviews at GeneTests: medical genetics information resource (database online). Seattle (WA): University of Washington; 1997–2011. Available at: http://www.genetests.org. Accessed November 6, 2012.

37. Kalachikov S, Evgrafov O, Ross B, et al. Mutations in LGI1 cause autosomal-dominant partial epilepsy with auditory features. Nat Genet 2002;30(3):335–41.

38. Panayiotopoulos CP. Benign childhood focal seizures and related epileptic syndromes. In: A clinical guide to the epileptic syndromes and their treatment. 2nd edition. London: Springer-Verlag; 2007. p. 285–318.

39. Strug LJ, Clarke T, Chiang T, et al. Centrotemporal sharp wave EEG trait in rolandic epilepsy maps to elongator protein complex 4 (ELP4). Eur J Hum Genet 2009;17:1171–81.

40. Ishii A, Miyajima T, Kuruhashi H, et al. KCNQ2 abnormality in BECTS: benign childhood epilepsy with centrotemporal spikes following benign neonatal seizures resulting from a mutation in KCNQ2. Epilepsy Res 2012;102(1–2):122–5.

41. Barkovich AJ, Guerrini R, Kuzniecky RI, et al. A developmental and genetic classification for malformations and cortical development: update 2012. Brain 2012;135:1348–69.

42. Hirtz D, Ashwal S, Berg A, et al. Practice parameter: evaluating a first nonfebrile seizure in children. Report of the quality standards subcommittee of the American Academy of Neurology, the Child Neurology Society, and the American Epilepsy Society. Neurology 2000;55:616–23.

43. Feero GW, Guttmacher AE. Genomic medicine-an updated primer. N Engl J Med 2010;362(21):2001–11.

44. Mefford HC, Batshaw ML, Hoffman EP. Genomics, intellectual disability and autism. N Engl J Med 2012;366(8):733–43.

45. Ottman R, Hirose S, Jain S, et al. Genetic testing in the epilepsies—report of the ILAE Genetics Commission. Epilepsia 2010;51(4):655–70.

46. Michelson DJ, Shevell MI, Sherr EH, et al. Evidence report: genetic and metabolic testing on children with global developmental delay: report of the Quality Standards Subcommittee of the American Academy of Neurology and the Practice Committee of the Child Neurology Society. Neurology 2011;77:1629–35.

47. De Ligt J, Willemsen MH, van Bon BW, et al. Diagnostic exome sequencing in persons with severe intellectual disability. N Engl J Med 2012;367(20):1921–9.

48. Striano P, Weber YG, Toliat MR, et al. GLUT1 mutations are a rare cause of familial idiopathic generalized epilepsy. Neurology 2012;78:557–62.

49. Richards CS, Bale S, Bellissimo DB, et al. ACMG recommendations for standards for interpretation and reporting of sequence variations: revisions 2007. Genet Med 2008;10(4):294–300.

50. Klassen T, Davis C, Goldman A, et al. Exome sequencing of ion channel genes reveals complex profiles confounding personal risk assessment in epilepsy. Cell 2011;145:1036–48.

51. Kwan P, Brodie MJ. Early identification of refractory epilepsy. N Engl J Med 2000;342:314–9.

52. Cavalleri GL, McCormack M, Alhusaini S, et al. Pharmacogenomics and epilepsy: the road ahead. Pharmacogenomics 2011;12(10):1429–47.

53. Chung WH, Hung SI, Hong HS, et al. Medical genetics: a marker for Stevens-Johnson syndrome. Nature 2004;428(6982):486.

54. Pandolfo M. Genetics of epilepsy. Semin Neurol 2011;3:506–18.

55. Shi X, Yasumoto S, Kurahashi H, et al. Clinical spectrum of SCN2A mutations. Brain Dev 2012;34:541–5.

56. GeneTests medical genetics information resource (database online). Seattle (WA): University of Washington; 1993–2012. Available at: http://www.genetests.org. Accessed November 6, 2012.

57. Falace A, Filipello F, La Padula V, et al. TBC1D24, an ARF6-interacting protein, is mutated in familial infantile myoclonic epilepsy. Am J Hum Genet 2010;87(3):365–70.

58. Scheffer IE, Turner SJ, Dibbens LM, et al. Epilepsy and mental retardation limited to females: an under-recognized disorder. Brain 2008;131(4):918–27.

59. Dibbens LM, Tarpey PS, Hynes K, et al. X-linked protocadherin 19 mutations cause female-limited epilepsy and cognitive impairment. Nat Genet 2008;40(6):776–81.

60. Yalcin O. Genes and molecular mechanisms involved in the epileptogenesis of idiopathic absence epilepsies. Seizure 2012;21:79–86.

61. Pal DK, Greenberg DA. Major susceptibility genes for common idiopathic epilepsies: ELP4 in rolandic epilepsy and BRD2 in juvenile myoclonic epilepsy. In: Noebels JL, Avoli M, Rogawski MA, et al, editors. Jasper's basic mechanisms of the epilepsies [internet]. 4th edition. Bethesda (MD): National Center for Biotechnology Information (US); 2012.

62. Grissar T, Lakaye B, de Nijs L, et al. Myoclonin1/EFHC1 in cell division, neuroblast migration, synapse/dendrite formation in juvenile myoclonic epilepsy. In: Noebels JL, Avoli M, Rogawski MA, et al, editors. Jasper's basic mechanisms of the epilepsies [internet]. 4th edition. Bethesda (MD): National Center for Biotechnology Information (US); 2012.

63. Ma S, Blair MA, Abou-Khalil B, et al. Mutations in the GABRA1 and EHFC1 genes are rare in familial juvenile myoclonic epilepsy. Epilepsy Res 2006;71(2–3):129–34.

64. Cossette P, Lui L, Brisebois K, et al. Mutation of GABRA1 is an autosomal dominant form of juvenile myoclonic epilepsy. Nat Genet 2002;31(2):184–9.

65. Escayg A, De Waard M, Lee DD, et al. Coding and noncoding variation of the human calcium-channel beta4-subunit gene CACNB4 in patients with idiopathic generalized epilepsy and episodic ataxia. Am J Hum Genet 2000;66(5):1531–9.

66. Suis A, Dedeken P, Goffin K, et al. Paroxysmal exercise-induced dyskinesia and epilepsy is due to mutations in SLC2A1, encoding the glucose transporter GLUT1. Brain 2008;131(7):1831–44.

67. Michelucci R, Pasini E, Riguzzi P, et al. Genetics of epilepsy and relevance to current practice. Curr Neurol Neurosci Rep 2012;12:445–55.
68. Hwang SK, Hirose S. Genetics of temporal lobe epilepsy. Brain Dev 2012;34: 609–16.
69. Berkovic SF, Serratosa JM, Phillips HA, et al. Familial partial epilepsy with variable foci: clinical features and linkage to chromosome 22q12. Epilepsia 2004; 45:1054–60.
70. Xiong L, Labuda M, Li DS, et al. Mapping of a gene determining familial partial epilepsy with variable foci to chromosome 22q11-q12. Am J Hum Genet 1999; 65(6):1698–710.
71. Azmanov DN, Zhelyazkova S, Radionova M, et al. Focal epilepsy of probable temporal lobe origin in a gypsy family showing linkage to a novel locus on 7p21.3. Epilepsy Res 2011;96:101–8.
72. Hedera P, Blair MA, Andermann E, et al. Familial mesial temporal lobe epilepsy maps to chromosome 4q13.2-q21.3. Neurology 2007;68(24):2107–12.
73. Baulac S, Picard F, Herman A, et al. Evidence for digenic inheritance in a family with both febrile convulsions and temporal lobe epilepsy implicating chromosomes 18qter and 1q25-q31. Ann Neurol 2001;49(6):786–92.
74. Claes L, Audenaert D, Deprez L, et al. Novel locus on chromosome 12q22-q23.3 responsible for familial temporal lobe epilepsy associated with febrile seizures. J Med Genet 2004;41(9):710–4.
75. Ropper AH, Samuels MA. Epilepsy and other seizure disorders. In: Adams and Victor's principles of neurology. 9th edition. New York: McGraw-Hill; 2009. p. 305–38.
76. Solomon BD, Gropman A. Holoprosencephaly overview (Last updated November 3, 2011). In: GeneReviews at GeneTests: medical genetics information resource (database online). Seattle (WA): University of Washington; 1997–2011. Available at: http://www.genetests.org. Accessed November 6, 2012.
77. Hehr U, Uyanik G, Aigner L, et al. DCX-related disorders (Last updated March 24, 2011). In: GeneReviews at GeneTests: medical genetics information resource (database online). Seattle (WA): University of Washington; 1997–2011. Available at: http://www.genetests.org. Accessed November 6, 2012.
78. Sheen VL, Bodell A, Walsh CA. X-Linked periventricular heterotopia (Last updated June 4, 2009). In: GeneReviews at GeneTests: medical genetics information resource (database online). Seattle (WA): University of Washington; 1997–2011. Available at: http://www.genetests.org. Accessed November 6, 2012.
79. Northrup H, Koenig MK, Au KS. Tuberous sclerosis complex (Last updated November 23, 2011). In: GeneReviews at GeneTests: medical genetics information resource (database online). Seattle (WA): University of Washington; 1997–2011. Available at: http://www.genetests.org. Accessed November 6, 2012.
80. Friedman JM. Neurofibromatosis 1 (Last updated May 3, 2012). In: GeneReviews at GeneTests: medical genetics information resource (database online). Seattle (WA): University of Washington; 1997–2011. Available at: http://www. genetests.org. Accessed November 6, 2012.
81. Gospe SM. Pyridoxine-dependent epilepsy (Last updated June 7, 2012). In: GeneReviews at GeneTests: medical genetics information resource (database online). Seattle (WA): University of Washington; 1997–2011. Available at: http://www.genetests.org. Accessed November 6, 2012.
82. Hamosh A, Gunter Scharer G, Van Hove J. Glycine encephalopathy (Last updated November 24, 2009). In: GeneReviews at GeneTests: medical genetics

information resource (database online). Seattle (WA): University of Washington; 1997–2011. Available at:. http://www.genetests.org. Accessed November 6, 2012.

83. Wolf B. Biotinidase deficiency (Last updated March 15, 2011). In: GeneReviews at GeneTests: medical genetics information resource (database online). Seattle (WA): University of Washington; 1997–2011. Available at: http://www.genetests.org. Accessed November 6, 2012.

84. Cowan TM, Blitzer MG, Wolf B, Working Group of the American College of Medical Genetics Laboratory Quality Assurance Committee. Technical standards and guidelines for the diagnosis of biotinidase deficiency. Genet Med 2010; 12(7):464–70.

85. Steinberg SJ, Raymond GV, Braverman NE, et al. Peroxisome biogenesis disorders, Zellweger syndrome spectrum (Last updated May 10, 2012). In: GeneReviews at GeneTests: medical genetics information resource (database online). Seattle (WA): University of Washington; 1997–2011. Available at: http://www.genetests.org. Accessed November 6, 2012.

86. Fluharty AL. Arylsulfatase A deficiency (Last updated August 25, 2011). In: GeneReviews at GeneTests: medical genetics information resource (database online). Seattle (WA): University of Washington; 1997–2011. Available at: http://www.genetests.org. Accessed November 6, 2012.

87. Wenger DA. Krabbe disease (Last updated March 31, 2011). In: GeneReviews at GeneTests: medical genetics information resource (database online). Seattle (WA): University of Washington; 1997–2011. Available at: http://www.genetests.org. Accessed November 6, 2012.

88. Sparks SE, Krasnewich DM. PMMG-CDG (CDG 1a) (Last updated April 21, 2011). In: GeneReviews at GeneTests: medical genetics information resource (database online). Seattle (WA): University of Washington; 1997–2011. Available at: http://www.genetests.org. Accessed February 2, 2012.

89. Saito K. Fukuyama congenital muscular dystrophy (Last updated May 10, 2012). In: GeneReviews at GeneTests: medical genetics information resource (database online). Seattle (WA): University of Washington; 1997–2011. Available at: http://www.genetests.org. Accessed November 6, 2012.

90. Sparks S, Quijano-Roy S, Harper A, et al. Congenital muscular dystrophy overview (Last updated August 23, 2012). In: GeneReviews at GeneTests: medical genetics information resource (database online). Seattle (WA): University of Washington; 1997–2011. Available at: http://www.genetests.org. Accessed November 6, 2012.

91. Mole SE, Williams RE. Neuronal ceroid-lipofuscinoses (Last updated March 2, 2010). In: GeneReviews at GeneTests: medical genetics information resource (database online). Seattle (WA): University of Washington; 1997–2011. Available at: http://www.genetests.org. Accessed November 6, 2012.

92. Lehesjoki A, Kälviäinen R. Unverricht-Lundborg disease (Last updated June 18, 2009). In: GeneReviews at GeneTests: medical genetics information resource (database online). Seattle (WA): University of Washington; 1997–2011. Available at: http://www.genetests.org. Accessed November 6, 2012.

93. Pennacchio LA, Bouley DM, Higgins KM, et al. Progressive ataxia, myoclonic epilepsy and cerebellar apoptosis in cystatin B-deficient mice. Nat Genet 1998;20:251–8.

94. Jansen AC, Andermann E. Progressive myoclonus epilepsy, lafora type (Last updated November 3, 2011). In: GeneReviews at GeneTests: medical genetics information resource (database online). Seattle (WA): University of Washington;

1997–2011. Available at: http://www.genetests.org. Accessed November 6, 2012.

95. Minassian BA, Lee JR, Herbrick JA, et al. Mutations in a gene encoding a novel protein tyrosine phosphatase cause progressive myoclonus epilepsy. Nat Genet 1998;20:171–4.

96. Chan EM, Young EJ, Ianzano L, et al. Mutations in NHLRC1 cause progressive myoclonus epilepsy. Nat Genet 2003;35:125–7.

97. Tsuji S. DRPLA (Last updated June 1, 2010). In: GeneReviews at GeneTests: medical genetics information resource (database online). Seattle (WA): University of Washington; 1997–2011. Available at: http://www.genetests.org. Accessed November 6, 2012.

98. Dimauro S, Hirano M. MELAS (Last updated October 14, 2010). In: GeneReviews at GeneTests: medical genetics information resource (database online). Seattle (WA): University of Washington; 1997–2011. Available at: http://www.genetests.org. Accessed November 6, 2012.

99. Cohen BH, Chinnery PF, Copelend WC. POLG-related disorders (Last updated October 11, 2012). In: GeneReviews at GeneTests: medical genetics information resource (database online). Seattle (WA): University of Washington; 1997–2011. Available at: http://www.genetests.org. Accessed November 6, 2012.

100. Dagli AI, Williams CA. Angelman syndrome (Last updated June 16, 2011). In: GeneReviews at GeneTests: medical genetics information resource (database online). Seattle (WA): University of Washington; 1997–2011. Available at: http://www.genetests.org. Accessed November 6, 2012.

101. Saul RA, Tarleton JC. FMR1-related disorders (Last updated April 26, 2012). In: GeneReviews at GeneTests: medical genetics information resource (database online). Seattle (WA): University of Washington; 1997–2011. Available at: http://www.genetests.org. Accessed November 6, 2012.

102. Christodoulou J. MECP2-related disorders (Last updated June 28, 2012). In: GeneReviews at GeneTests: medical genetics information resource (database online). Seattle (WA): University of Washington; 1997–2011. Available at: http://www.genetests.org. Accessed November 6, 2012.

103. Morris CA. Williams syndrome (Last updated April 21, 2006). In: GeneReviews at GeneTests: medical genetics information resource (database online). Seattle (WA): University of Washington; 1997–2011. Available at: http://www.genetests.org. Accessed November 6, 2012.

104. Battaglia A, Carey JC, South ST, et al. Wolf-Hirschhorn syndrome (Last updated June 17, 2010). In: GeneReviews at GeneTests: medical genetics information resource (database online). Seattle (WA): University of Washington; 1997–2011. Available at: http://www.genetests.org. Accessed November 6, 2012.

Clinical Neurogenetics: Stroke

Natalia S. Rost, MD, MPH

KEYWORDS

- Cerebrovascular disease • Genetics • Stroke subtype • Ischemic stroke
- Intracerebral hemorrhage • White matter hyperintensity • Phenotype
- Genome-wide association study

KEY POINTS

- Genetic methodology has undergone a major revolution over the past decade.
- The development of advanced genotyping and computational techniques has improved understanding of complex traits.
- Despite clear setbacks in the genetics of cerebrovascular disease and stroke, large-scale, systematic collaborations promise a much needed advance in the field.
- With light being already shed on the role of stroke subtype genetics, as well as shared contributions to disease-specific pathways, future discoveries may offer a greater scope and a more detailed assessment of the genetic spectrum of cerebrovascular disease.

INTRODUCTION

Stroke is one of the most serious neurologic disorders, affecting functionality and, often, at patients' prime. Despite recent improvement in stroke mortality, patients often face the prospect of substantial poststroke disability.[1,2] Use of intravenous (IV) tissue plasminogen activator (tPA), the only treatment of acute ischemic stroke (AIS) approved by the US Food and Drug Administration (FDA), is still limited[3] and its impact on poststroke outcomes is modest.[4] Development of novel stroke prevention strategies and therapeutics that are both safe and effective[5,6] is desperately needed to reduce stroke incidence and improve poststroke outcomes in order to alleviate the projected stroke morbidity estimates.

Recent successes in gene discovery for several complex disorders[7–9] may offer innovative approaches to unraveling complex causal pathways leading to a severe disorder such as stroke, and, with that, a promise of translational preventative and therapeutic advances. Stroke genetics have undergone a comprehensive reassessment in recent years, along with revolutionary advances in genotyping and

Dr Natalia S. Rost is supported by the National Institute of Neurological Disorders and Stroke (NINDS) (K23NS064052).
Department of Neurology, JP Kistler Stroke Research Center, Massachusetts General Hospital, 175 Cambridge Street, Suite 300, Boston, MA 02114, USA
E-mail address: nrost@partners.org

computational methodologies[10–12] that, in turn, have enabled whole-genome studies[13,14] and supported the evolution of functional genomics.[15,16] In stroke, genetic advances have been largely hindered to date by heterogeneity of the phenotype; however, recent efforts by an international network of stroke geneticists show progress in understanding the genetic architecture of stroke and other cerebrovascular disorders.[17,18] This article discusses the current concepts in stroke genetics and their future research and clinical implications.

STROKE AS A PHENOTYPE: DEFINITION AND VARIABILITY
Etiologic Stroke Subtypes

Understanding of etiologic stroke subtypes evolved considerably from their initial division by cerebral ischemia versus intracerebral hemorrhage (ICH) (**Fig. 1**). Ischemic stroke is defined as an infarction of central nervous system (CNS) tissue, which can be either symptomatic or silent.[19] Symptomatic ischemic strokes present with clinical signs of focal or global cerebral, spinal, or retinal dysfunction caused by CNS infarction, whereas silent strokes are documented by neuroimaging or neuropathologic findings that are otherwise asymptomatic in a given individual.[19] In some situations, clinical features alone (prolonged neurologic deficits consistent with a specific stroke syndrome and referable to a defined vascular territory involved by cerebral ischemia) render a diagnosis of an ischemic stroke despite the absence of neuroimaging evidence of infarct. In contrast, presence of a distinct ischemic injury on head computed tomography (CT) or brain magnetic resonance imaging (MRI) should prompt a detailed clinical investigation to determine whether the stroke is silent.

Definition of stroke as a phenotype of interest for genetic studies presents a challenge because of the heterogeneity of stroke subtypes (**Fig. 2**). The common consensus in stroke genetics is that stroke, per se, is not a disorder but a syndrome that arises as an acute manifestation of chronic cerebrovascular disease. In more

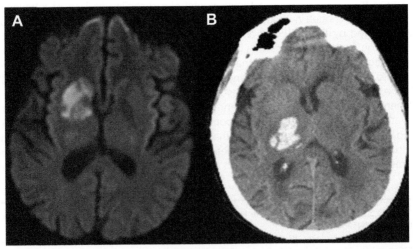

Fig. 1. Major stroke subtypes. Use of neuroimaging revolutionized diagnosis of etiologic stroke subtypes. Similarities in clinical syndromes caused by the injury to the same brain structures (right basal ganglia) can be differentiated using diffusion-weighted magnetic resonance imaging in ischemic stroke (*A*) versus computed tomography in ICH (*B*), even in the hyperacute phase of stroke.

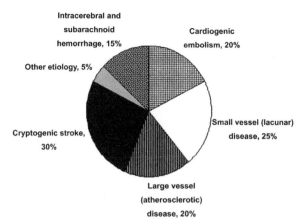

Fig. 2. Heterogeneity of stroke phenotype. Most strokes (~85%) are ischemic, some of which are considered cryptogenic, or of undetermined cause. Distribution of stroke subtypes, both ischemic and hemorrhagic, varies significantly based on demographic and population-based characteristics, likely because of the prevalence of the specific stroke risk factors.

than 80% of cases, these long-standing vascular abnormalities result in cerebral blood flow obstruction with consequent ischemia/infarct in the territory of the vascular occlusion, and in 15% to 20% of cases the vascular wall integrity is compromised to the extent of rupture resulting in ICH.[20] Additional phenotypic dilemmas arise when considering cardioembolic stroke subtype, when cerebral ischemia is present in the absence of any detectable disease of cerebrovascular vessels. Identifying the cause of each stroke subtype is critical for guiding individual therapeutic and preventative approaches in stroke management, and many classification systems have been used to date.[21] The most broadly accepted stroke subtype classification, Trial of Org 10172 in Acute Stroke Treatment (TOAST),[22,23] is being challenged by the new complexities in causative classification of stroke subtypes because of current and evolving advances in research methodology and diagnostic technology.[24,25] Instead, an automated evidence-based algorithm, the Causative Classification System (CCS) (http://ccs.martinos.org/), which harmonizes multiple aspects of the diagnostic stroke evaluation to identify the most likely mechanism of stroke, has recently been optimized and validated for large-scale stroke genetics studies in multicenter settings.[26]

Intermediate Cerebrovascular Phenotypes

Diagnosed cerebral ischemia and ICH are not the sole manifestations of cerebrovascular disease. MRI-detectable white matter hyperintensity (WMH), also known as leukoaraiosis,[27] cerebral microbleeds (CMBs),[28] cerebral microinfarcts,[29] Virchow-Robin spaces,[30] and superficial siderosis[31] are all considered manifestations of cerebrovascular disease. Whether overt or covert at the time of diagnosis, these cerebrovascular phenotypes have been linked to risk of stroke or ICH and are thought to be situated directly in the disease pathway, or so-called intermediate phenotypes **(Fig. 3)**.[32–34] Furthermore, because of their assumed proximity to causative genes compared with that of clinical stroke phenotypes, these intermediate phenotypes are presumed to have genetic architecture that is less complex and, as result, greater phenotype-genotype association amendable to advanced methods of genomic interrogation.[35,36]

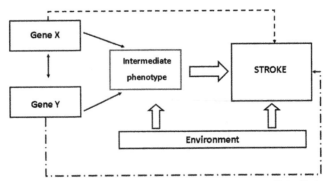

Fig. 3. Intermediate phenotype. An intermediate phenotype is a clinically important and measurable phenotype that is situated directly in the disease pathway (for example, WMH). It is thought to contribute to variation in the phenotype of interest (stroke) with greater effect size by being more proximal to causal genes (genes *X* and *Y*).

GENETIC DISORDERS ASSOCIATED WITH STROKE
Heritability of Stroke

Family history and twin studies suggest a genetic contribution to the risk of both ischemic stroke and ICH,[37–39] with variability affecting younger individuals[40] and specific stroke subtypes.[41–43] For ischemic stroke, concordance of nearly 60% has been reported in monozygotic twins compared with dizygotic twins, and a positive family history of stroke is associated with up to a two-thirds relative increase in ischemic stroke risk.[44] Compared with the general population, first-degree relatives of patients with hemorrhagic stroke have up to a 5-fold increase in relative risk of ICH[45] and a 3-fold to 7-fold increase in risk of subarachnoid hemorrhage.[46,47] However, estimates of heritability, or the proportion of phenotypic variability attributable to genetic variance for a particular trait, require complex statistical modeling and are often influenced by the research methodology and population-specific characteristics, including the frequently unaccounted for gene-environment interactions.

Known Monogenic Stroke Disorders

Several rare, singe-gene (or mendelian) disorders present with stroke as one of their clinical manifestation (**Table 1**).[48] Most of these monogenic disorders begin at an early age and affect multiple organ systems.[48,49] Diagnosis of mendelian syndromes manifesting with cerebrovascular disorders are particularly important in order to facilitate treatment and disease progression strategies, including genetic counseling to family members.[50,51] Furthermore, unraveling the mechanisms of disease responsible for monogenic stroke disorders may contribute to future understanding of the pathophysiology of sporadic stroke syndromes.[52]

COMPLEX GENETICS OF STROKE
Overview of Concepts and Methodology

Despite prior evidence of sporadic stroke heritability supported by familial studies, few genetic variants have been reliably identified in association with the risk, severity, or poststroke outcomes until now. Apart from specific single-gene disorders presenting with cerebrovascular syndromes (see **Table 1**), stroke is a complex genetic disorder influenced by a multitude of genetic variants that have a modest individual effect

Table 1
Monogenic disorders associated with stroke

Disorder	Mechanisms of Stroke	Other Clinical Features	Genetics
CADASIL	Small vessel arteriopathy	Depression, migraine headaches, cognitive decline, leukoaraiosis	*Notch3* gene; autosomal dominant
CARASIL	Small vessel arteriopathy	Dementia, leukoaraiosis, alopecia, spondylosis	*HTRA1* gene; autosomal recessive
Fabry disease	Small/large vessel arteriopathy; cardioembolism	Renal failure, angiokeratomas, cardiac failure and arrhythmias, neuropathy	*GAL* gene; X linked
Sickle cell disease	Small/large vessel arteriopathy; vasoocclusion	Anemia, pain crisis, seizures, infections	Beta globin gene; autosomal recessive
MELAS	Mitochondrial dysfunction	Myopathy, encephalopathy, lactic developmental delay	Multiple maternal mitochondrial DNA mutations
Homocystinuria	Large vessel arteriopathy, cervical artery dissection, cardioembolism	Premature atherosclerosis, lens dislocation, marfanlike features	*CBS* gene; autosomal recessive
Ehlers-Danlos type IV syndrome	Cervical artery dissection	Excessive soft tissue flexibility, large vessel dissections/rupture	*COL3A1*; autosomal dominant
Marfan syndrome	Cardioembolism; cervical artery dissection	Skeletal and soft tissue abnormalities, aortic dissection, ectopic lens	*FBN1* gene; autosomal dominant
HANAC	Small vessel arteriopathy	Nephropathy, leukoaraiosis, retinal arteriopathy, posttraumatic ICH, intracranial aneurysms	*COL4A1* gene; autosomal dominant
HCHWA	Hemorrhagic small vessel arteriopathy	Cerebral microbleeds, dementia, depression	*APP* (*Aβ*) gene; autosomal dominant
Moyamoya syndrome	Large vessel, nonatherosclerotic intracranial vasculopathy	Thoracic aneurysm and dissection, premature coronary artery disease, early ischemic stroke; ICH (adult)	*ACTA2* gene; autosomal dominant
HERNS	Small vessel arteriopathy	Retinopathy with visual impairment, nephropathy with hematuria, headaches	Chromosome 3p21 locus, gene unknown; autosomal recessive

Abbreviations: APP, amyloid precursor protein; CADASIL, cerebral autosomal dominant arteriopathy with subcortical infarcts and leukoencephalopathy; CARASIL, cerebral autosomal recessive arteriopathy with subcortical infarcts and leukoencephalopathy; CBS, cystathionine β-synthase; FBN, fibrillin; GAL, galactosidase; HANAC, hereditary angiopathy with nephropathy, aneurysm, and muscle cramps; HCHWA, hereditary cerebral hemorrhage with amyloidosis; HERNS, hereditary endotheliopathy with retinopathy, nephropathy, and stroke; HTRA, high-temperature requirement A serine peptidase; MELAS, mitochondrial myopathy, encephalopathy, lactic acidosis, and stroke.

size by increasing the risk of stroke when they are inherited together.[53] There have been 2 fundamentally different methodologies used to identify genetic variants thought to contribute to risk of disease: linkage analysis and association studies.[54]

Linkage analysis is traditionally used to study genetic variants within thoroughly assembled pedigrees. DNA of the family members affected by the disease or trait of interest is cross-tested for the presence of a specific genetic locus detected by calculating estimates of recombination frequency score (the logarithm [base 10] of odds): a measure of genetic linkage used in the creation of linkage maps.[55] In the past, genetic variants that have been discovered through linkage analysis were those tied to a significant risk of the disease when inherited, such as huntingtin (*HTT*) (chromosome 4p16.3) in Huntington disease[56] or *ANIB1* (chromosome 7q11.2) gene linked to cerebral aneurysms.[57] However, this methodology has not been successful in identifying genes with modest effects contributing to the development of complex disease phenotypes.

Genetic association studies have evolved over the past decade to address the limitations of linkage-based analysis. The major breakthrough in the last decade has been shifting the focus from the analysis of genetic association with preselected candidate genes implicated in any given disease pathway to an unbiased, genome-wide approach.[58] In most cases, inherently incomplete knowledge of disease biology led to candidate gene studies that yielded few substantial genetic discoveries.[59,60] The development of high-throughput genotyping techniques combined with advanced computational methods and rigorous statistical thresholds for significance has revolutionized genome-wide association (GWAS) analysis.[61] Unlike other methods, GWAS does not presuppose the location of the casual variant(s), which enables it to be a greatly powered method of genetic analysis.[61]

Genetic Architecture of Cerebrovascular Disorders

Ischemic stroke

Despite recent advances in genetics of complex disorders, the genetic architecture of sporadic ischemic stroke remains poorly understood. Plausible candidate gene pathways including inflammatory, coagulation/hemostasis, endothelial function, and renin-angiotensin-aldosterone pathways have been previously explored; however, few of these have withstood the test of independent replication or been confirmed by meta-analysis,[62] whereas others have been rejected through additional testing, as in the case of the phosphodiesterase 4D (*PDE4D*) variant.[63–65] In addition to phenotype-related challenges, insufficient statistical power and publication bias are recognized as obstacles to genetic discoveries in stroke.[33,66]

The Cohort for Heart and Aging Research in the Genomic Epidemiology (CHARGE) consortium conducted a GWAS analysis of incident ischemic stroke within population-based cohorts of stroke-free individuals. This large-scale analysis included 19,602 white people with 1544 incident strokes that developed over an average follow-up of 11 years.[67] An association between a chromosome 12p13 locus and incident ischemic stroke risk has been shown ($P<5 \times 10^{-8}$), and, when directly genotyped, rs12425791 was associated with an increased risk of total (ie, all types) and ischemic stroke, with hazard ratios of 1.30 (95% confidence interval [CI], 1.19–1.42) and 1.33 (95% CI, 1.21–1.47), respectively (yielding population-attributable risks of 11% and 12% in the discovery cohorts). In a replication cohort of 2430 black persons with 215 incident strokes (ischemic n = 191), another cohort of 574 black persons with 85 incident strokes (ischemic = 68), and 652 Dutch persons with ischemic stroke as well as 3613 unaffected persons, corresponding hazard ratios were 1.35 (95% CI, 1.01–1.79; $P = .04$) and 1.42 (95% CI, 1.06–1.91; $P = .02$) in the large cohort of black persons and 1.17 (95% CI, 1.01–1.37; $P = .03$) and 1.19 (95% CI, 1.01–1.41; $P = .04$) in the Dutch sample; the results of an underpowered analysis of the smaller black cohort were nonsignificant.[67] These findings have since undergone several replication attempts with highly variable results.[68–70] The largest validation effort of the chromosome 12p13 locus and risk of stroke did not replicate the association when tested in a series of hospital-based, case-control studies that involved nearly 9000 cases of ischemic stroke in subjects of predominantly European ancestry.[71]

GWAS of thoroughly phenotyped ischemic stroke completed to date confirmed the prior genetic discoveries in related disease processes and provided insights into disease pathways associated with carefully phenotyped stroke subtypes. In a large effort by the International Stroke Genetics Consortium, a chromosome 9p21 locus previously linked to coronary artery disease[72] showed a strong association with large vessel atherosclerotic stroke subtype, presumably through the vascular risk factors shared between coronary and cerebral artery disease.[73] This association remained significant (pooled odds ratio [OR] for the lead single nucleotide polymorphism [SNP] [rs1537378-C] of 1.21; 95% CI, 1.07–1.37; $P = .002$) after adjustment for the effects of demographics, population stratification, coronary artery disease, myocardial infarction, and other vascular factors, and was confirmed in independent analyses.[74] Genetic loci previously linked to atrial fibrillation, chromosome 4q25[75] and 16q22,[76] showed a strong association with the risk of cardioembolic stroke subtype[76,77] in patients with atrial fibrillation.

In the expanded effort to examine genome-wide variability associated with the risk of ischemic stroke, a meta-analysis of 15 cohorts with a combined total of 12,389 ischemic stroke cases and 62,004 controls of European ancestry has been conducted.[43] Replication of novel signals was completed in 13,347 cases and 29,083 controls. This study verified previous subtype-specific associations for cardioembolic stroke near *PITX2* ($P = 2.8 \times 10^{-16}$) and *ZFHX3* ($P = 2.28 \times 10^{-8}$), as well as for large vessel stroke at 9p21 locus ($P = 3.32 \times 10^{-5}$) and *HDAC9* ($P = 2.03 \times 10^{-12}$). Furthermore, it confirmed that the signal in each region could be attributed to 1 risk haplotype. An additional 12 novel loci associated with the risk of stroke at a nominal genome-wide significance ($P < 5 \times 10^{-6}$) have also been identified as potential candidate risk loci; however, none were reliably replicated in this analysis, likely because of insufficient statistical power.[43]

The progress to date shows that, along with the traditional genetic methods, genome-wide studies offer a promising and powerful approach to unraveling the genetic architecture of complex disorders such as ischemic stroke. Despite the persistent challenges posed by insufficient sample size, accuracy of phenotype ascertainment, and an inherent heterogeneity of the cerebrovascular disorders still limiting the pace of genetic discovery, a systematic, collaborative approach by the stroke genetics community is expected to yield additional results in the near future.

ICH

Similar efforts are ongoing to understand the complex genetic architecture of ICH.[78] Genetic susceptibility to the factors that predispose to intracerebral bleeding should be considered, including intrinsic cerebrovascular disease (such as vascular wall integrity, malformations) versus propensity for hematoma expansion, including both intrinsic (vascular wall or surrounding cerebral tissue properties) and extrinsic (hypocoagulability) factors. One indisputable genetic locus implicated in the ICH pathogenesis is apolipoprotein E (*APOE*). In addition to increasing the risk of recurrent lobar ICH,[79] the *APOE* ε2 and ε4 alleles increase risk of incident lobar ICH,[80] and the *APOE* ε2 allele has been associated with large baseline ICH volumes,[81] hematoma expansion,[82] and poor outcome[81] in lobar ICH. The *APOE* alleles are thought to exert their effect on the risk of ICH through previously suggested small cerebral vasculopathy (the *ε2* allele), ultimately leading to the diseased vessel rupture, as well as increased burden of amyloid deposition within the vessel wall (the *ε4* allele), as seen in cerebral amyloid angiopathy (CAA).[83] In CAA each allele is associated with characteristic pathologic changes.[84,85]

Additional insights into the shared contribution of common genetic variants to cerebral disorders have been gained from genetic studies of ICH and associated cerebrovascular disease. In a case-control genetic association study of 89 individuals with CAA-related ICH and 280 individuals with ICH unrelated to CAA compared with 324 ICH-free controls, a variant within the *CR1* gene (rs6656401), which is known to increase risk for Alzheimer disease, has been found to increase the risk of CAA-related ICH (OR, 1.61; 95% CI, 1.19–2.17; $P = 8.0 \times 10^{-4}$) as well as with risk of recurrent CAA-related ICH (hazard ratio, 1.35; 95% CI, 1.04–1.76; $P = .024$).[86] *CR1* is thought to influence β-amyloid deposition in brain tissue. In this study, adjustment for parenchymal amyloid burden did not cancel this effect, suggesting that, despite the correlation between parenchymal and vascular amyloid disorders, *CR1* acts independently on both processes, thus increasing risk of both Alzheimer disease and CAA.[86]

Another approach to deciphering the genetic contributions to a complex cerebrovascular phenotype, such as ICH, is to examine whether inherited variability in the vascular risk factor linked to ICH might play role in the overall disease risk. Hypertension is a potent risk factor for ICH, and several common variants have been linked to increased blood pressure levels. Although no individual hypertension-related SNP is anticipated to show an independent link to ICH, the cumulative burden of blood pressure–related SNPs has recently been shown to increase the risk of ICH and pre-ICH diagnosis of HTN.[87] In a prospective multicenter case-control study of 2272 subjects of European ancestry (1025 cases and 1247 controls), a genetic risk score comprising 39 SNPs previously reported to be associated with blood pressure levels was associated with increased risk of ICH (OR, 1.11; 95% CI, 1.02–1.21; $P = .01$) and the subset of ICH in deep regions (OR, 1.18; 95% CI, 1.07–1.30; $P = .001$), but not with the subset of lobar ICH. These findings suggest a potential cumulative genetic contribution from high blood pressure–related alleles in increasing risk of deep ICH as well as with clinically identified hypertension.[87]

Although discussion of intracranial aneurysms genetics is outside the scope of this article, a collaborative report by European and Japanese investigators has recently confirmed previously reported associations with the loci near *SOX17* (chromosome 8q11.23–q12.1; OR, 1.28; $P = 1.3 \times 10^{-12}$) and *CDKN2A-CDKN2B* (chromosome 9p21.3; OR, 1.31; $P = 1.5 \times 10^{-22}$), as well as reporting 3 new loci on chromosome 18q11.2 (OR, 1.22; $P = 1.1 \times 10^{-12}$), *STARD13-KL* on chromosome 13q13.1 (OR, 1.20; $P = 2.5 \times 10^{-9}$), and a gene-rich region on chromosome 10q24.32 (OR, 1.29; 1.2×10^{-9}) through a GWAS of 5891 cases and 14,181 controls.[88] Genetic contributions to subarachnoid hemorrhage are the subject of ongoing intense investigations.

WMH

MRI-detectable T2 and fluid-attenuated inversion recovery WMH, also seen as areas of hypoattenuation on CT (leukoaraiosis) are commonly reported as radiographic markers of cerebrovascular disease in the elderly.[89,90] In addition to being a powerful risk factor for ischemic stroke,[91] ICH,[92] severity of acute ischemia when it occurs,[93,94] as well as worse clinical outcomes after stroke,[95] a total WMH burden contributes to cognitive and functional disability of otherwise healthy aging adults through a multitude of cerebrovascular processes that are yet to be fully understood.[92,96–98] High heritability estimates for WMH in population-based studies[99,100] have led to a concerted, nearly decade-long effort to identify genetic factors for severe WMH[101]; however, until recently, no reliable loci have been identified. Among the CHARGE consortium participants, 7 community-based cohorts provided MRI-based WMH severity measurements on 9361 participants of European descent for a meta-analysis of GWAS data.[17] Six novel risk-associated SNPs in a single locus on chromosome 17q25 encompassing 6 known genes including *WBP2, TRIM65, TRIM47, MRPL38, FBF1,* and *ACOX1* have been identified. The most significant association was for rs3744028 ($P = 4.0 \times 10^{-9}$). Replication of the findings was completed in 3024 individuals from 2 additional cohorts ($p_{replication} = 1.3 \times 10^{-7}$). Variant alleles at these loci conferred a small increase in WMH burden (4%–8% of the overall mean WMH burden in the sample).[17]

In patients with stroke, WMH burden is strongly linked to severity of small vessel disease,[102,103] and the disease biology underlying its development and progression may vary significantly from that of WMH in otherwise healthy elderly people. In a multicenter, mitochondrial GWAS, 2284 ischemic stroke cases and 1728 controls from the International Stroke Genetics Consortium were genotyped for 64 mitochondrial SNPs.[18] Imputation resulted in 144 SNPs, which were tested in each cohort and in meta-analysis for ischemic stroke association. A genetic score comprising all mitochondrial variants showed an association with ischemic stroke in meta-analysis (OR, 1.13; $P<.0001$) and with WMH burden measured on MRI scans of 792 nested case individuals with ischemic stroke ($P = .037$).[18] These data suggest a type of shared genetic contribution that may help further elucidate the complex underlying biology of cerebrovascular disease. Large-scale collaborations intended to unravel the genetic architecture of WMH in patients with stroke are currently in progress.

FUTURE RESEARCH AND CLINICAL IMPLICATIONS

Genetic methodology has undergone a major revolution over the past decade. With the development of advanced genotyping and computational techniques, an understanding of complex traits has become more feasible than ever before. Furthermore, novel technologies including next-generation sequencing may prove to be more powerful still to fuel genetic discovery in stroke.[104] Despite clear setbacks in the genetics of cerebrovascular disease and stroke, preparations have been made for large-scale, systematic collaborations that promise a much needed advance in the field. With progress already being made on the role of stroke subtypes genetics, as well as shared contributions to disease-specific pathways, future discoveries may offer a greater scope and a more detailed assessment of the genetic spectrum of cerebrovascular disease. The main goals of cerebrovascular genetics remain to discover the multitude of risk factors that increase susceptibility to stroke or worse poststroke outcomes, to delineate their role in manifestation and pathogenesis of cerebral vessel disease, and to elucidate the pathways of discovery for novel genetics-based treatments that could deliver their preventative or therapeutic benefits on a personalized basis.

REFERENCES

1. Towfighi A, Saver JL. Stroke declines from third to fourth leading cause of death in the United States. Stroke 2011;42:2351–5.

2. Feigin VL, Lawes CM, Bennett DA, et al. Worldwide stroke incidence and early case fatality reported in 56 population-based studies: a systematic review. Lancet Neurol 2009;8:355.

3. Adeoye O, Hornung R, Khatri P, et al. Recombinant tissue-type plasminogen activator use for ischemic stroke in the United States. Stroke 2011;42:1952–5.

4. Tissue plasminogen activator for acute ischemic stroke. N Engl J Med 1995;333: 1581–8.

5. Jung KH. Challenges and pitfalls of stroke therapeutics research. Korean J Stroke 2011;13:11–5.

6. Lyden P. The future of basic science research and stroke: hubris and translational stroke research. Int J Stroke 2011;6:412.

7. Khor B, Gardet A, Xavier RJ. Genetics and pathogenesis of inflammatory bowel disease. Nature 2011;474:307.

8. Seddon JM, Reynolds R, Yu Y, et al. Risk models for progression to advanced age-related macular degeneration using demographic, environmental, genetic, and ocular factors. Ophthalmology 2011;118:2203.

9. Voight BF, Peloso GM, Orho-Melander M, et al. Plasma HDL cholesterol and risk of myocardial infarction: a mendelian randomisation study. Lancet 2012;380:572.

10. DePristo MA, Banks E, Poplin R, et al. A framework for variation discovery and genotyping using next-generation DNA sequencing data. Nat Genet 2011;43: 491.

11. 1000 Genomes Project Consortium, Abecasis GR, Altshuler D, Auton A, et al. A map of human genome variation from population-scale sequencing. Nature 2010;467:1061.

12. International HapMap 3 Consortium, Altshuler DM, Gibbs RA, Peltonen L, et al. Integrating common and rare genetic variation in diverse human populations. Nature 2010;467:52.

13. Voight BF, Scott LJ, Steinthorsdottir V, et al. Twelve type 2 diabetes susceptibility loci identified through large-scale association analysis. Nat Genet 2010;42:579.

14. Manning AK, Hivert M-F, Scott RA, et al. A genome-wide approach accounting for body mass index identifies genetic variants influencing fasting glycemic traits and insulin resistance. Nat Genet 2012;44:659.

15. Lage K, Greenway SC, Rosenfeld JA, et al. Genetic and environmental risk factors in congenital heart disease functionally converge in protein networks driving heart development. Proc Natl Acad Sci U S A 2012;109:14035–40.

16. Jostins L, Ripke S, Weersma RK, et al. Host-microbe interactions have shaped the genetic architecture of inflammatory bowel disease. Nature 2012;491:119.

17. Fornage M, Debette S, Bis JC, et al. Genome-wide association studies of cerebral white matter lesion burden: the charge consortium. Ann Neurol 2011;69(6): 928–39.

18. Anderson CD, Biffi A, Rahman R, et al, on behalf of the International Stroke Genetics Consortium. Common mitochondrial sequence variants in ischemic stroke. Ann Neurol 2011;69:471.

19. Easton JD, Saver JL, Albers GW, et al. Definition and evaluation of transient ischemic attack: a scientific statement for healthcare professionals from the American Heart Association/American Stroke Association Stroke Council; Council on Cardiovascular Surgery and Anesthesia; Council on Cardiovascular Radiology and Intervention; Council on Cardiovascular Nursing; and the Interdisciplinary Council on Peripheral Vascular Disease. Stroke 2009;40:2276–93.

20. Furie KL, Kasner SE, Adams RJ, et al. Guidelines for the prevention of stroke in patients with stroke or transient ischemic attack. Stroke 2011;42:227–76.

21. Ay H. Advances in the diagnosis of etiologic subtypes of ischemic stroke. Curr Neurol Neurosci Rep 2012;10:14.

22. Adams HP Jr, Bendixen BH, Kappelle LJ, et al. Classification of subtype of acute ischemic stroke. Definitions for use in a multicenter clinical trial. TOAST. Trial of Org 10172 in acute stroke treatment. Stroke 1993;24:35–41.

23. Low molecular weight heparinoid, ORG 10172 (danaparoid), and outcome after acute ischemic stroke: a randomized controlled trial. The Publications Committee for the Trial of ORG 10172 in Acute Stroke Treatment (TOAST) Investigators. JAMA 1998;279:1265–72.

24. Ay H, Benner T, Murat Arsava E, et al. A computerized algorithm for etiologic classification of ischemic stroke: the causative classification of stroke system. Stroke 2007;38:2979–84.

25. Saver JL, Warach S, Janis S, et al, for the National Institute of Neurological Disorders and Stroke Stroke Common Data Element Working Group. Standardizing the structure of stroke clinical and epidemiologic research data. Stroke 2012;43: 967–73.

26. Arsava EM, Ballabio E, Benner T, et al, On behalf of the International Stroke Genetics Consortium. The causative classification of stroke system: an international reliability and optimization study. Neurology 2010;75:1277–84.

27. Pantoni L, Garcia JH. Pathogenesis of leukoaraiosis: a review. Stroke 1997;28: 652–9.

28. Greenberg SM, Vernooij MW, Cordonnier C, et al. Cerebral microbleeds: a guide to detection and interpretation. Lancet Neurol 2009;8:165.

29. Smith EE, Schneider JA, Wardlaw JM, et al. Cerebral microinfarcts: the invisible lesions. Lancet Neurol 2012;11:272.

30. Adachi M, Hosoya T, Haku T, et al. Dilated Virchow-Robin spaces: MRI pathological study. Neuroradiology 1998;40:27.

31. Feldman HH, Maia LF, Mackenzie IR, et al. Superficial siderosis. Stroke 2008;39: 2894–7.

32. Pruissen DM, Kappelle LJ, Rosendaal FR, et al. Genetic association studies in ischaemic stroke. Cerebrovasc Dis 2009;27:290.

33. Meschia JF. Addressing the heterogeneity of the ischemic stroke phenotype in human genetics research. Stroke 2002;33:2770–4.

34. Meschia JF. Ischaemic stroke: one or several complex genetic disorders? Lancet Neurol 2003;2:459.

35. Carvajal-Carmona LG. Genetic dissection of intermediate phenotypes as a way to discover novel cancer susceptibility alleles. Curr Opin Genet Dev 2010;20:308.

36. Pendergrass SA, Brown-Gentry K, Dudek SM, et al. The use of phenome-wide association studies (PHEWAS) for exploration of novel genotype-phenotype relationships and pleiotropy discovery. Genet Epidemiol 2012;35:410.

37. Bak S, Gaist D, Sindrup SH, et al. Genetic liability in stroke. Stroke 2002;33: 769–74.

38. Liao D, Myers R, Hunt S, et al. Familial history of stroke and stroke risk. Stroke 1997;28:1908–12.

39. Touze E, Rothwell PM. Heritability of ischaemic stroke in women compared with men: a genetic epidemiological study. Lancet Neurol 2007;6:125.

40. Schulz UG, Flossmann E, Rothwell PM. Heritability of ischemic stroke in relation to age, vascular risk factors, and subtypes of incident stroke in population-based studies. Stroke 2004;35:819–24.

41. Nicolaou M, DeStefano AL, Gavras I, et al. Genetic predisposition to stroke in relatives of hypertensives. Stroke 2000;31:487–92.

42. Bevan S, Traylor M, Adib-Samii P, et al. Genetic heritability of ischemic stroke and the contribution of previously reported candidate gene and genomewide associations. Stroke 2012;43(12):3161–7.

43. Traylor M, Farrall M, Holliday EG, et al. Genetic risk factors for ischaemic stroke and its subtypes (the Metastroke Collaboration): a meta-analysis of genome-wide association studies. Lancet Neurol 2012;11:951.

44. Flossmann E, Schulz UG, Rothwell PM. Systematic review of methods and results of studies of the genetic epidemiology of ischemic stroke. Stroke 2004; 35:212–27.

45. Woo D, Sauerbeck LR, Kissela BM, et al. Genetic and environmental risk factors for intracerebral hemorrhage: preliminary results of a population-based study. Stroke 2002;33:1190–6 [discussion: 1190–6].

46. Kissela BM, Sauerbeck L, Woo D, et al. Subarachnoid hemorrhage. Stroke 2002;33:1321–6.

47. Feigin VL, Rinkel GJ, Lawes CM, et al. Risk factors for subarachnoid hemorrhage. Stroke 2005;36:2773–80.

48. Muqtadar H, Testai F. Single gene disorders associated with stroke: a review and update on treatment options. Curr Treat Options Cardiovasc Med 2012; 14:288–97.

49. Meschia JF, Brott TG, Brown RD Jr. Genetics of cerebrovascular disorders. Mayo Clin Proc 2005;80:122.

50. Dichgans M. A new cause of hereditary small vessel disease: angiopathy of retina and brain. Neurology 2003;60:8–9.

51. Opherk C, Peters N, Herzog J, et al. Long-term prognosis and causes of death in CADASIL: a retrospective study in 411 patients. Brain 2004;127:2533–9.

52. Dichgans M. Genetics of ischaemic stroke. Lancet Neurol 2007;6:149–61.

53. Altshuler D, Daly M, Kruglyak L. Guilt by association. Nat Genet 2000;26:135–7.

54. Rosand J, Altshuler D. Human genome sequence variation and the search for genes influencing stroke. Stroke 2003;34:2512–6.

55. Morton N. Sequential tests for the detection of linkage. Am J Hum Genet 1955;7: 277–318.

56. MacDonald ME, Ambrose CM, Duyao MP, et al. A novel gene containing a trinucleotide repeat that is expanded and unstable on Huntington's disease chromosomes. Cell 1993;72:971.

57. Onda H, Kasuya H, Yoneyama T, et al. Genomewide-linkage and haplotype-association studies map intracranial aneurysm to chromosome 7q11. Am J Hum Genet 2001;69:804.

58. The International HC. A haplotype map of the human genome. Nature 2005; 437(7063):1299–320.

59. Hirschhorn JN, Lohmueller K, Byrne E, et al. A comprehensive review of genetic association studies. Genet Med 2002;4:45–61.

60. Lohmueller KE, Pearce CL, Pike M, et al. Meta-analysis of genetic association studies supports a contribution of common variants to susceptibility to common disease. Nat Genet 2003;33:177–82.

61. Hirschhorn JN, Daly MJ. Genome-wide association studies for common diseases and complex traits. Nat Rev Genet 2005;6:95.

62. Casas JP, Hingorani AD, Bautista LE, et al. Meta-analysis of genetic studies in ischemic stroke: thirty-two genes involving approximately 18,000 cases and 58,000 controls. Arch Neurol 2004;61:1652.

63. Gretarsdottir S, Thorleifsson G, Reynisdottir ST, et al. The gene encoding phosphodiesterase 4D confers risk of ischemic stroke. Nat Genet 2003;35:131–8.

64. Bevan S, Dichgans M, Gschwendtner A, et al. Variation in the PDE4D gene and ischemic stroke risk: a systematic review and meta-analysis on 5200 cases and 6600 controls. Stroke 2008;39:1966–71.
65. Rosand J, Bayley N, Rost N, et al. Many hypotheses but no replication for the association between PDE4D and stroke. Nat Genet 2006;38:1091.
66. Meschia JF. Stroke genome-wide association studies: the large numbers imperative. Stroke 2010;41:579–80.
67. Ikram MA, Seshadri S, Bis JC, et al. Genomewide association studies of stroke. N Engl J Med 2009;360:1718–28.
68. Matsushita T, Umeno J, Hirakawa Y, et al. Association study of the polymorphisms on chromosome 12p13 with atherothrombotic stroke in the Japanese population. J Hum Genet 2010;55:473.
69. Ding H, Tu X, Xu Y, et al. No evidence for association of 12p13 SNPS rs11833579 and rs12425791 within NINJ2 gene with ischemic stroke in Chinese Han population. Atherosclerosis 2011;216:381.
70. Wan XH, Li SJ, Cheng P, et al. NINJ2 polymorphism is associated with ischemic stroke in Chinese Han population. J Neurol Sci 2011;308:67.
71. International Stroke Genetics Consortium and Wellcome Trust Case-Control Consortium 2. Failure to validate association between 12p13 variants and ischemic stroke. N Engl J Med 2010;362:1547–50.
72. McPherson R, Pertsemlidis A, Kavaslar N, et al. A common allele on chromosome 9 associated with coronary heart disease. Science 2007;316:1488–91.
73. Gschwendtner A, Bevan S, Cole J, et al, International Stroke Genetics Consortium. Sequence variants on chromosome 9p21.3 confer risk for atherosclerotic stroke. Ann Neurol 2009;65:531–9.
74. Anderson CD, Biffi A, Rost NS, et al. Chromosome 9p21 in ischemic stroke: population structure and meta-analysis. Stroke 2010;41:1123–31.
75. Gudbjartsson DF, Arnar DO, Helgadottir A, et al. Variants conferring risk of atrial fibrillation on chromosome 4q25. Nature 2007;448:353.
76. Gudbjartsson DF, Holm H, Gretarsdottir S, et al. A sequence variant in ZFHX3 on 16q22 associates with atrial fibrillation and ischemic stroke. Nat Genet 2009;41:876.
77. Gretarsdottir S, Thorleifsson G, Manolescu A, et al. Risk variants for atrial fibrillation on chromosome 4q25 associate with ischemic stroke. Ann Neurol 2008;64:402.
78. Rost NS, Greenberg SM, Rosand J. The genetic architecture of intracerebral hemorrhage. Stroke 2008;39:2166–73.
79. O'Donnell HC, Rosand J, Knudsen KA, et al. Apolipoprotein E genotype and the risk of recurrent lobar intracerebral hemorrhage [see comments]. N Engl J Med 2000;342:240–5.
80. Biffi A, Sonni A, Anderson CD, et al, on behalf of the International Stroke Genetics Consortium. Variants at APOE influence risk of deep and lobar intracerebral hemorrhage. Ann Neurol 2010;68:934.
81. Biffi A, Anderson CD, Jagiella JM, et al. APOE genotype and extent of bleeding and outcome in lobar intracerebral haemorrhage: a genetic association study. Lancet Neurol 2011;10:702–9. http://dx.doi.org/10.1016/S1474-4422(1011)70148-X.
82. Brouwers HB, Biffi A, Ayres AM, et al. Apolipoprotein E genotype predicts hematoma expansion in lobar intracerebral hemorrhage. Stroke 2012;43:1490–5.
83. Vinters HV. Cerebral amyloid angiopathy. A critical review. Stroke 1987;18:311–24.

84. Greenberg SM, Vonsattel JPG, Segal AZ, et al. Association of apolipoprotein E epsilon2 and vasculopathy in cerebral amyloid angiopathy. Neurology 1998;50: 961–5.

85. Alonzo NC, Hyman BT, Rebeck GW, et al. Progression of cerebral amyloid angiopathy: accumulation of amyloid-[latin sharp s]40 in affected vessels. J Neuropathol Exp Neurol 1998;57:353–9.

86. Biffi A, Shulman JM, Jagiella JM, et al. Genetic variation at CR1 increases risk of cerebral amyloid angiopathy. Neurology 2012;78:334–41.

87. Falcone GJ, Biffi A, Devan WJ, et al, on behalf of the International Stroke Genetics Consortium. Burden of risk alleles for hypertension increases risk of intracerebral hemorrhage. Stroke 2012;43:2877–83.

88. Yasuno K, Bilguvar K, Bijlenga P, et al. Genome-wide association study of intracranial aneurysm identifies three new risk loci. Nat Genet 2010;42:420.

89. de Leeuw FE, de Groot JC, Achten E, et al. Prevalence of cerebral white matter lesions in elderly people: a population based magnetic resonance imaging study. The Rotterdam Scan Study. J Neurol Neurosurg Psychiatry 2001;70:9–14.

90. Bernick C, Kuller L, Dulberg C, et al. Silent MRI infarcts and the risk of future stroke: the cardiovascular health study. Neurology 2001;57:1222–9.

91. Jeerakathil T, Wolf PA, Beiser A, et al. Stroke risk profile predicts white matter hyperintensity volume: the Framingham Study. Stroke 2004;35:1857–61.

92. Smith EE, Rosand J, Knudsen KA, et al. Leukoaraiosis is associated with warfarin-related hemorrhage following ischemic stroke. Neurology 2002;59: 193–7.

93. Ay H, Arsava EM, Rosand J, et al. Severity of leukoaraiosis and susceptibility to infarct growth in acute stroke. Stroke 2008;39:1409–13.

94. Rost NS, Fitzpatrick K, Biffi A, et al. White matter hyperintensity burden and susceptibility to cerebral ischemia. Stroke 2010;41:2807–11.

95. Arsava EM, Bayrlee A, Vangel M, et al. Severity of leukoaraiosis determines clinical phenotype after brain infarction. Neurology 2011;77:55–61.

96. de Groot JC, de Leeuw FE, Oudkerk M, et al. Cerebral white matter lesions and cognitive function: the Rotterdam Scan Study. Ann Neurol 2000;47:145–51.

97. de Groot JC, de Leeuw FE, Oudkerk M, et al. Cerebral white matter lesions and depressive symptoms in elderly adults. Arch Gen Psychiatry 2000;57:1071–6.

98. Smith EE. Leukoaraiosis and stroke. Stroke 2010;41:S139–43.

99. Carmelli D, DeCarli C, Swan GE, et al. Evidence for genetic variance in white matter hyperintensity volume in normal elderly male twins. Stroke 1998;29: 1177–81.

100. Atwood LD, Wolf PA, Heard-Costa NL, et al. Genetic variation in white matter hyperintensity volume in the Framingham Study. Stroke 2004;35:1609–13.

101. Assareh A, Mather KA, Schofield PR, et al. The genetics of white matter lesions. CNS Neurosci Ther 2010;17:525.

102. Rost NS, Rahman R, Sonni S, et al. Determinants of white matter hyperintensity volume in patients with acute ischemic stroke. J Stroke Cerebrovasc Dis 2010; 19:230–5.

103. Rost NS, Rahman RM, Biffi A, et al. White matter hyperintensity volume is increased in small vessel stroke subtypes. Neurology 2010;75:1670–7.

104. Cole JW, Stine OC, Liu X, et al. Rare variants in ischemic stroke: an exome pilot study. PLoS One 2012;7(4):e35591. http://dx.doi.org/10.1371/journal.pone.0035591.

Clinical Neurogenetics
Amyotrophic Lateral Sclerosis

Matthew B. Harms, MD[a],*, Robert H. Baloh, MD, PhD[b],*

KEYWORDS

- Amyotrophic lateral sclerosis • ALS • Genetics • Phenotypes

KEY POINTS

- ALS is increasingly genetically heterogeneous as studies have implicated more than 20 genes, at least half of which are definitively causative and represent moderate-penetrance to high-penetrance genes.
- Mutations in ALS genes are increasingly recognized in patients with no family history, emphasizing the incomplete ascertainment of familial links as well as the importance of genetic causes in even apparently sporadic cases.
- With a few notable exceptions, correlations between the mutated gene and the ALS phenotype are imprecise. Thus, sequencing approaches targeting the increasing number of ALS genes are required, including next-generation gene panels or whole-exome sequencing.

DEFINITION

Amyotrophic lateral sclerosis (ALS), also referred to as Lou Gehrig disease or motor neuron disease, is a fatal neurodegenerative disease characterized by the progressive loss of cortical, brainstem, and spinal cord motor neurons.

SYMPTOMS AND CLINICAL COURSE

The classic clinical symptoms of ALS arise from the progressive loss of both upper motor neurons (UMN) located in the cerebral cortex and lower motor neurons (LMN) located in brainstem nuclei or the anterior horn of the spinal cord. However,

This work was supported by National Institutes of Health (NIH) Grants NS055980 and NS069669 (R.H.B), and NS075094 (M.B.H.). R.H.B. holds a Career Award for Medical Scientists from the Burroughs Wellcome Fund.

[a] Neuromuscular Division, Department of Neurology, Hope Center for Neurological Disorders, Washington University School of Medicine, 660 South Euclid Avenue, St Louis, MO 63110, USA;
[b] Department of Neurology, Regenerative Medicine Institute, Cedars-Sinai Medical Center, 8730 Alden Drive, Los Angeles, CA 90048, USA
* Corresponding authors.
E-mail addresses: harmsm@neuro.wustl.edu; robert.baloh@csmc.edu

ALS is increasingly recognized as a multisystem neurodegenerative disease, in which motor neurons are particularly, but not exclusively, involved.[1–3] As a result, degeneration of nonmotor system neurons occurs and results in clinically recognizable symptoms.

- LMN degeneration produces
  - Muscle cramping and fasciculations, even before weakness occurs
  - Atrophy of affected muscles
  - Weakness
- UMN degeneration produces
  - Slowed movement and weakness in a pyramidal distribution
  - Uncoordinated movements, particularly of fine manipulation
  - Spastic tone
  - Increased deep tendon reflexes, sometimes with spread or clonus
  - Lost regulation of laughing and/or crying (pseudobulbar affect)
- Nonmotor system degeneration can produce
  - Executive dysfunction in most patients (loss of frontotemporal neurons)[4]
  - Frontotemporal dementia in ~5% (loss of frontotemporal neurons)[5,6]
  - Parkinsonism (basal ganglia)[7,8]
  - Sensory loss (dorsal root ganglia)[9,10]

ALS is commonly diagnosed according to the revised El Escorial criteria.[11,12] These criteria require:

- Evidence of LMN degeneration by clinical examination, neurophysiologic testing, or pathologic examination in 1 or more of 4 body regions (bulbar, cervical, thoracic, lumbar)
- Evidence of UMN degeneration by clinical examination
- Progressive spread of signs within a body region or to additional body regions
- Exclusion of causes other than ALS by appropriate testing (eg, laboratory, imaging, electrodiagnostic)

These criteria were initially developed for research purposes but are routinely applied in many neuromuscular clinics to specify the certainty of an ALS diagnosis according to definite, probable, and possible categories (**Table 1**).

The clinical phenotype of a given patient with ALS depends on the location, degree, and proportion of LMN, UMN, and nonmotor involvement. At one end of the spectrum are patients with progressive muscular atrophy (PMA) where only LMN involvement is

Table 1	
Revised El Escorial criteria for the classification of ALS diagnostic certainty	
Category	
Definite	UMN and LMN signs in the bulbar region and ≥2 other spinal regions OR UMN and LMN signs in 3 spinal regions with progression over 12 mo
Probable	UMN and LMN signs in ≥2 regions, with UMN signs above a region with LMN signs AND progression over 12 mo after diagnosis
Probable, laboratory supported	UMN and LMN signs in only 1 region, or UMN signs in only 1 region AND electromyographic evidence for LMN degeneration is present in ≥2 regions without another cause
Possible	UMN or LMN signs in only 1 region (ie, progressive bulbar palsy) UMN signs in ≥2 regions (ie, primary lateral sclerosis)

clinically apparent. Primary lateral sclerosis (PLS) occupies the other end, with UMN involvement as its defining feature. Current evidence suggests that most cases of PMA and PLS eventually progress to meet the criteria for ALS and are therefore diseases on the ALS spectrum.[13–16] Furthermore, sequencing studies highlight identical genetic causes.[17] Many lines of evidence also support ALS and frontotemporal dementia (FTD) as 2 ends of a clinical spectrum, including clinical observations, co-occurrence in patients, shared neuropathologic findings, and genetic causes in common (reviewed in Refs.[18,19]).

ALS phenotypes are frequently classified by the site of symptom onset. Two-thirds of patients have onset in the limbs (spinal onset), with an approximately equal distribution between upper and lower extremities.[20–22] The remaining one-third of patients first experience difficulties with speech or swallowing (bulbar onset). Regardless of the site of onset or initial phenotype, the relentless loss of motor system neurons leads to progressive paralysis and eventually to terminal respiratory failure. The rate of disease progression varies widely, but for a given patient seems fairly linear, possibly with faster rates of decline in early and late disease.[23] Median survival estimates center on 32 months[24] from symptom onset, but vary from 23 to 48 months.[25–29] However, 20% of patients survive 5 years and 10% are still living after a decade.[24] Across multiple studies, bulbar onset ALS is consistently found to be more common in women, shows a later age of onset, and is associated with a poorer prognosis.[4,30–32] An earlier age of onset, a family history of ALS, and presentation with PLS are consistent predictors of longer survival.[4,20,22] Studies suggest that improvements in supportive care, including earlier use of noninvasive ventilation are improving survival trends.[29,33] Riluzole is the only medication approved for the treatment of ALS and improves survival by 2 to 3 months.[34]

NATURE OF THE DISEASE

The incidence of ALS is generally consistent across diverse populations at 1 to 3 per 100,000,[35–42] producing a lifetime risk of 1 in 300 to 1000.[43,44] ALS is more common in men, typically by a ratio of 1.3,[20,30,45] but this gender gap may be disappearing as a result of a rising incidence of ALS among women.[44,46]

Beginning with the earliest descriptions of the disease, hereditary forms of ALS have been apparent[47] and prompted categorization into familial (FALS) and sporadic (SALS) forms. Most cases of FALS show autosomal dominant inheritance; X-linked and recessive patterns are rare. The prevalence of FALS is widely cited to be 10%, but this number depends greatly on the population sampled and the definition of FALS used (for which is there is currently no clear consensus[48]). For example, regional clinic-based series report FALS rates as high as 23%,[49,50] whereas prospective population-based analyses suggest the number may be closer to 5% with modest geographic variability.[51] It has been proposed that the definition of FALS should take into consideration a family history of other neurodegenerative diseases, including FTD (**Table 2**).[52]

CLINICAL FINDINGS
Physical Examination

Physical examination findings in early ALS are highly variable, and depend on the site of symptom onset in a given patient, the relative contributions of upper and lower motor neuron degeneration, and the degree of extramotor involvement. No examination findings reliably distinguish FALS from SALS, or definitively differentiate between specific genetic causes.

Table 2
Proposed classification of familial ALS

Category	Criteria
Definite	≥3 affected individuals OR 2 affected individuals with a segregating of genetic mutation
Probable	≥1 affected first-degree or second-degree relative(s)
Possible	An affected relative is more distant than second degree OR A sporadic patient is found to carry a known genetic mutation OR A first-degree relative has/had frontotemporal dementia, but not ALS

Data from Byrne S, Bede P, Elamin M, et al. Proposed criteria for familial amyotrophic lateral sclerosis. Amyotroph Lateral Scler 2011;12(3):157–9.

Other Diagnostic Modalities

Nerve conduction studies (NCS) and electromyography (EMG) play an important role in identifying the degree and extent of lower motor neuron loss in ALS. Furthermore, they are used to exclude important mimics of ALS, including radiculopathy, polyneuropathies, and multifocal motor neuropathy. Magnetic resonance imaging (MRI) and analysis of cerebrospinal fluid are also frequently used to rule out infectious polyradiculitis, carcinomatosis, lymphomatosis, and other mimics of ALS.

GENETIC BASIS OF DISEASE

Rapid advances in DNA sequencing technologies have accelerated the pace of gene discovery and revealed an impressive genetic heterogeneity in ALS. Mutations in more than 22 genes have now been described in patients with ALS or ALS-like phenotypes; more than half of these represent clear moderate-penetrance or high-penetrance causative genes (**Table 3**). Several themes have been highlighted by these discoveries:

1. Genotype-phenotype correlations are imprecise in most cases.
   As is often the case with adult-onset, autosomal dominant disease, the clinical manifestations of each gene and each specific mutation show broad clinical heterogeneity. Even within a given pedigree, the age of onset can span decades, the ALS phenotype can range from pure LMN syndrome to pure FTD, and the course of the disease can range from fast progression to prolonged survival. There are some identifiable broad trends in phenotypes (eg, *SOD1* mutations tend to have lower extremity onset with predominantly LMN manifestations, *TARDBP* mutations are more commonly upper extremity onset, *C9ORF72* expansions have an increased rate of bulbar onset and of accompanying FTD), but for each gene, many cases disprove the rules. As a result, it is usually difficult to predict which gene might be mutated in a given pedigree or patient.
2. Mutations in known ALS genes also explain a minority of patients with SALS.
   This fact is not surprising given that familial and sporadic ALS are virtually indistinguishable in the clinic and under the microscope, showing similar ranges of onset, survival, phenotype, and neuropathologic features. Mathematical models considering current demographic trends (eg, increasingly smaller family sizes),

predict that moderate-penetrance and even high-penetrance mutations would seem sporadic at approximately the same rate observed in empirical cohorts.[53]

3. In a surprising number of cases, more than 1 ALS-associated mutation may be found.

As the simultaneous sequencing of panels of ALS genes has increased with declining costs of sequencing, patients with mutations in more than 1 gene are being reported. Most commonly, the *C9ORF72* expansion is found alongside a second mutation, but co-occurrence has also been noted for other combinations of genes, including *FUS* with *ANG*,[54] *UBQLN2* with *TARDBP* or *OPTN*.[55] These cases are possible examples of oligogenic inheritance, in which clinical manifestations of disease are influenced by the presence of both mutations. At this point, however, the number of 2-hit cases is small and it is unclear whether second mutations influence penetrance, disease phenotype, or progression.

C9ORF72

In 2006, FALS pedigrees were first linked to chromosome 9p21,[56] with a notable co-occurrence of ALS and FTD. This pedigree and additional 9p21-linked ALS/FTD families were recently shown to carry a massive expansion of a hexanucleotide repeat in the first intron of *C9ORF72*.[57,58] Whereas normal individuals carry 2 to 30 of the GGGGCC repeat units, pathologic expansions are at least 700 to 2400 repeat units in length, show a tremendous degree of somatic variability, and seem to be larger in neuronal tissue than elsewhere.[59] As a result of a Northern European founder mutation, the prevalence of *C9ORF72* expansions is highest in white populations, which explains 37% of FALS, 25% of familial FTD, and ~6% of sporadic cases of ALS or FTD.[60] However, the mutation is found worldwide.[61]

The function of *C9ORF72* is currently unknown, but recent studies suggest it may function as a guanine exchange factor for Rab GTPases.[62,63] How a noncoding expansion in the gene causes neurodegeneration is not currently known, but emerging evidence supports the following:

- Loss of function: repeat expansions reduce allele-specific expression by as much as 50%.[57,64]
- Gain of function:
  - Repeat-containing RNA transcripts[57] form intranuclear foci, believed to sequester required RNA binding proteins and lead to disrupted gene expression and dysregulated alternative splicing, as is the case for myotonic dystrophy (reviewed in Ref.[65]).
  - Repeat-associated non–ATG-dependent translation (RANT) of the GGGGCC repeat itself produces repetitive dipeptides that aggregate in the cytoplasm of affected cells.[66,67]

The *C9ORF72* repeat expansion most commonly presents with ALS, ALS/FTD, or pure FTD, and is associated with an increased incidence of bulbar symptom onset, an earlier age of onset, and statistically shorter survival. The expansion has also been found in patients with other neurodegenerative syndromes, including Alzheimer disease, Parkinson disease, corticobasal degeneration, and ataxia.[68–71]

SOD1

In 1993, *SOD1,* encoding copper/zinc superoxide dismutase, was the first causative gene identified for ALS.[72] Since then, more than 160 mutations have been reported, involving almost every amino acid of the protein (http://alsod.iop.kcl.ac.uk/). *SOD1*

Table 3
Genetic causes of ALS

Gene	Frequency	Inheritance	Main Phenotype(s)	Other Features
C9ORF72	30%–50% of FALS; as high as 10% of SALS	AD	ALS-FTD = ALS only = FTD only	Parkinsonism, psychosis
SOD1	10%–20% of FALS; as high as 3% of SALS	AD (rare AR or de novo)	ALS; FTD is rare	Often LMN predominant; highly variable
TARDBP	0%–62% of FALS; as high as 2% of SALS	AD (rare AR)	ALS; ALS-FTD	Parkinsonism
FUS	1%–13% of FALS; as high as 2% of SALS	AD (rare AR and de novo)	ALS > FTD	Juvenile ALS; mutations reported in essential tremor
UBQLN2	0%–2.6% FALS; rare SALS cases reported	X-linked dominant	ALS-FTD; pure FTD in single patient thus far	Reduced penetrance in females; seen in patients with potential second mutations
ANG	Most common in Irish/Scottish populations	AD	ALS; rare FTD	Rare variants increased in Parkinson disease
OPTN	0%–4% FALS; rare SALS cases reported	AD, AR	ALS-FTD	Mutations also cause POAG
FIG4	2.8% FALS; 0%–1.6% SALS	AD	ALS, UMN predominant	Only 1 additional study reports sequencing FIG4, with 0/80 gene negative SALS
PFN1[123]	0%–2.6% FALS; single SALS report	AD	ALS	Only limb onset described thus far
VCP	0%–1% FALS; reported in SALS	AD	ALS; ALS-FTD	Mutations also cause IBMPFD
SETX	Rare	AD	Juvenile ALS; dHMN	Recessive mutations cause AOA2
VAPB	Rare in FALS; Novel or rare variants found; segregation not shown	AD	Late-onset SMA; ALS	P56S mutation with best evidence found in Brazilian kindreds

hnRNPA2B1	Single family	AD	ALS IBMPFD like	
hnRNPA1	Two families; 1 SALS	AD	ALS IBMPFD like	
DAO	Single FALS pedigree	AD	ALS	
TAF15	Novel or rare variants found in SALS	AD	ALS	N/A
EWSR1	Novel or rare variants found in SALS	AD	ALS	N/A
SQSTM1	Novel or rare variants found; segregation not shown	AD	ALS	Mutations also cause Paget disease
CHMP2B	Novel or rare variants found; segregation not shown	AD		
NEFH	Novel or rare variants found: segregation not shown	AD	ALS	
DCTN1	Novel or rare variants found; segregation not shown	AD	LMN disease, dHMN	Mutations also cause Perry syndrome
PRPH	Novel or rare variants found; segregation not shown	AD		
SPG11	Rare	AR	Juvenile ALS; HSP	
ALS2	Rare	AR	Juvenile ALS; juvenile PLS; infantile HSP	
SIGMAR1	1 consanguineous family reported	AR	Juvenile ALS	FALS cases later found to carry the C9ORF72 hexanucleotide expansion
ERLIN2	1 consanguineous family reported	AR	Juvenile PLS; HSP	

Abbreviations: AD, autosomal dominant; AOA2, ataxia with oculomotor apraxia type 2; AR, autosomal recessive; dHMN, distal hereditary motor neuropathy; FALS, familial ALS; FTD, frontotemporal dementia; HSP, hereditary spastic paraparesis; IBMPFD, inclusion body myopathy with Paget disease and frontotemporal dementia; LMN, lower motor neuron; N/A, not applicable; PLS, primary lateral sclerosis; POAG, primary open-angle glaucoma; SALS, sporadic ALS; SMA, spinal muscular atrophy; UMN, upper motor neuron.

mutations account for 15% to 20% of FALS pedigrees[73,74] and until the discovery of C9ORF72 was the most commonly identified gene in ALS. This likely remains true in many nonwhite populations, in which C9ORF72 is much less common.

Although SOD1 is the best studied of all ALS genes, our understanding of its pathogenic mechanism is incomplete. SOD1 is a ubiquitously expressed cytosolic protein known to neutralize superoxides. Several clearly pathogenic mutations have no effect on the dismutase activity of SOD1 and reduced enzyme activity shows no correlation with disease severity, suggesting that a gain-of-function mechanism most likely explains the pathogenesis.[75] Misfolding of SOD1 is likely to be important, with downstream disruption of mitochondrial function, oxidative stress, endosomal trafficking, and excitotoxicity (reviewed in Ref.[76]).

SOD1-associated ALS is clinically heterogeneous but shows several phenotypic trends that warrant mention. First, cognitive impairment is infrequent and FTD is rare.[77] Second, in most patients, UMN findings are minimal or absent and the clinical picture is dominated by LMN degeneration.[78] Third, because large numbers of patients with individual mutations have been studied, some genotype-phenotype correlations can be made: p.A5V (also called A4V) is associated with rapidly progressive disease, whereas other mutations (including p.G38R and p.D11Y) are uniformly slow.[79,80] A recessive form found in Scandinavia is caused by homozygous p.D91A mutations and causes a characteristic ascending paralysis as a result of LMN degeneration.[81]

TARDBP

One consistent pathologic finding in cases of ALS and FTD is the presence of heavily ubiquitinated neuronal cytoplasmic inclusions, which in 2006 were found to contain TDP-43, encoded by the TARDBP gene.[82] Mutations in TARDBP were soon found to cause ALS[83–85] and later, FTD.[86] TARDBP causes 3% to 5% of FALS and less than 1% of SALS, although founder mutations make it more common in some areas.[49]

TDP-43 is a DNA/RNA binding protein with broad roles in RNA metabolism,[87,88] including microRNA biogenesis.[89] Almost all pathogenic mutations affect the C-terminal glycine-rich domain, the function of which is still being uncovered. Mutations in this domain result in the translocation of TDP-43 from the nucleus to the cytoplasm, where it forms the hallmark aggregates. Whether it is nuclear depletion of TDP-43, cytoplasmic aggregation, or both that causes neurodegeneration is an area of active investigation using an expanding list of cellular and animal models.

Patients with TARDBP mutations have an earlier age of onset and longer disease duration,[90] but otherwise share the broad range of presentations with sporadic ALS. Upper extremity onset is the most common presentation, which may help differentiate from patients with SOD1 mutations.[90] Some patients have extrapyramidal involvement and rarely present with pure parkinsonism.[91,92] Co-occurrence of FTD with ALS is common, but pure FTD has also been reported.[86]

FUS

Not long after the discovery of TARDBP, linkage of ALS families to chromosome 16 revealed mutations in another RNA binding protein called FUS.[93,94] Broader screening of this gene in FALS cohorts has shown a frequency of 1% to 8% of Caucasian pedigrees,[95–97] but a much higher frequency (10%–13%) in Asian populations.[98–100] A similar trend is recognized in SALS, where the FUS mutation rate is 0% to 0.74%[95,101,102] among Caucasians but approaches 2% in Asian studies.[100,103] Most families show autosomal dominant transmission, but recessive inheritance[93] and de novo cases with juvenile onset and rapid progression are also reported.[104,105]

FUS is a member of the FET family of proteins along with EWSR1 and TAF15, which have also been implicated in ALS.[106,107] As with *TARDBP*, disease-associated mutations cluster in the C-terminal domain and cause mislocalization of FUS from the nucleus into the cytoplasm, where it is found in cytoplasmic aggregates.[93,94] The degree of impaired nuclear localization correlates with the age of onset for a given mutation.[108] *FUS* mutations, with their cytoplasmic redistribution are hypothesized to cause neurodegeneration by a combination of mechanisms focused on (1) loss of its normal functions in the nucleus (microRNA biosynthesis, gene expression regulation, alternative splicing) and (2) a toxic gain of function in the cytoplasm (stress granules, aggregation).

FUS mutations are associated with predominantly lower motor neuron symptoms[109] and most show incomplete penetrance.[110] In comparison with other causes of FALS (including *SOD1*), *FUS* mutation carriers show earlier onset and shorter survival.[54,111] Several specific mutations, especially p.P525L, typically arise de novo and have an early enough onset to be classified as juvenile ALS.[112] Truncation mutations resulting in deletion of the C-terminal nuclear localization domain also show more aggressive disease.[97] A broader set of phenotypes is also rarely associated with FUS mutations, including behavioral-variant FTD.[113] Mutations in FUS have also been reported in familial essential tremor, but screening of other cohorts has failed to find additional families.[114]

UBQLN2

Candidate gene sequencing in a large family with X-linked inheritance of ALS-FTD led to the recent identification of *UBQLN2* as a cause of ALS.[115] *UBQLN2* mutations are found in up to 2% of families without evidence of male-to-male transmission, but have proved to be rarer in other large FALS cohorts.[55,116–118] The earliest reported mutations all disrupt proline residues in a unique, but highly conserved, PXX domain.[115] Subsequent studies have uncovered a few additional families with PXX domain mutations and 2 Australian pedigrees have been reported with a pathogenic mutation adjacent to this domain.[119] Screening in patients with SALS has uncovered additional novel variants with a frequency of ~1%,[120] but most fall outside the PXX domain and their pathogenicity is currently uncertain.[116,121] Phenotypes associated with *UBQLN2* mutations include ALS, ALS with FTD, and juvenile-onset ALS.[115]

Ubiquilin 2 is 1 of 4 members of the ubiquitinlike family, with roles in delivering ubiquitinated proteins to the proteasome for degradation. *UBQLN2* alone has the unique PXX domain in which most mutations have been found, and it is hypothesized that this domain and its proline residues are important for the specificity of protein-protein interactions.[115] UBQLN2 localizes to the same neuronal cytoplasmic inclusions that stain for TDP-43, FUS, and OPTN, not just in the spinal cords of patients with *UBQLN2* mutations, but in all ALS patients studied.[115,122]

PFN1

Exome sequencing recently identified *PFN1* mutations in ALS.[123] Although this gene explained 1% to 2% of families in the initial study, its frequency is likely much lower; only 1 additional family[124] has been found despite screening in large ALS or FTD cohorts from around the world.[121,125–127] Furthermore, ~1 in 1000 patients with SALS screened has a p.E117G mutation,[123,128] but the pathogenicity status of this variant is currently unclear; it is found in control datasets at half the frequency of SALS but by functional studies seems to be a milder mutation.[123]

Profilin 1 is essential for the polymerization of monomeric G-actin into filamentous actin with roles in axonal integrity and axonal transport. These roles may be important to motor neuron degeneration because other cytoskeletal pathway genes are also implicated in ALS, including *DCTN1*, *NEFH*, *spastin* and *peripherin*. All ALS-associated mutations described to date are missense variants affecting amino acids in close proximity to actin binding residues. Not surprisingly, all but the milder p.E117G mutation show decreased actin binding, and when overexpressed, inhibit neurite outgrowth, reduce the size of axonal growth cones, and alter growth cone morphology.[123] Furthermore, the expression of mutated PFN1 in N2A cells and primary neuronal culture results in ubiquitinated cytosolic aggregates with TDP-43 colocalization, similar to those identified in patients with SALS.[123]

Fewer than 30 ALS patients with *PFN1* mutations have been reported to date. All have presented with limb onset and none have had significant cognitive impairment or FTD,[123,124] hinting at a consistent phenotype for *PFN1* mutations that may parallel *SOD1*-associated ALS.

ANG

Since angiogenin (*ANG*) was first examined as a candidate gene for ALS, numerous mutations have been reported in both familial and sporadic disease. However, many reported variants lack segregation evidence and are now recognized as rare variants in the population (eg, 1000 Genomes Project or the National Heart, Lung, and Blood Institute's Exome Variant Server). These ANG variants might function as low penetrance mutations, increasing the risk of developing ALS.[129] Recent work demonstrates that ALS-associated *ANG* mutations impair the formation of stress granules in neurons,[130] which is interesting in light of the recruitment of TDP-43 and FUS to stress granules. Clinical and neuropathologic features of *ANG*-associated ALS are typical of ALS in general, without discriminating features.[131]

OPTN

Study of Japanese patients with ALS identified mutations in *OPTN* as a rare cause of ALS, with both recessive and dominant-acting mutations.[132] Subsequent studies have revealed a few additional families and rare mutations in SALS.[133–135] Optineurin is found in TDP-43 positive neuronal aggregates in mutation carriers,[132] and can be seen in neuronal aggregates in non-*OPTN* ALS.[132] *OPTN*-associated ALS is heterogeneous in its presentation based on the limited number of patients reported to date, and no clear phenotype has yet been identified.

VCP

Mutations in valosin-containing protein (*VCP*) were first shown to cause inclusion body myopathy with Paget disease and frontotemporal dementia (IBMPFD).[136] Recently, however, it has been recognized that rarely, an ALS phenotype can also be seen.[137–141] A personal or family history of FTD, myopathy, Paget disease, or increased level of serum alkaline phosphatase (a biomarker for the presence of Paget disease) may serve as clues to this genetic cause.

SETX

Mutations in senataxin (*SETX*), a DNA/RNA helicase, were first associated with a juvenile-onset, slowly progressive form of ALS (ALS4).[142] Screening in patients with more typical ALS has uncovered a handful of additional novel or rare variants in SALS, but the pathogenicity of these variants remains unclear.[143,144]

VAPB

A founder mutation in *VAPB* (p.P56S) was first identified in Brazilian families with a spectrum of motor neuron degenerative phenotypes ranging from late-onset spinal muscular atrophy to rapidly progressive ALS.[145] Although a large number of FALS and SALS cases have been screened for this gene, only a handful of additional rare or novel variants have been uncovered but with unclear pathogenicity.[146–149]

Other Genes

Mutations in additional genes have also been found in patients with ALS, including *FIG4*,[150] *DAO*,[151] *hnRNPA2B1*,[152] *hnRNPA1*,[152] *SQSTM1/p62*,[153–156] and *DCTN1*.[157,158]

GENOMICS/RISK VARIANTS

With only 5% to 10% of cases of sporadic ALS harboring disease-associated mutations in known ALS genes,[159] the remainder of SALS is presumed to be a complex disease influenced by both genetic and environmental exposures. Efforts to identify genetic risk factors have largely focused on genome-wide and candidate gene association studies, with mixed success.

- *CYP27A1*[160]: Using gene expression and genotyping data from patients with SALS, single nucleotide polymorphisms (SNPs) affecting the expression of *CYP27A1* were recently identified as a small-effect risk factor for ALS. Validation studies have yet to be reported.
- Ataxin-2 intermediate length repeats: Full pathogenic expansions in the CAG repeat (>34 repeats) of *ATXN2* cause spinocerebellar ataxia type 2, a disorder sometimes accompanied by motor neuron degeneration. Investigations of CAG repeat length in SALS identified intermediate-sized repeats (27–33) as a risk factor.[161] Additional studies across multiple populations have confirmed this association,[162–169] although the strength of the association may be lower in some populations.[170] The link between intermediate repeats in ATXN2 and ALS seems to be due to an interaction with FUS[171] and TDP-43.[172]
- *UNC13A*: First identified by a genome-wide association study (GWAS) in 2009,[173] variation near *UNC13A* has been replicated as a risk for developing SALS,[174] and the minor allele at SNP rs12608932 shows a significant association with reduced survival in patients.[174,175] UNC13A is a presynaptic protein involved in regulating neurotransmitter release and it has been hypothesized that the increased risk could be caused by glutamate dysregulation and resulting excitotoxicity.[173]
- *DPP6*: DPP6 is a component of type A neuronal transmembrane potassium channels and was first associated with SALS in a GWAS of Irish patients,[176] and subsequently validated in other European populations.[177,178] However, since then, efforts to replicate the association in other populations have failed, leaving the status of this risk factor uncertain.[179–183]
- *ELP3:* A single study identified a risk for ALS in association with alleles of an RNA polymerase component, Elongation protein 3 (ELP3).[184] Although mutations in ELP3 cause neurodegeneration in a *Drosophila* model and increase interest as an ALS candidate gene, other GWASs have not identified this association.

EVALUATION AND MANAGEMENT
Strategies for Diagnosis

Obtaining a genetic diagnosis in ALS is challenging because of the overlapping phenotypes and genetic heterogeneity. Given the complicated implications of a genetic diagnosis, the decision to undertake testing warrants careful consideration by patients and their families. Referral to a knowledgeable genetic counselor may help patients make informed decisions. Five years ago, when causative mutations were identified in only 20% of familial cases, the usefulness of genetic testing was unclear. Now, however, a causative mutation is found in ~2/3 of pedigrees,[59] making testing more informative to patients and their at-risk relatives. Typically, the C9ORF72 repeat expansion is investigated first, because this is the most common mutation in Caucasian populations and cannot be detected using standard sequencing methods. If no expansion is present, direct sequencing of other common genes is usually pursued, either sequentially (typically starting with SOD1 followed by TARDBP and FUS) or as a panel. As sequencing costs decrease, next-generation sequencing methods are also becoming a cost-effective option. Whole-exome sequencing will screen for mutations in all known ALS genes, with the added benefit that data can be reanalyzed in the future as new genes are discovered. Historically, the yield of genetic testing in sporadic disease was low. Now, however, the realization that 6% to 10% of patients with apparently sporadic ALS carry C9ORF72 expansions is challenging this belief. Testing for the C9ORF72 expansion should be considered in SALS, especially if the patient or a close relative has dementia. Other genes are sufficiently rare that further testing is usually of limited usefulness.

Current Management and Therapeutic Options

Although riluzole is the only medication for ALS approved by the US Food and Drug Administration, there are numerous supportive therapies that likely improve quality of life and survival. These include noninvasive positive pressure ventilation[185,186] and nutritional support via placement of a gastric tube.[187] Most importantly, care in a multidisciplinary clinic setting has been shown to significantly improve prognosis,[188] and clinicians should strive to refer their patients to multidisciplinary ALS clinics if available.

SUMMARY

In the last 5 years, there has been a staggering expansion in our understanding of the genetics of ALS. With these insights, several key molecular pathways have been identified on which to focus basic science research and therapeutic efforts. The most notable include alterations in RNA metabolism and protein homeostasis. There is no doubt that the prospects for developing meaningful interventions for patients with ALS have never been better, providing hope for these patients and their caregivers.

REFERENCES

1. Geser F, Martinez-Lage M, Robinson J, et al. Clinical and pathological continuum of multisystem TDP-43 proteinopathies. Arch Neurol 2009;66(2):180–9.
2. Geser F, Brandmeir NJ, Kwong LK, et al. Evidence of multisystem disorder in whole-brain map of pathological TDP-43 in amyotrophic lateral sclerosis. Arch Neurol 2008;65(5):636–41.
3. Isaacs JD, Dean AF, Shaw CE, et al. Amyotrophic lateral sclerosis with sensory neuropathy: part of a multisystem disorder? J Neurol Neurosurg Psychiatry 2007;78(7):750–3.
4. Scotton WJ, Scott KM, Moore DH, et al. Prognostic categories for amyotrophic lateral sclerosis. Amyotroph Lateral Scler 2012;13(6):502–8.
5. Lomen-Hoerth C, Murphy J, Langmore S, et al. Are amyotrophic lateral sclerosis patients cognitively normal? Neurology 2003;60(7):1094–7.

6. Ringholz GM, Appel SH, Bradshaw M, et al. Prevalence and patterns of cognitive impairment in sporadic ALS. Neurology 2005;65(4):586–90.
7. Gilbert RM, Fahn S, Mitsumoto H, et al. Parkinsonism and motor neuron diseases: twenty-seven patients with diverse overlap syndromes. Mov Disord 2010;25(12):1868–75.
8. Pinkhardt EH, Sperfeld AD, Gdynia HJ, et al. The combination of dopa-responsive parkinsonian syndrome and motor neuron disease. Neurodegener Dis 2009;6(3):95–101.
9. Hammad M, Silva A, Glass J, et al. Clinical, electrophysiologic, and pathologic evidence for sensory abnormalities in ALS. Neurology 2007;69(24):2236–42.
10. Luigetti M, Conte A, Del Grande A, et al. Sural nerve pathology in ALS patients: a single-centre experience. Neurol Sci 2012;33(5):1095–9.
11. Brooks BR, Miller RG, Swash M, et al. El Escorial revisited: revised criteria for the diagnosis of amyotrophic lateral sclerosis. Amyotroph Lateral Scler Other Motor Neuron Disord 2000;1(5):293–9.
12. de Carvalho M, Dengler R, Eisen A, et al. Electrodiagnostic criteria for diagnosis of ALS. Clin Neurophysiol 2008;119(3):497–503.
13. Kim WK, Liu X, Sandner J, et al. Study of 962 patients indicates progressive muscular atrophy is a form of ALS. Neurology 2009;73(20):1686–92.
14. Kosaka T, Fu YJ, Shiga A, et al. Primary lateral sclerosis: upper-motor-predominant amyotrophic lateral sclerosis with frontotemporal lobar degeneration–immunohistochemical and biochemical analyses of TDP-43. Neuropathology 2012;32(4):373–84.
15. Pamphlett R. Study of 962 patients indicates progressive muscular atrophy is a form of ALS. Neurology 2010;74(23):1926 [author reply: 1926–7].
16. Visser J, van den Berg-Vos RM, Franssen H, et al. Disease course and prognostic factors of progressive muscular atrophy. Arch Neurol 2007;64(4):522–8.
17. van Blitterswijk M, Vlam L, van Es MA, et al. Genetic overlap between apparently sporadic motor neuron diseases. PLoS One 2012;7(11):e48983.
18. Ringholz GM, Greene SR. The relationship between amyotrophic lateral sclerosis and frontotemporal dementia. Curr Neurol Neurosci Rep 2006;6(5):387–92.
19. Fecto F, Siddique T. Making connections: pathology and genetics link amyotrophic lateral sclerosis with frontotemporal lobe dementia. J Mol Neurosci 2011;45(3):663–75.
20. Rosen AD. Amyotrophic lateral sclerosis. Clinical features and prognosis. Arch Neurol 1978;35(10):638–42.
21. Dietrich-Neto F, Callegaro D, Dias-Tosta E, et al. Amyotrophic lateral sclerosis in Brazil: 1998 national survey. Arq Neuropsiquiatr 2000;58(3A):607–15.
22. Haverkamp LJ, Appel V, Appel SH. Natural history of amyotrophic lateral sclerosis in a database population. Validation of a scoring system and a model for survival prediction. Brain 1995;118(Pt 3):707–19.
23. Gordon PH, Cheng B, Salachas F, et al. Progression in ALS is not linear but is curvilinear. J Neurol 2010;257(10):1713–7.
24. Murray B. Natural history and prognosis in amyotrophic lateral sclerosis. In: Mitsumoto HP, Gordon PH, editors. Amyotrophic lateral sclerosis. 1st edition. New York: Taylor & Francis; 2006. p. 227–55.
25. Juergens SM, Kurland LT, Okazaki H, et al. ALS in Rochester, Minnesota, 1925-1977. Neurology 1980;30(5):463–70.
26. Caroscio JT, Mulvihill MN, Sterling R, et al. Amyotrophic lateral sclerosis. Its natural history. Neurol Clin 1987;5(1):1–8.

27. Lee CT, Chiu YW, Wang KC, et al. Riluzole and prognostic factors in amyotrophic lateral sclerosis long-term and short-term survival: a population-based study of 1149 cases in Taiwan. J Epidemiol 2013;23(1):35–40.

28. Gordon PH, Salachas F, Lacomblez L, et al. Predicting survival of patients with amyotrophic lateral sclerosis at presentation: a 15-year experience. Neurodegener Dis 2013;12:81–90.

29. Czaplinski A, Yen AA, Simpson EP, et al. Slower disease progression and prolonged survival in contemporary patients with amyotrophic lateral sclerosis: is the natural history of amyotrophic lateral sclerosis changing? Arch Neurol 2006;63(8):1139–43.

30. The Scottish Motor Neuron Disease Register: a prospective study of adult onset motor neuron disease in Scotland. Methodology, demography and clinical features of incident cases in 1989. J Neurol Neurosurg Psychiatry 1992;55(7): 536–41.

31. Chancellor AM, Slattery JM, Fraser H, et al. The prognosis of adult-onset motor neuron disease: a prospective study based on the Scottish Motor Neuron Disease Register. J Neurol 1993;240(6):339–46.

32. Forbes RB, Colville S, Cran GW, et al. Unexpected decline in survival from amyotrophic lateral sclerosis/motor neurone disease. J Neurol Neurosurg Psychiatry 2004;75(12):1753–5.

33. Gordon PH, Salachas F, Bruneteau G, et al. Improving survival in a large French ALS center cohort. J Neurol 2012;259(9):1788–92.

34. Miller RG, Mitchell JD, Moore DH. Riluzole for amyotrophic lateral sclerosis (ALS)/motor neuron disease (MND). Cochrane Database Syst Rev 2012;(3):CD001447.

35. Annegers JF, Appel S, Lee JR, et al. Incidence and prevalence of amyotrophic lateral sclerosis in Harris County, Texas, 1985-1988. Arch Neurol 1991;48(6): 589–93.

36. McGuire V, Longstreth WT Jr, Koepsell TD, et al. Incidence of amyotrophic lateral sclerosis in three counties in western Washington state. Neurology 1996;47(2):571–3.

37. Traynor BJ, Codd MB, Corr B, et al. Incidence and prevalence of ALS in Ireland, 1995-1997: a population-based study. Neurology 1999;52(3):504–9.

38. Pradas J, Puig T, Rojas-Garcia R, et al. Amyotrophic lateral sclerosis in Catalonia: a population based study. Amyotroph Lateral Scler Frontotemporal Degener 2013;14(4):278–83.

39. Bandettini di Poggio M, Sormani MP, Truffelli R, et al. Clinical epidemiology of ALS in Liguria, Italy. Amyotroph Lateral Scler Frontotemporal Degener 2013; 14(1):52–7.

40. Abhinav K, Stanton B, Johnston C, et al. Amyotrophic lateral sclerosis in South-East England: a population-based study. The South-East England register for amyotrophic lateral sclerosis (SEALS Registry). Neuroepidemiology 2007; 29(1–2):44–8.

41. Sajjadi M, Etemadifar M, Nemati A, et al. Epidemiology of amyotrophic lateral sclerosis in Isfahan, Iran. Eur J Neurol 2010;17(7):984–9.

42. Vazquez MC, Ketzoian C, Legnani C, et al. Incidence and prevalence of amyotrophic lateral sclerosis in Uruguay: a population-based study. Neuroepidemiology 2008;30(2):105–11.

43. Johnston CA, Stanton BR, Turner MR, et al. Amyotrophic lateral sclerosis in an urban setting: a population based study of inner city London. J Neurol 2006; 253(12):1642–3.

44. McGuire Van LM. Epidemiology of ALS. In: Mitsumoto HP, Gordon PH, editors. Amyotrophic lateral sclerosis. 1st edition. New York: Taylor & Francis; 2006. p. 17–41.

45. Blasco H, Guennoc AM, Veyrat-Durebex C, et al. Amyotrophic lateral sclerosis: a hormonal condition? Amyotroph Lateral Scler 2012;13(6):585–8.

46. Logroscino G, Traynor BJ, Hardiman O, et al. Descriptive epidemiology of amyotrophic lateral sclerosis: new evidence and unsolved issues. J Neurol Neurosurg Psychiatry 2008;79(1):6–11.

47. Osler W. Heredity in progressive muscular atrophy as illustrated in Farr family of Vermont. Arch Med 1880;4:316–20.

48. Byrne S, Elamin M, Bede P, et al. Absence of consensus in diagnostic criteria for familial neurodegenerative diseases. J Neurol Neurosurg Psychiatry 2012;83(4): 365–7.

49. Chio A, Borghero G, Pugliatti M, et al. Large proportion of amyotrophic lateral sclerosis cases in Sardinia due to a single founder mutation of the TARDBP gene. Arch Neurol 2011;68(5):594–8.

50. Eisen A, Mezei MM, Stewart HG, et al. SOD1 gene mutations in ALS patients from British Columbia, Canada: clinical features, neurophysiology and ethical issues in management. Amyotroph Lateral Scler 2008;9(2):108–19.

51. Byrne S, Walsh C, Lynch C, et al. Rate of familial amyotrophic lateral sclerosis: a systematic review and meta-analysis. J Neurol Neurosurg Psychiatry 2011; 82(6):623–7.

52. Byrne S, Bede P, Elamin M, et al. Proposed criteria for familial amyotrophic lateral sclerosis. Amyotroph Lateral Scler 2011;12(3):157–9.

53. Al-Chalabi A, Lewis CM. Modelling the effects of penetrance and family size on rates of sporadic and familial disease. Hum Hered 2011;71(4):281–8.

54. Millecamps S, Salachas F, Cazeneuve C, et al. SOD1, ANG, VAPB, TARDBP, and FUS mutations in familial amyotrophic lateral sclerosis: genotype-phenotype correlations. J Med Genet 2010;47(8):554–60.

55. Gellera C, Tiloca C, Del Bo R, et al. Ubiquilin 2 mutations in Italian patients with amyotrophic lateral sclerosis and frontotemporal dementia. J Neurol Neurosurg Psychiatry 2013;84(2):183–7.

56. Morita M, Al-Chalabi A, Andersen PM, et al. A locus on chromosome 9p confers susceptibility to ALS and frontotemporal dementia. Neurology 2006;66(6): 839–44.

57. DeJesus-Hernandez M, Mackenzie IR, Boeve BF, et al. Expanded GGGGCC hexanucleotide repeat in noncoding region of C9ORF72 causes chromosome 9p-linked FTD and ALS. Neuron 2011;72(2):245–56.

58. Renton AE, Majounie E, Waite A, et al. A hexanucleotide repeat expansion in C9ORF72 is the cause of chromosome 9p21-linked ALS-FTD. Neuron 2011; 72(2):257–68.

59. Harms MB, Cady J, Zaidman C, et al. Lack of C9ORF72 coding mutations supports a gain of function for repeat expansions in amyotrophic lateral sclerosis. Neurobiol Aging 2013;34(9):2234.e13–9.

60. van Blitterswijk M, Dejesus-Hernandez M, Rademakers R. How do C9ORF72 repeat expansions cause amyotrophic lateral sclerosis and frontotemporal dementia: can we learn from other noncoding repeat expansion disorders? Curr Opin Neurol 2012;25(6):689–700.

61. Majounie E, Renton AE, Mok K, et al. Frequency of the C9orf72 hexanucleotide repeat expansion in patients with amyotrophic lateral sclerosis and frontotemporal dementia: a cross-sectional study. Lancet Neurol 2012;11(4):323–30.

62. Levine TP, Daniels RD, Gatta AT, et al. The product of C9orf72, a gene strongly implicated in neurodegeneration, is structurally related to DENN Rab-GEFs. Bioinformatics 2013;29(4):499–503.

63. Zhang D, Iyer LM, He F, et al. Discovery of novel DENN proteins: implications for the evolution of eukaryotic intracellular membrane structures and human disease. Front Genet 2012;3:283.

64. van der Zee J, Gijselinck I, Dillen L, et al. A pan-European study of the C9orf72 repeat associated with FTLD: geographic prevalence, genomic instability, and intermediate repeats. Hum Mutat 2013;34(2):363–73.

65. Echeverria GV, Cooper TA. RNA-binding proteins in microsatellite expansion disorders: mediators of RNA toxicity. Brain Res 2012;1462:100–11.

66. Mori K, Weng SM, Arzberger T, et al. The C9orf72 GGGGCC repeat is translated into aggregating dipeptide-repeat proteins in FTLD/ALS. Science 2013; 339(6125):1335–8.

67. Ash PE, Bieniek KF, Gendron TF, et al. Unconventional translation of C9ORF72 GGGGCC expansion generates insoluble polypeptides specific to c9FTD/ALS. Neuron 2013;77(4):639–46.

68. Harms M, Benitez BA, Cairns N, et al. C9orf72 hexanucleotide repeat expansions in clinical Alzheimer disease. JAMA Neurol 2013;1–6.

69. Majounie E, Abramzon Y, Renton AE, et al. Repeat expansion in C9ORF72 in Alzheimer's disease. N Engl J Med 2012;366(3):283–4.

70. Lindquist S, Duno M, Batbayli M, et al. Corticobasal and ataxia syndromes widen the spectrum of C9ORF72 hexanucleotide expansion disease. Clin Genet 2013;83(3):279–83.

71. Rollinson S, Halliwell N, Young K, et al. Analysis of the hexanucleotide repeat in C9ORF72 in Alzheimer's disease. Neurobiol Aging 2012;33(8):1846.e5–6.

72. Rosen DR, Siddique T, Patterson D, et al. Mutations in Cu/Zn superoxide dismutase gene are associated with familial amyotrophic lateral sclerosis. Nature 1993; 362(6415):59–62.

73. Chio A, Traynor BJ, Lombardo F, et al. Prevalence of SOD1 mutations in the Italian ALS population. Neurology 2008;70(7):533–7.

74. Battistini S, Giannini F, Greco G, et al. SOD1 mutations in amyotrophic lateral sclerosis. Results from a multicenter Italian study. J Neurol 2005;252(7):782–8.

75. Ratovitski T, Corson LB, Strain J, et al. Variation in the biochemical/biophysical properties of mutant superoxide dismutase 1 enzymes and the rate of disease progression in familial amyotrophic lateral sclerosis kindreds. Hum Mol Genet 1999;8(8):1451–60.

76. Ilieva H, Polymenidou M, Cleveland DW. Non-cell autonomous toxicity in neurodegenerative disorders: ALS and beyond. J Cell Biol 2009;187(6):761–72.

77. Wicks P, Abrahams S, Papps B, et al. SOD1 and cognitive dysfunction in familial amyotrophic lateral sclerosis. J Neurol 2009;256(2):234–41.

78. Cudkowicz ME, McKenna-Yasek D, Chen C, et al. Limited corticospinal tract involvement in amyotrophic lateral sclerosis subjects with the A4V mutation in the copper/zinc superoxide dismutase gene. Ann Neurol 1998;43(6):703–10.

79. Cudkowicz ME, McKenna-Yasek D, Sapp PE, et al. Epidemiology of mutations in superoxide dismutase in amyotrophic lateral sclerosis. Ann Neurol 1997;41(2): 210–21.

80. Del Grande A, Conte A, Lattante S, et al. D11Y SOD1 mutation and benign ALS: a consistent genotype-phenotype correlation. J Neurol Sci 2011;309(1–2):31–3.

81. Andersen PM, Forsgren L, Binzer M, et al. Autosomal recessive adult-onset amyotrophic lateral sclerosis associated with homozygosity for Asp90Ala

CuZn-superoxide dismutase mutation. A clinical and genealogical study of 36 patients. Brain 1996;119(Pt 4):1153–72.

82. Neumann M, Sampathu DM, Kwong LK, et al. Ubiquitinated TDP-43 in fronto-temporal lobar degeneration and amyotrophic lateral sclerosis. Science 2006; 314(5796):130–3.

83. Sreedharan J, Blair IP, Tripathi VB, et al. TDP-43 mutations in familial and sporadic amyotrophic lateral sclerosis. Science 2008;319(5870):1668–72.

84. Gitcho MA, Baloh RH, Chakraverty S, et al. TDP-43 A315T mutation in familial motor neuron disease. Ann Neurol 2008;63(4):535–8.

85. Kabashi E, Valdmanis PN, Dion P, et al. TARDBP mutations in individuals with sporadic and familial amyotrophic lateral sclerosis. Nat Genet 2008;40(5): 572–4.

86. Borroni B, Bonvicini C, Alberici A, et al. Mutation within TARDBP leads to fronto-temporal dementia without motor neuron disease. Hum Mutat 2009;30(11): E974–83.

87. Ayala YM, Pagani F, Baralle FE. TDP43 depletion rescues aberrant CFTR exon 9 skipping. FEBS Lett 2006;580(5):1339–44.

88. Ayala YM, Pantano S, D'Ambrogio A, et al. Human, Drosophila, and C. elegans TDP43: nucleic acid binding properties and splicing regulatory function. J Mol Biol 2005;348(3):575–88.

89. Ling SC, Albuquerque CP, Han JS, et al. ALS-associated mutations in TDP-43 increase its stability and promote TDP-43 complexes with FUS/TLS. Proc Natl Acad Sci U S A 2010;107(30):13318–23.

90. Corcia P, Valdmanis P, Millecamps S, et al. Phenotype and genotype analysis in amyotrophic lateral sclerosis with TARDBP gene mutations. Neurology 2012; 78(19):1519–26.

91. Quadri M, Cossu G, Saddi V, et al. Broadening the phenotype of TARDBP mu-tations: the TARDBP Ala382Thr mutation and Parkinson's disease in Sardinia. Neurogenetics 2011;12(3):203–9.

92. Rayaprolu S, Fujioka S, Traynor S, et al. TARDBP mutations in Parkinson's dis-ease. Parkinsonism Relat Disord 2013;19(3):312–5.

93. Kwiatkowski TJ Jr, Bosco DA, Leclerc AL, et al. Mutations in the FUS/TLS gene on chromosome 16 cause familial amyotrophic lateral sclerosis. Science 2009; 323(5918):1205–8.

94. Vance C, Rogelj B, Hortobagyi T, et al. Mutations in FUS, an RNA processing protein, cause familial amyotrophic lateral sclerosis type 6. Science 2009; 323(5918):1208–11.

95. Belzil VV, Valdmanis PN, Dion PA, et al. Mutations in FUS cause FALS and SALS in French and French Canadian populations. Neurology 2009;73(15):1176–9.

96. Damme PV, Goris A, Race V, et al. The occurrence of mutations in FUS in a Belgian cohort of patients with familial ALS. Eur J Neurol 2010;17(5):754–6.

97. Waibel S, Neumann M, Rosenbohm A, et al. Truncating mutations in FUS/TLS give rise to a more aggressive ALS-phenotype than missense mutations: a clinico-genetic study in Germany. Eur J Neurol 2013;20(3):540–6.

98. Suzuki N, Aoki M, Warita H, et al. FALS with FUS mutation in Japan, with early onset, rapid progress and basophilic inclusion. J Hum Genet 2010;55(4):252–4.

99. Tsai CP, Soong BW, Lin KP, et al. FUS, TARDBP, and SOD1 mutations in a Taiwa-nese cohort with familial ALS. Neurobiol Aging 2011;32(3):553.e13–21.

100. Zou ZY, Cui LY, Sun Q, et al. De novo FUS gene mutations are associated with juvenile-onset sporadic amyotrophic lateral sclerosis in China. Neurobiol Aging 2013;34(4):1312.e1–8.

101. Drepper C, Herrmann T, Wessig C, et al. C-terminal FUS/TLS mutations in familial and sporadic ALS in Germany. Neurobiol Aging 2011;32(3):548.e1–4.
102. Lai SL, Abramzon Y, Schymick JC, et al. FUS mutations in sporadic amyotrophic lateral sclerosis. Neurobiol Aging 2011;32(3):550.e1–4.
103. Kwon MJ, Baek W, Ki CS, et al. Screening of the SOD1, FUS, TARDBP, ANG, and OPTN mutations in Korean patients with familial and sporadic ALS. Neurobiol Aging 2012;33(5):1017.e17–23.
104. DeJesus-Hernandez M, Kocerha J, Finch N, et al. De novo truncating FUS gene mutation as a cause of sporadic amyotrophic lateral sclerosis. Hum Mutat 2010; 31(5):E1377–89.
105. Chio A, Calvo A, Moglia C, et al. A de novo missense mutation of the FUS gene in a "true" sporadic ALS case. Neurobiol Aging 2011;32(3):553.e23–6.
106. Couthouis J, Hart MP, Shorter J, et al. A yeast functional screen predicts new candidate ALS disease genes. Proc Natl Acad Sci U S A 2011;108(52):20881–90.
107. Couthouis J, Hart MP, Erion R, et al. Evaluating the role of the FUS/TLS-related gene EWSR1 in amyotrophic lateral sclerosis. Hum Mol Genet 2012;21(13): 2899–911.
108. Dormann D, Rodde R, Edbauer D, et al. ALS-associated fused in sarcoma (FUS) mutations disrupt Transportin-mediated nuclear import. EMBO J 2010;29(16): 2841–57.
109. Hewitt C, Kirby J, Highley JR, et al. Novel FUS/TLS mutations and pathology in familial and sporadic amyotrophic lateral sclerosis. Arch Neurol 2010;67(4): 455–61.
110. Blair IP, Williams KL, Warraich ST, et al. FUS mutations in amyotrophic lateral sclerosis: clinical, pathological, neurophysiological and genetic analysis. J Neurol Neurosurg Psychiatry 2010;81(6):639–45.
111. Waibel S, Neumann M, Rabe M, et al. Novel missense and truncating mutations in FUS/TLS in familial ALS. Neurology 2010;75(9):815–7.
112. Baumer D, Hilton D, Paine SM, et al. Juvenile ALS with basophilic inclusions is a FUS proteinopathy with FUS mutations. Neurology 2010;75(7):611–8.
113. Huey ED, Ferrari R, Moreno JH, et al. FUS and TDP43 genetic variability in FTD and CBS. Neurobiol Aging 2012;33(5):1016.e9–17.
114. Parmalee N, Mirzozoda K, Kisselev S, et al. Genetic analysis of the FUS/TLS gene in essential tremor. Eur J Neurol 2013;20(3):534–9.
115. Deng HX, Chen W, Hong ST, et al. Mutations in UBQLN2 cause dominant X-linked juvenile and adult-onset ALS and ALS/dementia. Nature 2011; 477(7363):211–5.
116. Daoud H, Suhail H, Szuto A, et al. UBQLN2 mutations are rare in French and French-Canadian amyotrophic lateral sclerosis. Neurobiol Aging 2012;33(9): 2230.e1–5.
117. Millecamps S, Corcia P, Cazeneuve C, et al. Mutations in UBQLN2 are rare in French amyotrophic lateral sclerosis. Neurobiol Aging 2012;33(4):839.e1–3.
118. van Doormaal PT, van Rheenen W, van Blitterswijk M, et al. UBQLN2 in familial amyotrophic lateral sclerosis in The Netherlands. Neurobiol Aging 2012;33(9): 2233.e7–8.
119. Williams KL, Warraich ST, Yang S, et al. UBQLN2/ubiquilin 2 mutation and pathology in familial amyotrophic lateral sclerosis. Neurobiol Aging 2012; 33(10):2527.e3–10.
120. Synofzik M, Maetzler W, Grehl T, et al. Screening in ALS and FTD patients reveals 3 novel UBQLN2 mutations outside the PXX domain and a pure FTD phenotype. Neurobiol Aging 2012;33(12):2949.e13–7.

121. Dillen L, Van Langenhove T, Engelborghs S, et al. Explorative genetic study of UBQLN2 and PFN1 in an extended Flanders-Belgian cohort of frontotemporal lobar degeneration patients. Neurobiol Aging 2013;34(6):1711.e1–5.

122. Brettschneider J, Van Deerlin VM, Robinson JL, et al. Pattern of ubiquilin pathology in ALS and FTLD indicates presence of C9ORF72 hexanucleotide expansion. Acta Neuropathol 2012;123(6):825–39.

123. Wu CH, Fallini C, Ticozzi N, et al. Mutations in the profilin 1 gene cause familial amyotrophic lateral sclerosis. Nature 2012;488(7412):499–503.

124. Ingre C, Landers JE, Rizik N, et al. A novel phosphorylation site mutation in profilin 1 revealed in a large screen of US, Nordic, and German amyotrophic lateral sclerosis/frontotemporal dementia cohorts. Neurobiol Aging 2012;34(6): 1708.e1–6.

125. Zou ZY, Sun Q, Liu MS, et al. Mutations in the profilin 1 gene are not common in amyotrophic lateral sclerosis of Chinese origin. Neurobiol Aging 2013;34(6): 1713.e5–6.

126. Lattante S, Le Ber I, Camuzat A, et al. Mutations in the PFN1 gene are not a common cause in patients with amyotrophic lateral sclerosis and frontotemporal lobar degeneration in France. Neurobiol Aging 2012;34(6):1709.e1–2.

127. Daoud H, Dobrzeniecka S, Camu W, et al. Mutation analysis of PFN1 in familial amyotrophic lateral sclerosis patients. Neurobiol Aging 2013;34(4):1311.e1–2.

128. Tiloca C, Ticozzi N, Pensato V, et al. Screening of the PFN1 gene in sporadic amyotrophic lateral sclerosis and in frontotemporal dementia. Neurobiol Aging 2013;34(5):1517.e9–10.

129. van Es MA, Schelhaas HJ, van Vught PW, et al. Angiogenin variants in Parkinson disease and amyotrophic lateral sclerosis. Ann Neurol 2011;70(6):964–73.

130. Thiyagarajan N, Ferguson R, Subramanian V, et al. Structural and molecular insights into the mechanism of action of human angiogenin-ALS variants in neurons. Nat Commun 2012;3:1121.

131. Kirby J, Highley JR, Cox L, et al. Lack of unique neuropathology in amyotrophic lateral sclerosis associated with p.K54E angiogenin (ANG) mutation. Neuropathol Appl Neurobiol 2013;39(5):562–71.

132. Maruyama H, Morino H, Ito H, et al. Mutations of optineurin in amyotrophic lateral sclerosis. Nature 2010;465(7295):223–6.

133. van Blitterswijk M, van Vught PW, van Es MA, et al. Novel optineurin mutations in sporadic amyotrophic lateral sclerosis patients. Neurobiol Aging 2012;33(5): 1016.e1–7.

134. Del Bo R, Tiloca C, Pensato V, et al. Novel optineurin mutations in patients with familial and sporadic amyotrophic lateral sclerosis. J Neurol Neurosurg Psychiatry 2011;82(11):1239–43.

135. Iida A, Hosono N, Sano M, et al. Optineurin mutations in Japanese amyotrophic lateral sclerosis. J Neurol Neurosurg Psychiatry 2012;83(2):233–5.

136. Watts GD, Wymer J, Kovach MJ, et al. Inclusion body myopathy associated with Paget disease of bone and frontotemporal dementia is caused by mutant valosin-containing protein. Nat Genet 2004;36(4):377–81.

137. Johnson JO, Mandrioli J, Benatar M, et al. Exome sequencing reveals VCP mutations as a cause of familial ALS. Neuron 2010;68(5):857–64.

138. Koppers M, van Blitterswijk MM, Vlam L, et al. VCP mutations in familial and sporadic amyotrophic lateral sclerosis. Neurobiol Aging 2012;33(4):837.e7–13.

139. DeJesus-Hernandez M, Desaro P, Johnston A, et al. Novel p.Ile151Val mutation in VCP in a patient of African American descent with sporadic ALS. Neurology 2011;77(11):1102–3.

140. Williams KL, Solski JA, Nicholson GA, et al. Mutation analysis of VCP in familial and sporadic amyotrophic lateral sclerosis. Neurobiol Aging 2012;33(7): 1488.e15–6.
141. Tiloca C, Ratti A, Pensato V, et al. Mutational analysis of VCP gene in familial amyotrophic lateral sclerosis. Neurobiol Aging 2012;33(3):630.e1–2.
142. Chen YZ, Bennett CL, Huynh HM, et al. DNA/RNA helicase gene mutations in a form of juvenile amyotrophic lateral sclerosis (ALS4). Am J Hum Genet 2004; 74(6):1128–35.
143. Zhao ZH, Chen WZ, Wu ZY, et al. A novel mutation in the senataxin gene identified in a Chinese patient with sporadic amyotrophic lateral sclerosis. Amyotroph Lateral Scler 2009;10(2):118–22.
144. Hirano M, Quinzii CM, Mitsumoto H, et al. Senataxin mutations and amyotrophic lateral sclerosis. Amyotroph Lateral Scler 2011;12(3):223–7.
145. Nishimura AL, Mitne-Neto M, Silva HC, et al. A mutation in the vesicle-trafficking protein VAPB causes late-onset spinal muscular atrophy and amyotrophic lateral sclerosis. Am J Hum Genet 2004;75(5):822–31.
146. Kirby J, Hewamadduma CA, Hartley JA, et al. Mutations in VAPB are not associated with sporadic ALS. Neurology 2007;68(22):1951–3.
147. Conforti FL, Sprovieri T, Mazzei R, et al. Sporadic ALS is not associated with VAPB gene mutations in Southern Italy. J Negat Results Biomed 2006;5:7.
148. Chen HJ, Anagnostou G, Chai A, et al. Characterization of the properties of a novel mutation in VAPB in familial amyotrophic lateral sclerosis. J Biol Chem 2010;285(51):40266–81.
149. Kabashi E, El Oussini H, Bercier V, et al. Investigating the contribution of VAPB/ALS8 loss of function in amyotrophic lateral sclerosis. Hum Mol Genet 2013; 22(12):2350–60.
150. Chow CY, Landers JE, Bergren SK, et al. Deleterious variants of FIG4, a phosphoinositide phosphatase, in patients with ALS. Am J Hum Genet 2009;84(1):85–8.
151. Mitchell J, Paul P, Chen HJ, et al. Familial amyotrophic lateral sclerosis is associated with a mutation in D-amino acid oxidase. Proc Natl Acad Sci U S A 2010; 107(16):7556–61.
152. Kim HJ, Kim NC, Wang YD, et al. Mutations in prion-like domains in hnRNPA2B1 and hnRNPA1 cause multisystem proteinopathy and ALS. Nature 2013; 495(7442):467–73.
153. Fecto F, Yan J, Vemula SP, et al. SQSTM1 mutations in familial and sporadic amyotrophic lateral sclerosis. Arch Neurol 2011;68(11):1440–6.
154. Rubino E, Rainero I, Chio A, et al. SQSTM1 mutations in frontotemporal lobar degeneration and amyotrophic lateral sclerosis. Neurology 2012;79(15): 1556–62.
155. Hirano M, Nakamura Y, Saigoh K, et al. Mutations in the gene encoding p62 in Japanese patients with amyotrophic lateral sclerosis. Neurology 2013;80(5): 458–63.
156. Teyssou E, Takeda T, Lebon V, et al. Mutations in SQSTM1 encoding p62 in amyotrophic lateral sclerosis: genetics and neuropathology. Acta Neuropathol 2013;125(4):511–22.
157. Puls I, Jonnakuty C, LaMonte BH, et al. Mutant dynactin in motor neuron disease. Nat Genet 2003;33(4):455–6.
158. Munch C, Sedlmeier R, Meyer T, et al. Point mutations of the p150 subunit of dynactin (DCTN1) gene in ALS. Neurology 2004;63(4):724–6.
159. Chio A, Calvo A, Mazzini L, et al. Extensive genetics of ALS: a population-based study in Italy. Neurology 2012;79(19):1983–9.

160. Diekstra FP, Saris CG, van Rheenen W, et al. Mapping of gene expression reveals CYP27A1 as a susceptibility gene for sporadic ALS. PLoS One 2012; 7(4):e35333.
161. Elden AC, Kim HJ, Hart MP, et al. Ataxin-2 intermediate-length polyglutamine expansions are associated with increased risk for ALS. Nature 2010; 466(7310):1069–77.
162. Lee T, Li YR, Ingre C, et al. Ataxin-2 intermediate-length polyglutamine expansions in European ALS patients. Hum Mol Genet 2011;20(9):1697–700.
163. Van Damme P, Veldink JH, van Blitterswijk M, et al. Expanded ATXN2 CAG repeat size in ALS identifies genetic overlap between ALS and SCA2. Neurology 2011;76(24):2066–72.
164. Ross OA, Rutherford NJ, Baker M, et al. Ataxin-2 repeat-length variation and neurodegeneration. Hum Mol Genet 2011;20(16):3207–12.
165. Soraru G, Clementi M, Forzan M, et al. ALS risk but not phenotype is affected by ataxin-2 intermediate length polyglutamine expansion. Neurology 2011;76(23): 2030–1.
166. Daoud H, Belzil V, Martins S, et al. Association of long ATXN2 CAG repeat sizes with increased risk of amyotrophic lateral sclerosis. Arch Neurol 2011;68(6): 739–42.
167. Gispert S, Kurz A, Waibel S, et al. The modulation of amyotrophic lateral sclerosis risk by ataxin-2 intermediate polyglutamine expansions is a specific effect. Neurobiol Dis 2012;45(1):356–61.
168. Gellera C, Ticozzi N, Pensato V, et al. ATAXIN2 CAG-repeat length in Italian patients with amyotrophic lateral sclerosis: risk factor or variant phenotype? Implication for genetic testing and counseling. Neurobiol Aging 2012;33(8): 1847.e15–21.
169. Lahut S, Omur O, Uyan O, et al. ATXN2 and its neighbouring gene SH2B3 are associated with increased ALS risk in the Turkish population. PLoS One 2012; 7(8):e42956.
170. Chen Y, Huang R, Yang Y, et al. Ataxin-2 intermediate-length polyglutamine: a possible risk factor for Chinese patients with amyotrophic lateral sclerosis. Neurobiol Aging 2011;32(10):1925.e1–5.
171. Farg MA, Soo KY, Warraich ST, et al. Ataxin-2 interacts with FUS and intermediate-length polyglutamine expansions enhance FUS-related pathology in amyotrophic lateral sclerosis. Hum Mol Genet 2013;22(4):717–28.
172. Hart MP, Gitler AD. ALS-associated ataxin 2 polyQ expansions enhance stress-induced caspase 3 activation and increase TDP-43 pathological modifications. J Neurosci 2012;32(27):9133–42.
173. van Es MA, Veldink JH, Saris CG, et al. Genome-wide association study identifies 19p13.3 (UNC13A) and 9p21.2 as susceptibility loci for sporadic amyotrophic lateral sclerosis. Nat Genet 2009;41(10):1083–7.
174. Diekstra FP, van Vught PW, van Rheenen W, et al. UNC13A is a modifier of survival in amyotrophic lateral sclerosis. Neurobiol Aging 2012;33(3):630.e3–8.
175. Chio A, Mora G, Restagno G, et al. UNC13A influences survival in Italian amyotrophic lateral sclerosis patients: a population-based study. Neurobiol Aging 2013;34(1):357.e1–5.
176. Cronin S, Berger S, Ding J, et al. A genome-wide association study of sporadic ALS in a homogenous Irish population. Hum Mol Genet 2008;17(5):768–74.
177. Del Bo R, Ghezzi S, Corti S, et al. DPP6 gene variability confers increased risk of developing sporadic amyotrophic lateral sclerosis in Italian patients. J Neurol Neurosurg Psychiatry 2008;79(9):1085.

178. van Es MA, van Vught PW, Blauw HM, et al. Genetic variation in DPP6 is associated with susceptibility to amyotrophic lateral sclerosis. Nat Genet 2008;40(1): 29–31.

179. Cronin S, Tomik B, Bradley DG, et al. Screening for replication of genome-wide SNP associations in sporadic ALS. Eur J Hum Genet 2009;17(2):213–8.

180. Chio A, Schymick JC, Restagno G, et al. A two-stage genome-wide association study of sporadic amyotrophic lateral sclerosis. Hum Mol Genet 2009;18(8): 1524–32.

181. Fogh I, D'Alfonso S, Gellera C, et al. No association of DPP6 with amyotrophic lateral sclerosis in an Italian population. Neurobiol Aging 2011;32(5):966–7.

182. Li XG, Zhang JH, Xie MQ, et al. Association between DPP6 polymorphism and the risk of sporadic amyotrophic lateral sclerosis in Chinese patients. Chin Med J (Engl) 2009;122(24):2989–92.

183. Kwee LC, Liu Y, Haynes C, et al. A high-density genome-wide association screen of sporadic ALS in US veterans. PLoS One 2012;7(3):e32768.

184. Simpson CL, Lemmens R, Miskiewicz K, et al. Variants of the elongator protein 3 (ELP3) gene are associated with motor neuron degeneration. Hum Mol Genet 2009;18(3):472–81.

185. Mustfa N, Walsh E, Bryant V, et al. The effect of noninvasive ventilation on ALS patients and their caregivers. Neurology 2006;66(8):1211–7.

186. Lechtzin N, Scott Y, Busse AM, et al. Early use of non-invasive ventilation prolongs survival in subjects with ALS. Amyotroph Lateral Scler 2007;8(3):185–8.

187. Spataro R, Ficano L, Piccoli F, et al. Percutaneous endoscopic gastrostomy in amyotrophic lateral sclerosis: effect on survival. J Neurol Sci 2011;304(1–2): 44–8.

188. Traynor BJ, Alexander M, Corr B, et al. Effect of a multidisciplinary amyotrophic lateral sclerosis (ALS) clinic on ALS survival: a population based study, 1996-2000. J Neurol Neurosurg Psychiatry 2003;74(9):1258–61.

Clinical Neurogenetics
Autism Spectrum Disorders

Sunil Q. Mehta, MD, PhD[a],*, Peyman Golshani, MD, PhD[b]

KEYWORDS

- Autism • Autism spectrum disorders • Genetic testing • Chromosomal microarray

KEY POINTS

- Autism spectrum disorders (ASDs) are defined by difficulties in social communication, language delay, and repetitive or restricted interests.
- The behavioral symptoms of ASDs manifest early in life and there are numerous screening tools to help clinicians identify patients.
- Although most cases of ASDs are idiopathic, there are syndromic forms of ASDs in which the behavioral deficits of autism are accompanied by other medical comorbidities.
- Chromosomal microarray testing is a recommended method for identifying syndromic forms of ASD and informing parents about potential medical problems as well as helping with family planning.

INTRODUCTION

Autism spectrum disorders (ASDs) are a prevalent disorder of childhood that affects an estimated 1 of 88 children in the United States.[1] Consequently, a wide range of medical practitioners, including pediatricians, pediatric neurologists, and child psychiatrists, are likely to encounter new cases. In this article, current recommendations concerning genetic testing in the routine evaluation of ASDs are summarized, a case study is presented to illustrate the utility of such a workup and what is currently known about the genetics and pathophysiology is reviewed.

ASD is an umbrella term defined by the Diagnostic and Statistical Manual (DSM-IV TR) that encompasses a range of disorders that have behavioral deficits in 3 core domains: social interaction, repetitive behaviors/restricted interests, and language.

Definition

- Patients with ASDs have deficits in 3 core domains:
  1. Social interaction
  2. Repetitive behavior/restricted interests

---

[a] Department of Psychiatry and Biobehavioral Sciences, David Geffen School of Medicine, University of California, Los Angeles, CA, USA; [b] Department of Neurology, David Geffen School of Medicine, University of California, Los Angeles, CA, USA
* Corresponding author.
E-mail address: SMehta@mednet.ucla.edu

Neurol Clin 31 (2013) 951–968
http://dx.doi.org/10.1016/j.ncl.2013.04.009
0733-8619/13/$ – see front matter Published by Elsevier Inc.

neurologic.theclinics.com

3. Language

- Symptoms must be present before age 3. However, parent report of historical data before age 3 can be used to make the diagnosis later in life.

- Patients with deficits in all 3 domains significant enough to cause functional impairments have autistic disorder or autism

- Patients with deficits in social interaction and repetitive behavior/restricted interests but not language before age 2 have Asperger syndrome

- Patients with deficits in one or more domains that are significant enough to cause functional impairments but do not meet criteria for Autism or Asperger syndrome are diagnosed with pervasive developmental disorder not otherwise specified (PDD NOS)

- Some patients with ASDs may show a period of normal development before showing regression in motor, social, or cognitive skills

- Patients with Rett syndrome or childhood disintegrative disorder may meet criteria for autism, but more frequently only have deficits in 1 or 2 of the core domains or may develop these deficits after the age cutoff. For this reason, Rett and childhood disintegrative disorder are considered pervasive developmental disorders.

In next revision of the DSM (DSM-V), the definition of ASDs will be altered such that patients with autism, Asperger syndrome, and PDD NOS will all carry the diagnosis of ASD. These patients will be differentiated from each other with the use of modifiers to the ASD diagnosis, such as ASD with intact language and mild repetitive behavior or ASD with severe intellectual disability and language deficits. In addition, patients with deficits in social interaction and/or language but not repetitive behavior/restricted interests will receive a new diagnosis of social communication disorder.

SYMPTOMS AND CLINICAL COURSE

Patients with ASDs typically come in for an evaluation because of parental concern about a child's communication, lack of developmental milestones, or problematic behavior (tantrums, social conflict). Although there are research efforts to diagnose cases of ASDs in infancy,[2,3] current diagnostic tools are validated in toddlers and most children still do not receive a diagnosis until age 4 or later.[1] If left untreated, the behavioral deficits associated with ASDs do not improve with age. ASDs are a very clinically heterogeneous group of disorders with the behavioral deficits varying greatly from patient to patient. However, there are certain medical comorbidities that occur frequently enough with ASDs to be clinically relevant.

Medical comorbidities

- Sleep Disturbances

Parental surveys indicate that 50% to 80% of patients with ASDs have sleep problems, which may be treated with a combination of environmental modifications and medications.[4]

- Head Circumference

The rate of macrocephaly among patients with ASDs is between 17% and 20%, compared with 3% in the general population.[5,6] In addition, there is evidence that the rate of brain growth during the first year of life is greater in patients with ASDs compared with the general population.[7,8]

- Seizures

Seizures are more common in syndromic forms of ASDs (up to 60%) but can also occur in idiopathic ASDs at a rate of 5% to 10%.[9,10]

- Gastrointestinal Problems

Patients with ASDs have a higher rate of gastrointestinal problems than the general population, with the most common complaints being constipation (33%) and food selectivity (24%).[11]

- Intellectual Disability

Between 34% and 55% of patients with ASDs have intellectual disability (IQ<70).[12–14]

PSYCHIATRIC COMORBIDITIES

Diagnosing psychiatric comorbidities in children with ASDs is difficult for several reasons. In some cases, dual diagnoses are explicitly forbidden by the DSM-IV diagnostic criteria (such as for ASDs and attention deficit-hyperactivity disorder). However, the major barriers to diagnosing psychiatric comorbidities in children with ASDs are that behaviors displayed by children with ASDs can meet the criteria for different diagnoses (for example, social difficulties could be due to the core deficit in ASD, social anxiety disorder, depressed mood, or all of the above; inattention in the classroom could be because of an inability to focus, or a restricted interest in an internal or external stimuli) and internal states such as anxiety or sadness may manifest themselves very differently in patients with ASD (particularly those with impaired language) compared with neurotypical children, which is not to say that psychiatric comorbidities do not exist in patients with ASDs. A study of adults with ASD (who are likely to manifest their psychiatric symptoms in a more uniform way) suggests that patients with ASDs have almost twice as many psychiatric comorbidities than non-ASD controls seeking psychiatric treatment.[15] In both children and adults, it is common clinical practice to treat psychiatric symptoms in ASD (ie, stimulants for inattention or antipsychotics for aggression, **Table 4**) regardless of whether a patient meets criteria for a separate psychiatric disorder.

NATURE OF THE DISEASE

There is considerable evidence that both environmental and genetic factors play a role in the cause of ASDs. Environmental factors known to increase the risk of ASDs include prematurity,[16] prenatal infections such as rubella,[17,18] and advanced parental age.[19–21] One environmental factor that has been intensely studied and shown not to have a causative role in ASDs is vaccinations. Suspicion about the link between ASDs and vaccines was fueled by parental observation of the temporal coincidence between when an infant received the MMR vaccine and when the symptoms of ASD became apparent. A prominent study in the *Lancet* validated these concerns but was later found to be fraudulent.[22–24] Several subsequent studies looking for correlation between vaccination and ASD incidence in different populations have all shown no link.[25–28] Although the percentage of risk for ASDs caused by genetics versus the percentage caused by environmental factors is still being debated, there is no doubt that ASDs are highly heritable. The most recent twin studies have shown a concordance rate of 39% to 58% among monozygotic twins and 24% to 31% among dizygotic twins, suggesting a heritability of 0.7.[29,30] A recent large-scale survey of younger siblings of patients with ASDs found that 20% of these siblings would go on to develop ASDs.[31] The high heritability of ASDs indicates a role for genetic testing.

CLINICAL FINDINGS (CASE STUDY)

Patient X was referred by his pediatrician to the autism evaluation clinic at a tertiary care medical center after his parents noticed that he was not developing language and had repetitive behavior.

Chief complaint: Seen in clinic at age 2 years, 6 months; brought in by parents who were concerned about language delay as well as repetitive speech and behavior.

Developmental History: The patient was the result of full-term, uneventful pregnancy. He was born via emergency C-section due to large cranial size (birth weight 9 lbs, 8 oz). The patient and his mother were in hospital for 2 days after birth. No problems eating or sleeping as an infant were reported. No medical problems as an infant were reported.

Allergies: none.

Medications: none.

Family History: No significant family history. The patient has one neurotypical younger sister.

Milestones: Sat unaided at 7 months, walking by 14 months, began using single words at 10 months. At 30 months, the patient was using simple phrases, but in a repetitive manner.

Physical examination: normal male toddler.

Diagnostic testing: Vineland Adaptive Behavior Scales II—standard score 84 (14th percentile); Mullen Scales of Early Learning–Learning composite 85 (16th percentile), classification range—average; the patient did not show significant fine or gross motor delays on subscales of the above tests. Autism Diagnostic Observation Schedule Module 1—showed significant deficits in verbal and nonverbal communication and play. The patient's play was repetitive and he did not use toys as independent agents. He had poor response to joint attention cues and did not smile reciprocally.

The patient was diagnosed with autism.

Imaging: none.

Genetic testing: The patient had Fragile X testing and chromosomal microarray testing using a genome-wide SNP array. Fragile X testing was normal but the chromosomal microarray showed a 611-kb heterozygous deletion at chromosome 16p11.2. Subsequent testing of the family showed that this was a de novo copy number variant (CNV).

In the case of Patient X, the chromosomal microarray testing was informative because deletions at 16p11.2 have been strongly associated with ASDs and childhood obesity.[32] In practice, most clinicians will also order separate tests for Fragile X syndrome in the case of male patients with ASD and intellectual disability and MECP2 testing for female patients with motor stereotypes and regression because chromosomal microarray testing will miss these single-gene disorders. Although their child was already clinically diagnosed with autism at the time of genetic testing, knowing the precise nature of the responsible genetic lesion will allow the parents and pediatrician of Patient X to monitor and possibly prevent the medical comorbidity (obesity) associated with his syndrome. Furthermore, the discovery that Patient X had a de novo mutation (not inherited from either parent) had important implications for future family planning for his parents because it lowered the risk of siblings of Patient X having ASDs.

GENETICS

Given the high heritability of ASD, there was hope that causative mutations would be found quickly, as had been the case for other neurologic diseases such as Huntington and Parkinson. Unfortunately, relatively few human genetic studies on ASDs could be replicated, partly due to the clinical heterogeneity of ASDs, and partly to nonstandard and evolving technology for identifying linked mutations. To solve the problem of clinical heterogeneity, 2 large collections of ASD patients and families were created by consortia of parents, advocates, and researchers. The Autism Genetic Resource Exchange is a collection of multiplex (more than one sibling with an ASD) families, whereas the Simons Simplex Collection has about 2700 families in which only one child has an ASD. In each of these collections, patients have been diagnosed and phenotyped using the same instruments. Although tremendous effort has been spent on performing large-scale linkage studies and genome-wide association scans for ASDs, only 2 regions of interest (7q[33] and 17q11-21[34]) have been replicated with linkage studies and only one region (an intergenic region between the cell adhesion genes *CDH9* and *CDH10*) achieved genome-wide significance in genome-wide association scans studies.[35] These types of studies are designed to find common variants in the population that contribute to the development of ASDs. Their relative lack of success suggests that common genetic variants with large effect sizes that influence ASDs may not exist. However, a meta-analysis of these data suggests that there could be many common variants with small effect sizes that additively contribute to the development of ASDs.[36]

Although CNVs (deletions, insertions, duplications) in the genome are thought to only account for 5% to 10% of cases of ASDs,[37,38] studies identifying CNVs associated with ASDs have been remarkably consistent and have helped to identify candidate genes that may play a role in the pathophysiology of ASDs.[39–41] These studies have shown that most CNVs associated with ASDs in simplex families (only one child has ASD) are de novo events and, while patients with ASDs have the same overall rate of CNVs as controls, the CNVs in patients are far more likely to affect gene function. Recent exome sequencing efforts found a similar result in simplex ASD families for rare single nucleotide variants in that the overall mutation rate for patients and controls were the same, but ASD patients were far more likely to have deleterious mutations in brain expressed genes.[42] These and other studies have implicated a large number of genes as potential causes of ASDs. Some estimates place the number of autism-related genes to be between 384 and 821.[43] There are now public databases that have compiled the available evidence linking the currently known candidate genes to ASDs cases (for example, see http://gene.sfari.org).

Although the studies mentioned above have concentrated on patients with idiopathic ASD, syndromic ASDs (where the behavioral features of the ASD are part of a larger syndrome of symptoms) are also associated with structural chromosomal variation.[37] **Table 1** lists the most common genetic syndromes that have ASD as a component. The penetrance of the ASD phenotype in these syndromes is highly variable, suggesting that genes outside the region causing the syndrome also play a role.

DISEASE PATHOLOGY

Large longitudinal studies of head circumference and magnetic resonance imaging (MRI)-based measurements of brain volume demonstrate that subjects with autism on average show mildly reduced head size at birth and a sudden accelerated rate of brain growth between 1 to 2 months and 6 to 14 months of age compared with typical controls.[7,44] This accelerated brain growth preferentially affects frontal, temporal, and cingulate cortices.[45] Subcortical structures are also affected: in fact, the extent of enlargement of the amygdala in toddlers correlates strongly with the level social and communication impairment, measured later in life.[46] This period of accelerated brain growth is followed by growth arrest such that in adolescence head and

Table 1
Genetic syndromes with ASD as a component

ASD-related Syndrome	Reference
1q21 duplication	68
3p deletion/duplication	69,70
7q35-q36 (cortical dysplasia, focal epilepsy)	71,72
10q23 (Cowden syndrome/BRRS)	73
11p15 (Beckwith-Weidemann syndrome)	74
11q13 (Smith-Lemli-Opitz syndrome)	75
12p13 (Timothy syndrome)	76
15q11-q13 duplication (maternal)	77
15q11 deletion	78
15q13 maternal deletion (Angelman syndrome)	79,80
15q11-q13 paternal deletion (Prader-Willi syndrome)	81
16p11 deletion	37,82,83
17p11 (Potocki-Lupski syndrome)	84
Trisomy 21 (Down syndrome)	85
22q11 deletion (DiGeorge syndrome/VCFS)	86,87
22q13 deletion	88
Xp27 (Fragile X syndrome)	89

brain volumes are similar in autistic and typical subjects.[47] That this period of accelerated growth precedes the onset of autism-related behaviors suggests that divergence in trajectory of brain development in autism is well established soon after birth and may be used as a biomarker for early diagnosis in some patients. Extending these studies into late adulthood using MRI-based brain volume measurements confirms the earlier findings but also indicates that there may be accelerated decline in brain volume in autistic subjects after adolescence into middle age.[48] Undoubtedly the ultimate cause of the autism syndrome will dictate the trajectory in brain development. This finding is readily apparent in a recent study where it was shown that autistic subjects with de novo PTEN and CHD8 mutations were macrocephalic, whereas those with DYRK1 mutations were microcephalic.[49] Future longitudinal MRI-based studies will need to be combined with genome sequencing to determine whether brain development trajectory can be more informative in the context of genetic information.

Autopsy studies examining neuronal number in far smaller numbers of autistic subjects and typical controls suggest that increased brain volume found in the MRI-based studies is partly caused by a large (67%) increase in cell counts in the prefrontal cortex.[50] The increased cell counts in dorsolateral prefrontal cortex were more severe (79%) than changes in the medial prefrontal cortex (mPFC) (29%), suggesting that brain subregion-specific changes may mediate the behavioral impairments.[51] Conversely, early studies from 4 autopsy samples show diminished numbers of Purkinje neurons,[52] again highlighting the regional specificity in cell counts. Studies of somatic, dendritic, or axonal structure in autopsy samples are much more limited. One study found reduced Purkinje cell size in a small number of samples from autistic subjects and controls, but even in these few samples there was great heterogeneity.[53] In autopsy samples from Fragile X syndrome patients, a mental retardation syndrome with a high comorbidity with autistic behavior, long tortuous immature-appearing spines associated with shorter synapses have been observed, suggesting that at least in this syndrome, pathologic immaturity or dysmaturity of the circuit may cause cognitive and behavioral impairments.[54]

Finally, in addition to abnormalities in neuronal cell number and cell structure, changes in microglia have also been found. These studies suggest that an inflammatory component could potentially play a role in a subset of patients, although it is not clear whether the changes in microglia are causal or secondary to other factors. Microglia are closer to neurons in the prefrontal cortex of autistic subjects compared with typical controls.[55] Furthermore, in some samples from autistic subjects, there is increased microglial density and microglial activation.[56,57]

EVALUATION AND MANAGEMENT

The diagnosis of an ASD can be made by any trained clinician who, through careful history taking and observation, determines that a patient meets the DSM-IV criteria for an ASD. In practice, this inserted considerable subjectivity to the diagnosis and added to the genuine clinical heterogeneity of the ASD population. In particular, patients on the milder end of the spectrum were either missed or had a delayed diagnosis. Therefore, several screening tools were developed to help primary care clinicians know when to refer a patient for further testing to confirm an ASD diagnosis (**Table 2**). The individual screening tools have not been rigorously compared with each other and it is largely a matter of personal preference among clinicians as to which tool best fits their practice model. The current gold standards for the diagnosis of ASDs are the Autism Diagnostic Observation Schedule[58] and Autism Diagnostic Interview,[59] which are commonly administered by psychologists, psychiatrists, neurologists, or developmental pediatricians with specialized training in these instruments.

Once diagnosed, the primary treatments for ASDs are behavioral interventions. A large body of research indicates that early intervention (starting at toddlerhood) produced better outcomes (for review, see Ref.[60]). **Table 3** lists commonly used evidence-based behavioral interventions for ASDs. Like with the screening tools, there have been very few head-to-head comparisons between the different types of therapies. In clinical practice, the resources available in a given community for a particular patient dictate what type of therapy a child receives far more often than clinician preference. However, when advocating for patients with ASDs, general guidelines for clinicians are that evidence-based therapies are better than non-evidence-based therapies; therapy in multiple settings (home and school) is better than single-setting therapy; longer therapy is better than shorter therapy; and earlier therapy is better than later therapy. Ideally, assessments should be made across all domains of development (cognitive, social, language, motor, occupational) in a patient with an ASD and therapy should be offered in all of the domains in which the patient has deficits.

Although risperidone and aripiprazole are currently the only FDA-approved medications for irritability and aggression in ASDs, other psychotropic agents have been investigated and shown very mild benefit (see **Table 4**). In addition, patients with ASDs may be more sensitive than neurotypical peers to dosage and side effects of common psychotropic medications that limit their tolerability. However, given the burden of psychiatric comorbidities in patients with ASD, clinicians are likely to continue to use these non-FDA-approved medications. In these cases, a careful and conservative approach to dosing and side-effect monitoring is warranted.

THE ROLE OF GENETIC TESTING

Once a patient has been diagnosed with an ASD, genetic testing can play an important and informative role in shaping future treatment and management. As in the case of

Table 2
Diagnostic screening tools

Screening Tool	Child's Age (mo)	Method of Administration (Time Required for Completion)	Citation
ITC	6–24	Parent-completed survey (5–10 min)	90
M-CHAT	16–48	Parent-completed survey (5–10 min)	91
Q-CHAT	18–24	Parent-completed survey (5–10 min)	92
STAT	24–35	Clinician administered test (20 min) Requires workshop training	93
PDDST-II Primary care Screener 1	12–48	Parent-completed survey (10–15 min)	
SCQ	48 and above	Parent questionnaire (5–10 min)	94
Social Responsiveness Scale	48 and above	Parent and teacher survey (5–10 min)	95
First Year Inventory	12–24	Parent-completed survey	96
Early Childhood Inventory-4	36–60	Parent and teacher completed survey (10–20 min)	97
Child Symptom Inventory-4	72–144	Parent- and teacher-completed survey	98
AQ-Child	48–122	Parent-completed survey (50 questions)	99
ABC	18–122	Parent or teacher survey (10–20 min)	100
AOSI	6–18	Clinician observation (20 min)	2
ADOS-G	All ages	Standardized observation method (40–60 min)	101

Abbreviations: ABC, Autism Behavior Checklist; ADOS-G, Autism Diagnostic Observation Schedule-Generic; AOSI, Autism Observation Scale for Infants; AQ, Autism Spectrum Quotient; ITC, Infant-Toddler Checklist; M-CHAT, Modified Checklist for Autism in Toddlers; PDDST, Pervasive Developmental Disorders Screening Test; Q-CHAT, Quantitative Checklist for Autism in Toddlers; SCQ, Social Communication Questionnaire (formerly known as the Autism Sreeening Questionaiare); STAT, Screening Tool for Autism in Two Year Olds.

Patient X, identifying if the patient has syndromic or idiopathic ASD can warn families of potential medical comorbidities and allow for more intensive screening. In many of the syndromes listed in **Table 1**, the behavioral features of ASDs are the first components of the syndrome that are readily apparent. Furthermore, determining if an ASD-associated mutation is inherited or de novo can have profound implications for family planning. The American College of Medical Genetics recommends chromosomal microarray testing (CMA) as a first-line test in the evaluation of ASDs.[61] Studies have shown that CMA has a much higher yield than the G-band karyotyping that is currently recommended by the American Academy of Pediatrics and American Academy of Neurology.[62,63] CMAs can find small deletions or duplications in the genome (CNVs), but limitations of this technology include incomplete coverage of the genome (depending on the platform used) as well as that CNVs are common in the general population and most are not associated with illness. Therefore, most clinical

Table 3
Behavioral treatments

Type	Method	Description	Evidence for Efficacy	Citation
Early intensive behavioral Intervention (EIBI)	UCLA/Lovaas method	Intensive individualized therapy, 25 h per wk × 1 y	RCT: 28 children randomized to intensive therapy vs Parent-based therapy. Results: Intensive therapy outperformed on measures of intelligence, visual-spatial skills, language, and academics, but not adaptive functioning or behavioral problems	102
EIBI	Early Start Denver Method (ESDM)	Intensive ABA based therapy with developmental and relationship based approaches	RCT: 48 autistic children (18–30 mo in age) randomized to ESDM vs Community-based therapy. Results: ESDM group showed bigger improvements in IQ, language ability, adaptive behavior than controls. More subjects in ESDM changed diagnosis from autism to PDD-NOS	103
EIBI	Nova Scotia (NS) EIBI	Parent training and naturalistic one-to-one behavior intervention using Pivotal Response Treatment	Prospective Observational Trial: 45 autistic children observed for 12 mo. Large gains in expressive and receptive language. Decrease in behavioral problems. Decrease in autism related symptoms for children with IQ >50	104
Targeted Behavioral Therapy	Preschool-based joint attention (JA) intervention	Preschool teachers trained to implement targeted therapies to engage JA	RCT: 61 autistic children randomized to JA + preschool program vs only preschool program. The treatment group initiated more JA with teachers and more joint engagement with parents	105
Targeted Behavioral Therapy	Preschool-based interpersonal synchrony	Classroom-based training in joint attention, affect sharing, socially engaged imitation	RCT: 50 toddlers (21–33 mo old) randomized to interpersonal synchrony supplementation vs standard therapy. Improvements in socially engaged imitation with eye contact	106
Targeted Behavioral Therapy	Joint attention and symbolic play	Brief (30 min) joint attention or symbolic play interventions	RCT: 58 autistic children randomized to JA intervention vs symbolic play vs standard therapy. JA group showed improvement in JA. Symbolic play group showed more diverse and higher levels of play	107

Abbreviation: RCT, randomized controlled trial.

Table 4
Pharmacologic treatments

Drug Class	Drug	Evidence (Double Blind Randomized Control Trials)	Citation
D2 receptor blocker	Risperidone	101 autistic children with irritability (tantrums, aggression, or self-injurious behavior) randomized to risperidone vs placebo. 69% in treatment group showed a decrease in irritability compared with 12% in the placebo group. Improvement in restricted repetitive behaviors but not social or communicative impairments	108,109
D2 receptor blocker	Risperidone	79 autistic children with behavioral problems randomized to risperidone vs placebo. 64% improvement in irritability score vs 31% in placebo group	110
D2 receptor blocker	Risperidone	39 autistic children randomized to risperidone vs placebo. The 63% showed improvement in the Childhood Autism Rating Scale and 89% showed improvement in the Children's Global Assesment Scale	111
D2 receptor partial agonist	Aripiprazole	218 children with autism randomized to increasing doses of aripiprazole vs placebo. Treatment group showed a 12%–14% improvement on the Aberrant Behavior Checklist vs 8% improvement in placebo group	112
D2 receptor partial agonist	Aripiprazole	98 children with autism randomized to increasing doses of aripiprazole vs placebo. Treatment group showed greater improvements on the aberrant behavior checklist and Clinical Global impression improvement with 67% showing much improvement after treatment with aripiprazole vs 16% after treatment with placebo	113
Norepinephrine-dopamine reuptake inhibitor	Methylphenidate	Cross-over design. 78 autistic children received 3 wk of methylphenidate and 1 wk of placebo (in random order). There was a decrease in hyperactivity (49% percent of children responded to medication) but effect smaller than typically developing children and autistic children more sensitive to side effects	114

(continued on next page)

Table 4
(continued)

Drug Class	Drug	Evidence (Double Blind Randomized Control Trials)	Citation
Selective serotonin reuptake inhibitor	Fluvoxamine	30 autistic adults randomized to fluvoxamine vs placebo. 53% of treatment group responded with improvements in repetitive thoughts and behaviors, as well as language.	[115]
Selective serotonin reuptake inhibitor	Fluoxetine	37 autistic adults randomized to fluoxetine vs placebo. Treatment group showed decrease in repetitive behaviors or obsessive-compulsive features (50% responders with fluoxetine, 0% with placebo)	[116]

laboratories will reference periodically updated databases of CNVs known to be associated with disease when issuing a result (for examples, see Refs.[64,65]). It is important for clinicians to note that a normal or negative CMA result does not exclude the possibility of a genetic factor in a given patient's ASD. There are commercial enterprises that offer genome sequencing to patients, including those with ASDs (for examples, see www.23andme.com and www.illumina.com), although the utility of such services for patients with ASDs has yet to be determined. Clinical exome sequencing is now offered by several academic institutions throughout the United States and has shown utility in the diagnosis of intellectual disability.[66] It could be clinically useful in cases of ASD as well. The problem of separating normal variation from pathologic mutation present in CMAs is magnified for sequence data and, currently, relatively few mutations implicated in ASDs have been shown to be deleterious in a biologic system. Still, in the near future, it is likely that sequencing will supplant CMAs as the primary means of genetic testing once the informational challenges are overcome, raising the exciting possibility of individualized pharmacologic treatments for ASDs. The clinical

Table 5
Syndrome-specific treatments

Drug Class	Drug	Syndrome	Evidence	Citation
mTOR inhibitor	Rapamycin	Tuberous sclerosis	Effective for astrocytomas and angiomyolipomas. Effects on autism related symptoms unknown	[117,118]
mGluR5 antagonist	Fenobam	Fragile X	Open-label single-dose trial in 12 Fragile X subjects. Hints of improved communication and eye contact	[119]
Mood stabilizer	Lithium	Fragile X	Open-label treatment trial in 15 FXS subjects. Treatment resulted in improvements in multiple behavioral domains	[120]

Abbreviation: mGluR5, metabotropic glutamate receptor 5.

heterogeneity of ASDs has long led researchers to surmise that ASDs were not one disorder, but many different neurodevelopmental disorders with similar behavioral features.[67] The work on candidate genes and syndromic forms of ASDs has led to trials of drugs that target biochemical pathways in those syndromes (**Table 5**). Within the next decade, clinicians should be able to offer individualized behavioral and pharmacologic treatments to a significant proportion of their patients with ASDs based on genomic data.

SUMMARY

ASDs are a clinically heterogeneous set of conditions that are defined by difficulties in social communication, language delay, and repetitive or restricted interests. The behavioral symptoms of ASDs manifest early in life and there are numerous screening tools to help clinicians identify patients. Studies on the disease pathologic abnormality suggest that neural development is adversely affected in ASDs and this can be caused by a combination of genetic factors and the in utero environment. There are syndromic forms of ASDs in which the behavioral deficits of autism are accompanied by other medical comorbidities. These syndromic forms of ASD are often associated with structural genetic changes, or CNVs. Chromosomal microarray testing is a recommended method for identifying syndromic forms of ASD and informing parents about potential medical problems as well as helping with family planning. In the future, genomic sequencing will help guide therapeutic choices for patients with ASDs, but several barriers exist. The technical barrier of obtaining sequence data at low cost is rapidly being overcome, but the bio-informatic challenge of using that information remains. The problem of determining which genetic changes are pathologic and which are normal variation is currently being researched for ASDs. Animal model systems are helping identify which biochemical pathways are important in ASDs and clinical trials on pharmacologic agents that target those pathways are ongoing. A future is envisioned whereby genetic sequencing can help determine an individualized program of behavioral and pharmacologic therapy for each patient with an ASD.

REFERENCES

1. Autism and Developmental Disabilities Monitoring Network Surveillance Year 2008 Principal Investigators, Centers for Disease Control and Prevention. Prevalence of autism spectrum disorders–Autism and Developmental Disabilities Monitoring Network, 14 sites, United States, 2008. MMWR Surveill Summ 2012;61(3):1–19.
2. Bryson SE, Zwaigenbaum L, McDermott C, et al. The Autism Observation Scale for Infants: scale development and reliability data. J Autism Dev Disord 2008; 38(4):731–8.
3. Wolff JJ, Gu H, Gerig G, et al. Differences in white matter fiber tract development present from 6 to 24 months in infants with autism. Am J Psychiatry 2012;169(6):589–600.
4. Kotagal S, Broomall E. Sleep in children with autism spectrum disorder. Pediatr Neurol 2012;47(4):242–51.
5. Fombonne E, Roge B, Claverie J, et al. Microcephaly and macrocephaly in autism. J Autism Dev Disord 1999;29(2):113–9.
6. Lainhart JE, Bigler ED, Bocian M, et al. Head circumference and height in autism: a study by the Collaborative Program of Excellence in Autism. Am J Med Genet A 2006;140(21):2257–74.

7. Courchesne E, Carper R, Akshoomoff N. Evidence of brain overgrowth in the first year of life in autism. JAMA 2003;290(3):337–44.
8. Hazlett HC, Poe M, Gerig G, et al. Magnetic resonance imaging and head circumference study of brain size in autism: birth through age 2 years. Arch Gen Psychiatry 2005;62(12):1366–76.
9. Bolton PF, Carcani-Rathwell I, Hutton J, et al. Epilepsy in autism: features and correlates. Br J Psychiatry 2011;198(4):289–94.
10. Tuchman R, Rapin I. Epilepsy in autism. Lancet Neurol 2002;1(6):352–8.
11. Ibrahim SH, Voigt RG, Katusic SK, et al. Incidence of gastrointestinal symptoms in children with autism: a population-based study. Pediatrics 2009;124(2): 680–6.
12. Charman T, Pickles A, Simonoff E, et al. IQ in children with autism spectrum disorders: data from the Special Needs and Autism Project (SNAP). Psychol Med 2011;41(3):619–27.
13. Icasiano F, Hewson P, Machet P, et al. Childhood autism spectrum disorder in the Barwon region: a community based study. J Paediatr Child Health 2004; 40(12):696–701.
14. Kawamura Y, Takahashi O, Ishii T. Reevaluating the incidence of pervasive developmental disorders: impact of elevated rates of detection through implementation of an integrated system of screening in Toyota, Japan. Psychiatry Clin Neurosci 2008;62(2):152–9.
15. Joshi G, Wozniak J, Petty C, et al. Psychiatric comorbidity and functioning in a clinically referred population of adults with autism spectrum disorders: a comparative study. J Autism Dev Disord 2013;43(6):1314–25.
16. Lampi KM, Lehtonen L, Tran PL, et al. Risk of autism spectrum disorders in low birth weight and small for gestational age infants. J Pediatr 2012;161(5):830–6.
17. Chess S. Autism in children with congenital rubella. J Autism Child Schizophr 1971;1(1):33–47.
18. Deykin EY, MacMahon B. Viral exposure and autism. Am J Epidemiol 1979; 109(6):628–38.
19. Croen LA, Najjar DV, Fireman B, et al. Maternal and paternal age and risk of autism spectrum disorders. Arch Pediatr Adolesc Med 2007;161(4):334–40.
20. Durkin MS, Maenner MJ, Newschaffer CJ, et al. Advanced parental age and the risk of autism spectrum disorder. Am J Epidemiol 2008;168(11):1268–76.
21. Shelton JF, Tancredi DJ, Hertz-Picciotto I. Independent and dependent contributions of advanced maternal and paternal ages to autism risk. Autism Res 2010;3(1):30–9.
22. Retraction–Ileal-lymphoid-nodular hyperplasia, non-specific colitis, and pervasive developmental disorder in children. Lancet 2010;375(9713):445.
23. Deer B. How the case against the MMR vaccine was fixed. BMJ 2011;342: c5347.
24. Wakefield AJ, Murch SH, Anthony A, et al. Ileal-lymphoid-nodular hyperplasia, non-specific colitis, and pervasive developmental disorder in children. Lancet 1998;351(9103):637–41.
25. Baird G, Pickles A, Simonoff E, et al. Measles vaccination and antibody response in autism spectrum disorders. Arch Dis Child 2008;93(10):832–7.
26. Honda H, Shimizu Y, Rutter M. No effect of MMR withdrawal on the incidence of autism: a total population study. J Child Psychol Psychiatry 2005;46(6): 572–9.
27. Smeeth L, Cook C, Fombonne E, et al. MMR vaccination and pervasive developmental disorders: a case-control study. Lancet 2004;364(9438):963–9.

28. Uno Y, Uchiyama T, Kurosawa M, et al. The combined measles, mumps, and rubella vaccines and the total number of vaccines are not associated with development of autism spectrum disorder: the first case-control study in Asia. Vaccine 2012;30(28):4292–8.

29. Hallmayer J, Cleveland S, Torres A, et al. Genetic heritability and shared environmental factors among twin pairs with autism. Arch Gen Psychiatry 2011; 68(11):1095–102.

30. Lichtenstein P, Carlstrom E, Rastam M, et al. The genetics of autism spectrum disorders and related neuropsychiatric disorders in childhood. Am J Psychiatry 2010;167(11):1357–63.

31. Ozonoff S, Young GS, Carter A, et al. Recurrence risk for autism spectrum disorders: a Baby Siblings Research Consortium Study. Pediatrics 2011;128(3): e488–95.

32. Zufferey F, Sherr EH, Beckmann ND, et al. A 600 kb deletion syndrome at 16p11.2 leads to energy imbalance and neuropsychiatric disorders. J Med Genet 2012;49(10):660–8.

33. Badner JA, Gershon ES. Regional meta-analysis of published data supports linkage of autism with markers on chromosome 7. Mol Psychiatry 2002;7(1): 56–66.

34. Cantor RM, Kono N, Duvall JA, et al. Replication of autism linkage: fine-mapping peak at 17q21. Am J Hum Genet 2005;76(6):1050–6.

35. Wang K, Zhang H, Ma D, et al. Common genetic variants on 5p14.1 associate with autism spectrum disorders. Nature 2009;459(7246):528–33.

36. Klei L, Sanders SJ, Murtha MT, et al. Common genetic variants, acting additively, are a major source of risk for autism. Mol Autism 2012;3(1):9.

37. Marshall CR, Noor A, Vincent JB, et al. Structural variation of chromosomes in autism spectrum disorder. Am J Hum Genet 2008;82(2):477–88.

38. Sebat J, Lakshmi B, Malhotra D, et al. Strong association of de novo copy number mutations with autism. Science 2007;316(5823):445–9.

39. Levy D, Ronemus M, Yamrom B, et al. Rare de novo and transmitted copy-number variation in autistic spectrum disorders. Neuron 2011;70(5):886–97.

40. Pinto D, Pagnamenta AT, Klei L, et al. Functional impact of global rare copy number variation in autism spectrum disorders. Nature 2010;466(7304):368–72.

41. Sanders SJ, Ercan-Sencicek AG, Hus V, et al. Multiple recurrent de novo CNVs, including duplications of the 7q11.23 Williams syndrome region, are strongly associated with autism. Neuron 2011;70(5):863–85.

42. Sanders SJ, Murtha MT, Gupta AR, et al. De novo mutations revealed by whole-exome sequencing are strongly associated with autism. Nature 2012;485(7397): 237–41.

43. O'Roak BJ, Vives L, Girirajan S, et al. Sporadic autism exomes reveal a highly interconnected protein network of de novo mutations. Nature 2012;485(7397): 246–50.

44. Courchesne E, Karns CM, Davis HR, et al. Unusual brain growth patterns in early life in patients with autistic disorder: an MRI study. Neurology 2001; 57(2):245–54.

45. Schumann CM, Bloss CS, Barnes CC, et al. Longitudinal magnetic resonance imaging study of cortical development through early childhood in autism. J Neurosci 2010;30(12):4419–27.

46. Schumann CM, Barnes CC, Lord C, et al. Amygdala enlargement in toddlers with autism related to severity of social and communication impairments. Biol Psychiatry 2009;66(10):942–9.

47. Thomas MS, Knowland VC, Karmiloff-Smith A. Mechanisms of developmental regression in autism and the broader phenotype: a neural network modeling approach. Psychol Rev 2011;118(4):637–54.
48. Courchesne E, Campbell K, Solso S. Brain growth across the life span in autism: age-specific changes in anatomical pathology. Brain Res 2011;1380:138–45.
49. O'Roak BJ, Vives L, Fu W, et al. Multiplex targeted sequencing identifies recurrently mutated genes in autism spectrum disorders. Science 2012;338(6114): 1619–22.
50. Courchesne E, Mouton PR, Calhoun ME, et al. Neuron number and size in prefrontal cortex of children with autism. JAMA 2011;306(18):2001–10.
51. Eyler LT, Pierce K, Courchesne E. A failure of left temporal cortex to specialize for language is an early emerging and fundamental property of autism. Brain 2012;135(Pt 3):949–60.
52. Ritvo ER, Freeman BJ, Scheibel AB, et al. Lower Purkinje cell counts in the cerebella of four autistic subjects: initial findings of the UCLA-NSAC Autopsy Research Report. Am J Psychiatry 1986;143(7):862–6.
53. Fatemi SH, Halt AR, Realmuto G, et al. Purkinje cell size is reduced in cerebellum of patients with autism. Cell Mol Neurobiol 2002;22(2):171–5.
54. Wisniewski KE, Segan SM, Miezejeski CM, et al. The Fra(X) syndrome: neurological, electrophysiological, and neuropathological abnormalities. Am J Med Genet 1991;38(2–3):476–80.
55. Morgan JT, Chana G, Abramson I, et al. Abnormal microglial-neuronal spatial organization in the dorsolateral prefrontal cortex in autism. Brain Res 2012;1456: 72–81.
56. Morgan JT, Chana G, Pardo CA, et al. Microglial activation and increased microglial density observed in the dorsolateral prefrontal cortex in autism. Biol Psychiatry 2010;68(4):368–76.
57. Vargas DL, Nascimbene C, Krishnan C, et al. Neuroglial activation and neuroinflammation in the brain of patients with autism. Ann Neurol 2005;57(1):67–81.
58. Lord C, Rutter M, Goode S, et al. Autism diagnostic observation schedule: a standardized observation of communicative and social behavior. J Autism Dev Disord 1989;19(2):185–212.
59. Lord C, Rutter M, Le Couteur A. Autism Diagnostic Interview-Revised: a revised version of a diagnostic interview for caregivers of individuals with possible pervasive developmental disorders. J Autism Dev Disord 1994;24(5):659–85.
60. Dawson G, Burner K. Behavioral interventions in children and adolescents with autism spectrum disorder: a review of recent findings. Curr Opin Pediatr 2011; 23(6):616–20.
61. Miller DT, Adam MP, Aradhya S, et al. Consensus statement: chromosomal microarray is a first-tier clinical diagnostic test for individuals with developmental disabilities or congenital anomalies. Am J Hum Genet 2010;86(5):749–64.
62. McGrew SG, Peters BR, Crittendon JA, et al. Diagnostic yield of chromosomal microarray analysis in an autism primary care practice: which guidelines to implement? J Autism Dev Disord 2012;42(8):1582–91.
63. Shen Y, Dies KA, Holm IA, et al. Clinical genetic testing for patients with autism spectrum disorders. Pediatrics 2010;125(4):e727–35.
64. GeneTests Medical Genetics Information Resource (database online). 2012. Available at: www.genetests.org. Accessed December 18, 2012.
65. Firth HV, Richards SM, Bevan AP, et al. DECIPHER: database of chromosomal imbalance and phenotype in humans using ensembl resources. Am J Hum Genet 2009;84(4):524–33.

66. de Ligt J, Willemsen MH, van Bon BW, et al. Diagnostic exome sequencing in persons with severe intellectual disability. N Engl J Med 2012;367(20):1921–9.

67. Geschwind DH, Levitt P. Autism spectrum disorders: developmental disconnection syndromes. Curr Opin Neurobiol 2007;17(1):103–11.

68. Mefford HC, Sharp AJ, Baker C, et al. Recurrent rearrangements of chromosome 1q21.1 and variable pediatric phenotypes. N Engl J Med 2008;359(16):1685–99.

69. Fernandez T, Morgan T, Davis N, et al. Disruption of contactin 4 (CNTN4) results in developmental delay and other features of 3p deletion syndrome. Am J Hum Genet 2004;74(6):1286–93.

70. Glessner JT, Wang K, Cai G, et al. Autism genome-wide copy number variation reveals ubiquitin and neuronal genes. Nature 2009;459(7246):569–73.

71. Jackman C, Horn ND, Molleston JP, et al. Gene associated with seizures, autism, and hepatomegaly in an Amish girl. Pediatr Neurol 2009;40(4):310–3.

72. Strauss KA, Puffenberger EG, Huentelman MJ, et al. Recessive symptomatic focal epilepsy and mutant contactin-associated protein-like 2. N Engl J Med 2006;354(13):1370–7.

73. Varga EA, Pastore M, Prior T, et al. The prevalence of PTEN mutations in a clinical pediatric cohort with autism spectrum disorders, developmental delay, and macrocephaly. Genet Med 2009;11(2):111–7.

74. Kent L, Bowdin S, Kirby GA, et al. Beckwith Weidemann syndrome: a behavioral phenotype-genotype study. Am J Med Genet B Neuropsychiatr Genet 2008;147B(7):1295–7.

75. Tierney E, Nwokoro NA, Porter FD, et al. Behavior phenotype in the RSH/Smith-Lemli-Opitz syndrome. Am J Med Genet 2001;98(2):191–200.

76. Splawski I, Timothy KW, Sharpe LM, et al. Ca(V)1.2 calcium channel dysfunction causes a multisystem disorder including arrhythmia and autism. Cell 2004;119(1):19–31.

77. Cook EH Jr, Lindgren V, Leventhal BL, et al. Autism or atypical autism in maternally but not paternally derived proximal 15q duplication. Am J Hum Genet 1997;60(4):928–34.

78. Ben-Shachar S, Lanpher B, German JR, et al. Microdeletion 15q13.3: a locus with incomplete penetrance for autism, mental retardation, and psychiatric disorders. J Med Genet 2009;46(6):382–8.

79. Bonati MT, Russo S, Finelli P, et al. Evaluation of autism traits in Angelman syndrome: a resource to unfold autism genes. Neurogenetics 2007;8(3):169–78.

80. Peters SU, Beaudet AL, Madduri N, et al. Autism in Angelman syndrome: implications for autism research. Clin Genet 2004;66(6):530–6.

81. Descheemaeker MJ, Govers V, Vermeulen P, et al. Pervasive developmental disorders in Prader-Willi syndrome: the Leuven experience in 59 subjects and controls. Am J Med Genet A 2006;140(11):1136–42.

82. Kumar RA, KaraMohamed S, Sudi J, et al. Recurrent 16p11.2 microdeletions in autism. Hum Mol Genet 2008;17(4):628–38.

83. Weiss LA, Shen Y, Korn JM, et al. Association between microdeletion and microduplication at 16p11.2 and autism. N Engl J Med 2008;358(7):667–75.

84. Potocki L, Bi W, Treadwell-Deering D, et al. Characterization of Potocki-Lupski syndrome (dup(17)(p11.2p11.2)) and delineation of a dosage-sensitive critical interval that can convey an autism phenotype. Am J Hum Genet 2007;80(4):633–49.

85. Lowenthal R, Paula CS, Schwartzman JS, et al. Prevalence of pervasive developmental disorder in Down's syndrome. J Autism Dev Disord 2007;37(7):1394–5.

86. Fine SE, Weissman A, Gerdes M, et al. Autism spectrum disorders and symptoms in children with molecularly confirmed 22q11.2 deletion syndrome. J Autism Dev Disord 2005;35(4):461–70.

87. Vorstman JA, Morcus ME, Duijff SN, et al. The 22q11.2 deletion in children: high rate of autistic disorders and early onset of psychotic symptoms. J Am Acad Child Adolesc Psychiatry 2006;45(9):1104–13.

88. Manning MA, Cassidy SB, Clericuzio C, et al. Terminal 22q deletion syndrome: a newly recognized cause of speech and language disability in the autism spectrum. Pediatrics 2004;114(2):451–7.

89. Hatton DD, Sideris J, Skinner M, et al. Autistic behavior in children with fragile X syndrome: prevalence, stability, and the impact of FMRP. Am J Med Genet A 2006;140A(17):1804–13.

90. Wetherby AM, Brosnan-Maddox S, Peace V, et al. Validation of the Infant-Toddler Checklist as a broadband screener for autism spectrum disorders from 9 to 24 months of age. Autism 2008;12(5):487–511.

91. Robins DL, Fein D, Barton ML, et al. The Modified Checklist for Autism in Toddlers: an initial study investigating the early detection of autism and pervasive developmental disorders. J Autism Dev Disord 2001;31(2):131–44.

92. Allison C, Baron-Cohen S, Wheelwright S, et al. The Q-CHAT (Quantitative CHecklist for Autism in Toddlers): a normally distributed quantitative measure of autistic traits at 18-24 months of age: preliminary report. J Autism Dev Disord 2008;38(8):1414–25.

93. Stone WL, Coonrod EE, Ousley OY. Brief report: screening tool for autism in two-year-olds (STAT): development and preliminary data. J Autism Dev Disord 2000; 30(6):607–12.

94. Berument SK, Rutter M, Lord C, et al. Autism screening questionnaire: diagnostic validity. Br J Psychiatry 1999;175:444–51.

95. Constantino JN, Davis SA, Todd RD, et al. Validation of a brief quantitative measure of autistic traits: comparison of the social responsiveness scale with the autism diagnostic interview-revised. J Autism Dev Disord 2003;33(4):427–33.

96. Reznick JS, Baranek GT, Reavis S, et al. A parent-report instrument for identifying one-year-olds at risk for an eventual diagnosis of autism: the first year inventory. J Autism Dev Disord 2007;37(9):1691–710.

97. DeVincent C, Gadow KD, Strong G, et al. Screening for autism spectrum disorder with the Early Childhood Inventory-4. J Dev Behav Pediatr 2008; 29(1):1–10.

98. Gadow KD, Schwartz J, Devincent C, et al. Clinical utility of autism spectrum disorder scoring algorithms for the child symptom inventory-4. J Autism Dev Disord 2008;38(3):419–27.

99. Auyeung B, Baron-Cohen S, Wheelwright S, et al. The Autism Spectrum Quotient: Children's Version (AQ-Child). J Autism Dev Disord 2008;38(7): 1230–40.

100. Rellini E, Tortolani D, Trillo S, et al. Childhood Autism Rating Scale (CARS) and Autism Behavior Checklist (ABC) correspondence and conflicts with DSM-IV criteria in diagnosis of autism. J Autism Dev Disord 2004;34(6):703–8.

101. Lord C, Risi S, Lambrecht L, et al. The autism diagnostic observation schedule-generic: a standard measure of social and communication deficits associated with the spectrum of autism. J Autism Dev Disord 2000;30(3):205–23.

102. Smith T, Groen AD, Wynn JW. Randomized trial of intensive early intervention for children with pervasive developmental disorder. Am J Ment Retard 2000;105(4): 269–85.

103. Dawson G, Rogers S, Munson J, et al. Randomized, controlled trial of an intervention for toddlers with autism: the Early Start Denver Model. Pediatrics 2010; 125(1):e17–23.

104. Smith IM, Koegel RL, Koegel LK, et al. Effectiveness of a novel community-based early intervention model for children with autistic spectrum disorder. Am J Intellect Dev Disabil 2010;115(6):504–23.

105. Kaale A, Smith L, Sponheim E. A randomized controlled trial of preschool-based joint attention intervention for children with autism. J Child Psychol Psychiatry 2012;53(1):97–105.

106. Landa RJ, Holman KC, O'Neill AH, et al. Intervention targeting development of socially synchronous engagement in toddlers with autism spectrum disorder: a randomized controlled trial. J Child Psychol Psychiatry 2011;52(1):13–21.

107. Kasari C, Freeman S, Paparella T. Joint attention and symbolic play in young children with autism: a randomized controlled intervention study. J Child Psychol Psychiatry 2006;47(6):611–20.

108. McCracken JT, McGough J, Shah B, et al. Risperidone in children with autism and serious behavioral problems. N Engl J Med 2002;347(5):314–21.

109. McDougle CJ, Scahill L, Aman MG, et al. Risperidone for the core symptom domains of autism: results from the study by the autism network of the research units on pediatric psychopharmacology. Am J Psychiatry 2005;162(6):1142–8.

110. Shea S, Turgay A, Carroll A, et al. Risperidone in the treatment of disruptive behavioral symptoms in children with autistic and other pervasive developmental disorders. Pediatrics 2004;114(5):e634–41.

111. Nagaraj R, Singhi P, Malhi P. Risperidone in children with autism: randomized, placebo-controlled, double-blind study. J Child Neurol 2006;21(6):450–5.

112. Marcus RN, Owen R, Kamen L, et al. A placebo-controlled, fixed-dose study of aripiprazole in children and adolescents with irritability associated with autistic disorder. J Am Acad Child Adolesc Psychiatry 2009;48(11):1110–9.

113. Owen R, Sikich L, Marcus RN, et al. Aripiprazole in the treatment of irritability in children and adolescents with autistic disorder. Pediatrics 2009;124(6):1533–40.

114. Research Units on Pediatric Psychopharmacology Autism Network. Randomized, controlled, crossover trial of methylphenidate in pervasive developmental disorders with hyperactivity. Arch Gen Psychiatry 2005;62(11):1266–74.

115. McDougle CJ, Naylor ST, Cohen DJ, et al. A double-blind, placebo-controlled study of fluvoxamine in adults with autistic disorder. Arch Gen Psychiatry 1996;53(11):1001–8.

116. Hollander E, Soorya L, Chaplin W, et al. A double-blind placebo-controlled trial of fluoxetine for repetitive behaviors and global severity in adult autism spectrum disorders. Am J Psychiatry 2012;169(3):292–9.

117. Bissler JJ, McCormack FX, Young LR, et al. Sirolimus for angiomyolipoma in tuberous sclerosis complex or lymphangioleiomyomatosis. N Engl J Med 2008; 358(2):140–51.

118. Franz DN, Belousova E, Sparagana S, et al. Efficacy and safety of everolimus for subependymal giant cell astrocytomas associated with tuberous sclerosis complex (EXIST-1): a multicentre, randomised, placebo-controlled phase 3 trial. Lancet 2013;381(9861):125–32.

119. Berry-Kravis E, Hessl D, Coffey S, et al. A pilot open label, single dose trial of fenobam in adults with fragile X syndrome. J Med Genet 2009;46(4):266–71.

120. Berry-Kravis E, Sumis A, Hervey C, et al. Open-label treatment trial of lithium to target the underlying defect in fragile X syndrome. J Dev Behav Pediatr 2008; 29(4):293–302.

Clinical Neurogenetics
Dystonia From Phenotype to Genotype

Jeffrey L. Waugh, MD, PhD[a,b,*], Nutan Sharma, MD, PhD[a]

KEYWORDS

- Dystonia • Myoclonus • Parkinsonism • Paroxysmal dyskinesia

KEY POINTS

- Dystonia is a movement disorder characterized by abnormal or twisting movements and postures, often elicited by specific tasks or positions.
- Characterizing a patient with idiopathic dystonia on 4 axes helps to produce a limited list of genetic tests: age of onset; site of onset; rate of progression; a multigeneration family history.
- Primary dystonias, dystonia-plus syndromes, paroxysmal dyskinesias (which have dystonia with other movement disorders), and secondary dystonias can all result from single-gene defects.
- Treatment of dystonia should be tailored to the age of the patient, the extent and site of symptoms, and the likelihood of progression.

INTRODUCTION
Definition

Dystonia is a movement disorder marked by twisting movements or fixed postures that may be intermittent or continuous. Often, dystonia is elicited by specific actions, usually highly skilled movements such as writing or playing a musical instrument. For most dystonic conditions, symptoms are stable over weeks to months, and spread (if it occurs) is slow, over months to years. Dystonia is a clinical diagnosis supported by genetic or neuroimaging studies.

This work was supported by the Bachmann-Strauss, Silverman Family Fellowship (JW); the American Academy of Neurology Clinical Research Training Fellowship (JW); and NINDS P50 NS037409 (NS).

[a] Department of Neurology, Massachusetts General Hospital, Harvard Medical School, MA, USA; [b] Department of Neurology, Boston Children's Hospital, MA, USA
* Corresponding author. Department of Neurology, Boston Children's Hospital, Fegan 11, 300 Longwood Avenue, Boston, MA 02115.
E-mail address: jeff.waugh@childrens.harvard.edu

http://dx.doi.org/10.1016/j.ncl.2013.04.002
0733-8619/13/$ – see front matter © 2013 Elsevier Inc. All rights reserved.
neurologic.theclinics.com

Symptoms and Clinical Course

There are many genetic causes of dystonia (**Figs. 1** and **2, Table 1**), making it difficult to identify a specific disorder at initial presentation. The onset and evolution of symptoms offer many clues to a genetic diagnosis; all patients should be characterized on the following axes:

Age at onset: preadolescent, young-adult (12–27 years), and late-adult onset. Although each genetic cause of dystonia has some variability in age of onset, the mean ages are distinct (see **Fig. 1, Table 1**).

Pace of single episodes: paroxysmal onset over seconds to minutes, slow evolution during each day, provocation by particular attempted movements (possibly

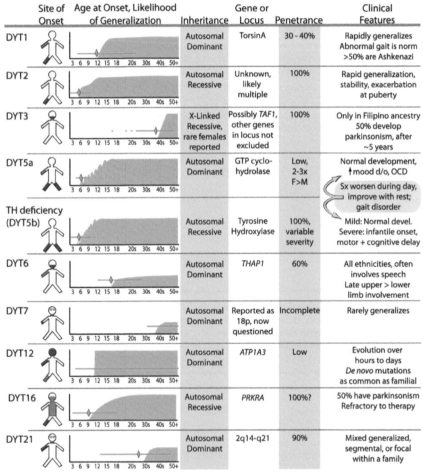

Site of Onset	Age at Onset, Likelihood of Generalization	Inheritance	Gene or Locus	Penetrance	Clinical Features
DYT1		Autosomal Dominant	TorsinA	30 - 40%	Rapidly generalizes Abnormal gait is norm >50% are Ashkenazi
DYT2		Autosomal Recessive	Unknown, likely multiple	100%	Rapid generalization, stability, exacerbation at puberty
DYT3		X-Linked Recessive, rare females reported	Possibly *TAF1*, other genes in locus not excluded	100%	Only in Filipino ancestry 50% develop parkinsonism, after ~5 years
DYT5a		Autosomal Dominant	GTP cyclo-hydrolase	Low, 2-3x F>M	Normal development, ↑mood d/o, OCD
					Sx worsen during day, improve with rest; gait disorder
TH deficiency (DYT5b)		Autosomal Recessive	Tyrosine Hydroxylase	100%, variable severity	Mild: Normal devel. Severe: infantile onset, motor + cognitive delay
DYT6		Autosomal Dominant	*THAP1*	60%	All ethnicities, often involves speech Late upper > lower limb involvement
DYT7		Autosomal Dominant	Reported as 18p, now questioned	Incomplete	Rarely generalizes
DYT12		Autosomal Dominant	*ATP1A3*	Low	Evolution over hours to days *De novo* mutations as common as familial
DYT16		Autosomal Recessive	*PRKRA*	100%?	50% have parkinsonism Refractory to therapy
DYT21		Autosomal Dominant	2q14-q21	90%	Mixed generalized, segmental, or focal within a family

Fig. 1. Syndromes with dystonia as the presenting or a predominant feature; primary dystonias or dystonia-plus syndromes that commonly begin with dystonia are listed. The most common sites of dystonia onset are indicated on the homunculus in red, with less-common sites of onset in pink. The distribution in age of onset is indicated by a blue bar, with mean age indicated by a blue diamond, and rare but reported outliers indicated by extralinear blue dashes. Typical rates of progression and likelihood of generalization are indicated by yellow plots. Note that homunculi and plots represent the most common clinical presentations, but variations on these axes are not uncommon.

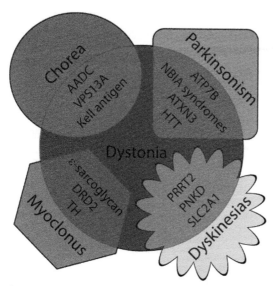

Fig. 2. Movement disorders with dystonia as a secondary or lesser feature. Mutations of the noted genes lead to syndromes in which dystonia follows another movement disorder, or in which dystonia is generally a less severe symptom. These dystonia-plus or paroxysmal dyskinetic syndromes typically onset in childhood, although the rapid-onset dystonia-parkinsonism syndromes may begin at any age. For each of the noted genes, a unique pattern of clinical presentation and progression aids in diagnosis. All gene designations are defined in the legend for **Table 1** with the following exceptions: Kell blood group antigen: mutation causes McLeod chorea-acanthocytosis syndrome; DRD-2, dopamine receptor D_2; NBIA, neurodegeneration with brain iron accumulation; TH, tyrosine hydroxylase; PRRT2, proline rich transmembrane protein 2; PNKD, paroxysmal nonkinesigenic dyskinesia; SLC2A1, solute carrier family 2, facilitated glucose transporter member 1, also knows as GLUT1.

many or no times in a particular day), or slow but inexorable progression are each prototypic patterns. Diurnal variation and relief with sleep strongly suggest the diagnosis of a dopa-responsive dystonia, a must-not-miss diagnosis in children. Note that the pace of dystonic episodes may differ from the progression of the disease as a whole.

Isolated versus mixed: dystonia can be the sole or predominant movement disorder (primary dystonias) or can be clearly secondary to a neurologic injury (eg, stroke, hemorrhage, resection) or a neurodegenerative syndrome, including heritable metabolic diseases that result in neurologic injury (secondary dystonias). The primary dystonias are subdivided into pure dystonia, dystonia-plus syndromes (in which dystonia is less prominent than another movement disorder, **Fig. 2**), and the paroxysmal dyskinesias (in which a variety of abnormal movements, including dystonia, briefly intrude on otherwise-normal motor function).

Distribution: dystonia begins in 1 body part but may spread; the pattern and timing of spread are key features in distinguishing between genetic causes of dystonia (see **Fig. 1, Table 1**).

- Focal: limited to 1 body area, such as the hand or larynx
- Segmental: involving 2 or more contiguous body regions (eg, hand-arm-neck; blepharospasm-orolingual)
- Generalized: (involving both legs or the trunk plus 1 leg) plus at least 1 other area

Table 1
Monogenic secondary dystonias. Many genetic disorders can result in dystonia as a secondary symptom, and dystonia can be the presenting symptom for some disorders. The age at onset, site of onset, and relationship of dystonia to other symptoms are helpful in developing a limited differential diagnosis. Note that disorders with dystonia as the sole or a dominant feature are listed in Figs. 1 and 2. Disorders are categorized by mean age of onset but may present at ages other than those listed

Disorder	Relationship of Dystonia to Other Features	Gene or Locus	Inheritance
Onset Before 2 y of Life			
Aromatic L-amino acid decarboxylase deficiency	Frequently present, usually involves orofacial muscles and may follow other symptoms: hypotonia, developmental delay, oculogyric crises, autonomic storms, central apnea, irritability. Diurnal variation in symptoms	DDC	R
Glutaric academia type I	Dystonia follows an acute encephalopathic crisis prompted by metabolic stress. Dystonia is often progressive with subsequent crises	GCDH	R
Leigh disease	Dystonia, chorea, and ataxia are common, always with rapidly progressive developmental regression	Many	M or R
NBIA2A and NBIA2B, PLAN, infantile neuroaxonal dystrophy (INAD)	PLA2G6 mutations cause a wide array of phenotypes: psychomotor regression and ataxia with eye movement abnormalities, optic atrophy (INAD); early developmental delay and hypotonia, progressing to myoclonic epilepsy, ataxia, chorea, and dystonia (PLAN); adult-onset dystonia-parkinsonism	PLA2G6	R
Methylmalonic aciduria	Dystonia is common and may be transient, with metabolic crises, persistent after basal ganglia infarction, difficult to treat	MUT or its cofactors	R
Lesch-Nyhan disease	Psychomotor retardation typically precedes dystonia/chorea	HPRT	XLR
Pelizaeus-Merzbacher	Oculomotor movement abnormalities are a common presenting feature. Hypotonia progressing to spasticity is an early sign, chorea > dystonia later	PLP1	XLR, rare in F carriers
Rett syndrome	Dystonia occurs late and most likely affects the legs	MECP2	XL D

(continued on next page)

Table 1
(continued)

Disorder	Relationship of Dystonia to Other Features	Gene or Locus	Inheritance
Onset Between 2 and 10 y of Age			
Wilson disease	Uncommon finding, usually following psychomotor decline and chorea	ATP7B	R
Leber optic neuropathy, Marsden variant	Dystonia often precedes optic atrophy and may be the sole feature, even in families with optic-only or mixed presentations are present	MTNDs 1, 3, 4, 6	M
Ataxia telangiectasia	Dystonia or chorea develop in ~90%, well after ataxia is evident	ATM	R
Fucosidosis	Lower extremity dystonia described in a single patient	FUCA1	R
PKAN, PANK-2 deficiency, NBIA I	May present with gait abnormalities, psychomotor decline, chorea, or dystonia Late generalized dystonia is universal, prominent jaw/tongue dystonia	PANK2	R
Tay-Sachs	Dystonia or chorea are rare and late findings	HEXA	R
Huntington-like 3	Dystonia presents early, often with chorea and ataxia	4p 15.3	R
Niemann-Pick C, type I and II	Type I: ataxia and myoclonus are common, dystonia less so Type II: chorea and facial dyskinesias common, dystonia rare	NPC1, NPC2/HE1	R
Woodhouse-Sakati syndrome	Cognitive impairment often present in childhood, with later development of other syndromic features. Dystonia, chorea are both common	DCAF17	R
Mohr-Tranebjaerg dystonia deafness syndrome	Progressive deafness after 2 y of life, later dystonia	TIMM8A/ DDP1	XLR, mild symptoms in F
Onset in Adolescence and Beyond			
SCA3, Machado-Joseph disease type 1	Usually follows ataxia, but dystonia may rarely be the presenting feature. Slowly progressive. Dystonia severity correlates with $(CAG)_n$ length	ATXN3	DwA
SCA7	Dystonia, chorea are atypical, usually years after ataxia. Highly variable between/within families. Onset usually in midlife, occasionally in teens	ATXN7	DwA

(continued on next page)

Table 1
(*continued*)

Disorder	Relationship of Dystonia to Other Features	Gene or Locus	Inheritance
SCA17	Focal dystonia is the presenting symptom in rare kindreds. Typically dystonia, chorea follow ataxia, dysphagia, or psychiatric symptoms	*TBP*	DwA, low penetrance
Huntington disease	Dystonia is common but not universal. <18 y are more likely to manifest as the Westphal variant, with hypokinetic rigidity instead of chorea	*HTT (IT-15)*	DwA, full penetrance
Neuroferrinopathy, NBIA3	Presents with chorea > focal limb dystonia > parkinsonism. Typical onset is 20–35 y; onset in teens has been reported	*FTL*	D
PARK9, Kufor-Rakeb syndrome	Parkinsonism is primary, rapidly progressive, frequently develop moderate dystonia or myoclonus	*ATP13A2*	R
PARK2	Focal dystonias, especially of the feet, follow onset of parkinsonism	*PRKN*	R
Choreoacanthocytosis	Chorea is near-universal; dystonia, tics, parkinsonism are less common. Onset is usually in 20s–40s. XL form (McLeod) typically without dystonia	*VPS13A* (chorein)	R, rare cases of D
Idiopathic basal ganglia calcification, familial Fahr disease	Follows motor and neuropsychiatric decline, often coexists with ataxia or parkinsonism. Most present in 20s–40s, but infantile onset has been reported, with severe developmental delay and epilepsy	Unknown, some links to 14q	R
Friedreich ataxia	Multiple movement disorders can occur as first symptom or follow ataxia: postural tremor is the most common, dystonia is common, chorea is atypical	*FXN*	R

Abbreviations: D, dominantly inherited; DwA, dominantly inherited with anticipation; M, mitochondrial inheritance pattern; R, recessively inherited; XL, X-linked; XLD, X-linked dominant.

Gene abbreviations: ATM, ataxia telangiectasia mutated; *ATP13A2*, adenosine triphosphatase (ATPase) type 13A2; *ATP7B*, ATPase, Cu++ transporting, β polypeptide; *ATXN3*, ataxin 3; *ATXN7*, ataxin 7; *DCAF17*, DDB1, and CUL4 associated factor 17, previously known as *C2ORF37*; *DDC*, dopa decarboxylase; *DDP1*, deafness dystonia protein 1; *FTL*, ferritin light chain; *FUCA1*, fucosidase, α-L-1, tissue; *FXN*, frataxin; *GCDH*, glutaryl-coenzyme A (CoA) dehydrogenase; *HEXA*, hexosaminidase A; *HPRT*, hypoxanthine-guanine phosphoribosyltransferase; *HTT (IT-15)*, huntingtin; *MECP2*, methyl CpG binding protein 2; *MTND*, mitochondrial NADH dehydrogenase, various subunits; *MUT*, methylmalonyl CoA mutase; *NPC1*, Niemann-Pick disease, type C1; *NPC2/HE1*, Niemann-Pick disease, type C2, originally named *HE1*; *PANK2*, pantothenate kinase 2; *PLA2G6*, phospholipase A2, group VI; *PLP1*, proteolipid protein 1; *PRKN*, parkin; *TBP*, TATA box binding protein; *TIMM8A*, translocase of inner mitochondrial membrane 8 homologue A, also known as *DDP1*; *VPS13A*, vacuolar protein sorting 13 homologue A.

Nature of Disease

Dystonia is the third most common movement disorder,[1] after essential tremor and Parkinson disease. The types and causes of dystonia are variable, and monogenic primary dystonias are rare. Most patients with dystonia have no clear genetic association: in adults, idiopathic cervical dystonia predominates, and in children, approximately 90% of dystonia is seen within the context of cerebral palsy. Whereas in some of these children, cerebral palsy results from a genetic cause (see **Table 1**), in most, anoxic or ischemic causes are likely responsible. Approximately 1% of children with cerebral palsy develop dystonia,[2] sometimes with onset of dystonia delayed by decades.

CLINICAL FINDINGS
Physical Examination

- Reproducible, abnormal postures or joint positions
- Task or position sensitivity, with many common tasks performed without limitation (eg, normal finger/hand use in all areas except writing); it is essential to examine the patient during tasks that elicit the abnormal movement
- Dystonic movements may appear bizarre and eliciting factors may be idiosyncratic
- Cocontraction of opposing muscle groups, overflow of movement from a desired action to surrounding muscles
- Mirroring of movements or activation of dystonia by contralateral limb movement
- Presence of a sensory trick (aka geste antagoniste): an idiosyncratic sensory stimulus that provides temporary relief of dystonia
- A sense of pull or drift into stereotyped abnormal positions
- Late in untreated disease, joint contracture is possible
- Tremor, if present, typically resolves if the affected body area is allowed to move to its position of comfort
- Use of standardized scales, such as the Burke-Fahn-Marsden Scale for generalized dystonia or the Toronto Western Spasmodic Torticollis Rating Scale, is helpful in determining treatment response and disease progression

---

Clinical scenarios that should prompt genetic testing

- Limb-onset dystonia in early adolescence: test torsinA (DYT1), especially with Ashkenazi ancestry

- Cervical/cranial onset in midadolescence: test THAP1 (DYT6), especially with strained speech (spasmodic dysphonia)

- Normal gait in the morning, disabled by the evening: give levodopa; if symptoms improve, then test guanosine triphosphate (GTP) cyclohydrolase 1 (DYT5a); if negative, test tyrosine hydroxylase (DYT5b)

- Mixed myoclonus and dystonia with onset throughout childhood: test ε-sarcoglycan (DYT11), especially if symptoms are alcohol responsive in family members

- Onset of dystonia ± parkinsonism over hours to days: test ATP1A3 (DYT12), especially if symptoms progress in a rostral to caudal fashion[3]

- Paroxysmal dystonia ± chorea triggered by:

  1. Sudden movement: test PRRT2 (DYT10), especially if there is a family history of complex migraines or benign seizures/chorea in infancy[4]

  2. Caffeine or alcohol: test PNKD (DYT8), especially if symptoms are rare but last many minutes to hours

  3. Exertion or if the ratio of cerebrospinal fluid/serum glucose is less than 0.5, test SLC2A1 (DYT18), especially in families with unexplained cognitive delay or seizure disorder[5]

Imaging

In the primary dystonias, standard T1-weighted and T2-weighted magnetic resonance imaging (MRI) is normal. For many secondary dystonias (eg, pantothenate kinase-associated neurodegeneration, Wilson disease), unique patterns of atrophy or toxic accumulation are a great aid in diagnosing the underlying syndrome. For this reason, we advocate obtaining a routine MRI scan in all cases of young-onset dystonia. For patients with mixed dystonia-parkinsonism, it may be necessary to differentiate between juvenile Parkinson disease, late-onset dopa-responsive dystonia, and other secondary dystonias. Single-photon emission computed tomography (SPECT) using a ligand for the dopamine transporter (DAT) readily distinguishes between dopa-responsive dystonia (normal scan) and neurodegenerative Parkinson disease (decreased binding in the caudate and putamen). SPECT is most useful in cases in which dystonia is the predominant feature and is less able to distinguish dystonic tremor from other causes of tremor.[6]

Although not yet available as a clinical tool, imaging techniques that assess functional connectivity have potential to both improve diagnosis of idiopathic dystonias and elucidate general mechanisms that underlie diverse types of dystonia. Using either positron emission tomography or functional MRI, brain regions that covary during the control of movement have been identified as nodes in motor control networks. These networks are altered in both genotype-specific and phenotype-specific ways: unique patterns distinguish DYT1 from DYT6 and affected from nonmanifesting gene carriers.[7] Dystonia-specific alterations in white matter tracts within the motor control network suggest that (just as with genetically defined syndromes) idiopathic focal dystonias also have phenotype-specific structural changes, which may be pathologic.[8] It may soon be possible to use the pattern of activation within motor control networks as a common variable to categorize patients with idiopathic dystonias, a critical step in the process of identifying new dystonia-related genes.

Other Diagnostic Modalities

Dystonia remains a clinical diagnosis aided by genetic testing (**Fig. 3**) and imaging (see preceding section). Several modalities have adjunctive usefulness in difficult cases, although none of these methods is sufficiently validated to form the primary basis for diagnosis.

Electromyography
Electromyography shows coactivation of agonist-antagonist muscles, can detect dystonic activation in clinically unaffected muscles, and aids in targeting involved muscles during botulinum toxin injections.[9]

Transcranial magnetic stimulation
Transcranial magnetic stimulation shows reduced intracortical and surround inhibition in dystonia. Parallel studies in brainstem and spine with similar reduction in inhibition suggest that this finding is a general feature of dystonic physiology, which predisposes to the abnormal movements.[10–12]

Polysomnography
Multiple types of focal and segmental dystonia, sleep efficiency, and proportion of sleep spent in rapid eye movement are reduced, and awakenings are more frequent. These findings are independent of dystonia severity and may be a nonmotor endophenotype of multiple types of dystonia.[13]

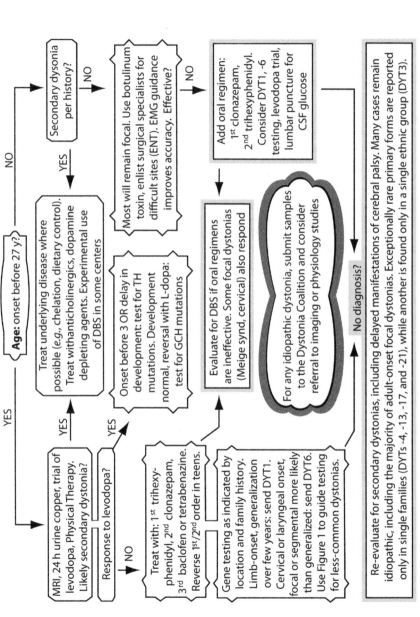

Fig. 3. An algorithm for diagnosis and treatment of dystonia. Patients with a variety of primary dystonias can be managed using these general guidelines. Secondary dystonias may be similarly managed, although it is difficult to predict responsiveness and prognosis. In most patients, careful examination and a detailed family history yield a limited differential diagnosis and allow focused genetic testing. CSF, cerebrospinal fluid; DBS, deep brain stimulation; EMG, electromyography; ENT, ear, nose, and throat specialists.

Sensory discrimination testing
For both visual and tactile stimuli, patients with a variety of focal dystonias require a higher stimulus intensity to distinguish between 2 stimuli (sensitivity of 85%–97%).[14]

Impaired motor learning
DYT1 mutation carriers (both manifesting and nonmanifesting) learn motor sequencing tasks less well than either normal controls or DYT6 mutation carriers.[15]

DISEASE PATHOLOGY

Classically, dystonia and other movement disorders were believed to arise from basal ganglia injury (in secondary cases) or derangement in the dopamine system (primary cases). It is now appreciated that any lesion within the motor control network (cortex, internal capsule, basal ganglia, thalamus, brainstem, cerebellum) can produce a movement disorder. The concept of derangement within a network, rather than injury to a discrete anatomic site, now informs much of the current understanding of the origins of dystonia.

Despite the caveat that it is likely networks, not individual nodes or neurons, that are disordered in dystonia, it remains likely that dysfunctional dopamine signaling plays a role in the development of dystonia. Dopaminergic derangement within the caudate and putamen is a probable contributor to most cases of dystonia.

- Disorders of dopamine synthesis (GTP cyclohydrolase 1 deficiency, DYT5a; tyrosine hydroxylase deficiency, DYT5b; aromatic amino acid decarboxylase deficiency) or transport[16] produce mixed movement disorders with prominent dystonia.
- Mutation of the dopamine receptor 2 (DRD2) is a rare cause of myoclonus-dystonia.[17]
- In basal ganglia encephalitis, anti-DRD2 antibodies correlate with a mixed movement disorder that includes dystonia.[18]
- Limited evidence suggests that specific polymorphisms in the dopamine receptor subtype 5 significantly increase the risk of developing cervical dystonia within families.[19,20]
- Murine models of DYT1, the best-characterized primary dystonia, reveal a variety of abnormalities in dopamine signaling, including reduced number of tyrosine hydroxylase-positive neurons in the substantia nigra, a deficit in amphetamine-stimulated dopamine release, and increased dopamine turnover.[21–24]

Even in genetic secondary dystonias with molecular pathology distinct from dopamine metabolism, selective toxicity of dopamine neurons has been shown.

- In a cellular model of Lesch-Nyhan disease, differentiation into dopaminergic neurons and sprouting of neurites is impaired.[25]
- In a cell-based model of Wilson disease, free copper ions complex with dopamine and these adducts induce caspase-mediated apoptosis, a potential mechanism for the relatively selective injury to the lentiform nuclei.[26]

Thus, although the cause of dystonia is more complicated than just dopamine dysfunction, accumulating evidence suggests that dopamine dysfunction is a common mechanism in diverse types of dystonia.

Recent work has raised the possibility that the cerebellum may be as important as the basal ganglia in the pathogenesis of dystonia. The cerebellum is implicated in many of the imaging studies noted earlier, with abnormalities in resting activation, functional connectivity, and volume of both gray and white matter structures (reviewed by Carbon and Eidelberg[27] and Neychev and colleagues[28]). Observations in humans are unable to tease apart the effect of any 1 nucleus on the greater motor control network. However, animal studies suggest that abnormalities isolated to the cerebellum can induce dystonia. An animal model of rapid-onset dystonia-parkinsonism (DYT12) suggests that abnormally increased firing in the cerebellum entrains basal ganglia circuits and induces dystonia; lesioning the cerebellar output nuclei or cerebellothalamic connections abolishes the induced-dystonia.[29] Similarly, in a mouse model of dystonia that restricts disease to the cerebellar Purkinje cells (using combined neurosurgical and genetic techniques), a range of focal to generalized dystonia can be produced by enlarging the area of cerebellar cortex that is affected.[30] Although these models do not exonerate the basal ganglia in the generation of dystonia, they suggest that a more nuanced understanding of motor control networks is necessary to understand and effectively treat dystonia.

GENETICS

The genetic causes of dystonia are many and varied (see **Figs. 1** and **2**, **Table 1**). Single-gene defects can produce primary or secondary dystonia, as well as mixed or paroxysmal movement disorders. Dystonia can be inherited through dominant, recessive, X-linked, or mitochondrial mechanisms. Penetrance is incomplete for many single-gene dystonic syndromes, making it difficult to determine the pattern of inheritance or prognosis for other family members. Recognition of these difficulties has led researchers to form extrainstitutional biorepositories of DNA and standardized clinical assessment tools (see **text box**).

Many patients and families have concerns about the effects that an abnormal genetic test has for other family members and the implications for access to health and other types of insurance. In the United States, the Genetic Information Nondiscrimination Act of 2008 made it illegal to discriminate based on genetic diagnoses for the purposes of employment or health insurance. However, this law does not prevent genetic discrimination in the sale of disability, long-term care, and life insurance

---

Resources to advance research in dystonia

We encourage patients to participate in research efforts to understand the genetic, molecular, and physiologic underpinnings of dystonia. Such studies include:

- The Dystonia Coalition (http://rarediseasesnetwork.epi.usf.edu/dystonia), a repository of both DNA and standardized clinical assessments

- The registry of all dystonia clinical trials ongoing in the United States (http://clinicaltrials.gov/search/term=Dystonias)

- The Dystonia International Patient Registry (http://www.dipregistry.com), a clearinghouse that provides researchers with deidentified clinical information on groups of patients with dystonia. No DNA samples are collected.

Educational resources and support for patients and families may be found here:

- The Dystonia Medical Research Foundation (http://www.dystonia-foundation.org)

- The Bachmann-Strauss Dystonia and Parkinson Foundation (http://www.dystonia-parkinson.org)

- The Worldwide Education and Awareness of Movement Disorders Web site (http://www.WeMove.org) provides clinically sound and up-to-date information on dystonia and other movement disorders.

policies. A few states have added additional antidiscrimination laws, but these are a patchwork of protections that leave many patients at risk of noninsurability. Before undergoing genetic testing, it is helpful to discuss these complex issues with a dedicated genetic counselor or geneticist. Recommendations for genetic testing in dystonia must also take into account the population from which the patient is derived: in patients with primary torsion dystonia, the DYT1 ΔGAG mutation is found in 2.7% in northern China,[31] 17% in Italy,[32] and 49% in Manhattan.[33] As in most areas of life, what one finds depends on where one looks.

Molecular Pathogenesis

How do dystonia-related mutations produce their effects on the motor control system? This mechanism is unclear, but interactions between genes with mutations that predispose to dystonia suggest that common molecular end points may result in the common final pathway of dystonia. A 3 base pair deletion (ΔGAG) in the torsinA gene results in DYT1 dystonia. The precise role of torsinA in the cell, and the way in which it causes dysfunction when mutated, is not known. However, there is growing evidence that it is involved in (1) processing of proteins through the secretory pathway; and (2) regulation of structure and movement of the nuclear envelope and endoplasmic reticulum.[34,35] Mutations in the transcription factor Thanatos-associated protein 1 (THAP1) lead to DYT6 dystonia (see **Table 1**). The promoter region for torsinA contains 2 sequences targeted by THAP1[36,37]; wild-type THAP1 is predicted to function as a transcriptional repressor, decreasing expression of torsinA. Thus, mutant THAP1 may produce pathologically increased levels of torsinA, thereby impairing protein trafficking through the endoplasmic reticulum and decreasing the surface expression of both the DAT and the D_2 dopamine receptor.[38]

It is also possible that dystonia-inducing mutations can interact to influence the clinical phenotype. Patients who harbor both torsinA and ε-sarcoglycan (DYT11) mutations seem to have onset of motor symptoms at the younger end of the normal range for disease and to have higher penetrance than family members with only 1 of these mutations.[39,40] These dual-mutation individuals are rare, and it is unclear if their clinical details can be applied to other individuals. However, mice carrying both torsinA and ε-sarcoglycan mutations develop motor control deficits at a younger age than littermates with only 1 of the 2 mutations.[41]

MEDICAL MANAGEMENT OF DYSTONIA

Many patients may be managed solely with oral medications (see **Fig. 3**, **Table 2**). For any patient with dystonia onset before the age of 27 years, we recommend a trial of levodopa even in cases without the diurnal variation seen in classic dopa-responsive dystonia. All of the medications described in **Table 2** may cause sedation and cognitive blunting, but these side effects are not shared equally across the group. Patients who do not tolerate a given agent may find relief, with fewer side effects, from another of these medications. For focal dystonias (especially those limited to the head and neck) and limited segmental dystonias, botulinum toxin injection is often sufficient therapy in isolation. Although it is not our practice to use botulinum toxin in generalized dystonia, we acknowledge that some practitioners find it a useful adjunct to oral medications in such cases.

SURGICAL MANAGEMENT OF DYSTONIA

Deep brain stimulation of the internal segment of the globus pallidus (GPi-DBS) is an effective treatment of many patients with primary dystonias: youth-onset generalized

Table 2
Medications commonly used to treat dystonia. Familiarity with these 6 agents allows a practitioner to treat most children and adults presenting with a diverse array of dystonias. This list reflects the availability of agents in the United States and should not limit the judicious use of other available agents

Agent	Population	Target Dose, Titration
Levodopa-carbidopa (Sinemet, generics)	Any patient younger than 26y, older patients with diurnal variation symptoms merit a trial of levodopa. Rare cases of DYT1 are dopa-responsive. Cranial and cervical dystonia, ineffective.	Start at 1 mg/kg/day div TID, increase by 1 mg/kg/d weekly. If patient will respond, most will do so at modest doses; some respond only at 10 mg/kg/d for one month
Benzodiazepines - Clonazepam - Diazepam	Mildly effective in all types of dystonia, especially helpful in focal dystonias (blepharospasm) and mixed disorders with tremor or myoclonus	Clonazepam: Child - start 0.25mg qHS, target 1–4 mg div TID. Adult - start 1 mg qHS, increase by 1-2 mg q7d, max dose 20 mg/day
Baclofen (Liorisol, Gablofen, generics)	Generalized > segmental, child > adult. Oral, intrathecal routes are effective, the latter with less sedation/cognitive blunting	Oral: Start 2.5–5 mg qHS, add 2.5 mg q5d to a max dose of 80 mg/d. Dose can be divided TID or QID
Trihexyphenidyl (Artane)	Generalized dystonia, especially in children, who tolerate high doses better than adults. Anticholinergic side effects often limit clinical utility	Start 1 mg/d, increase by 1mg q3-5d As doses are added change to TID Titrate to relief, max dose 200 mg/d
Tetrabenazine (Xenazine)	Generalized or segmental dystonia, especially useful in tardive and secondary dystonia	Start 12.5–25 mg, increase by same dose q5d to a max dose of 200 mg/d divided TID or QID. Titrate to relief
Botulinum toxin A (3 equivalent preparations in the US)	Adults or children with focal or mild segmental dystonia, especially cranial, cervical, laryngeal, and hand dystonia	Dependent on size of muscle and severity - empiric treatment q3 months is required, typical doses of 50–400 units per session.

dystonia (DYT1,[42] possibly less effective for DYT6,[43,44] and variably effective in those without identified mutations[45]), myoclonus-dystonia (DYT11),[46] cervical dystonia,[47,48] and craniofacial dystonia (Meige syndrome).[49–51] We and other colleagues who care for children with primary generalized dystonia often recommend GPi-DBS within 2 years of onset, with the goal of reducing loss of mobility and joint deformity. There is limited evidence to suggest that in DYT1, implanting DBS earlier in the disease course leads to greater recovery of function.[52,53] Although early estimates of DBS efficacy topped 80%, these were carefully screened and optimized patient populations; a realistic assessment of all primary dystonias suggests a lower efficacy of approximately 50%.[54]

Historically, secondary dystonias were considered poor candidates for DBS, with only a 20% to 25% improvement in mean disability scores and one-third of patients having no improvement at 2 to 3 years after surgery.[55] More recent reports suggest that with careful selection of subject and type of dystonia, DBS may be effective for secondary dystonias, especially tardive dystonia,[56–58] anoxic brain injury without structural lesions,[59] and NBIA (neurodegeneration with brain iron accumulation) disorders (see **Table 1**).[60–62] Similarly, idiopathic focal hand dystonia was initially considered unlikely to benefit from DBS, but small series and single-case reports have reported efficacy (in the ventro-oralis nucleus of the thalamus).[63,64] Although clinical outcome of DBS are greatest in DYT1 dystonia, for other primary and some secondary dystonias, there is reason for optimism. Further research into alternative DBS targets and stimulation parameters may provide further improvements for these populations.

SUMMARY

Dystonia is a neurologic disorder notable for abnormal postures and patterns of movement, often of a twisting or jerky character. Although abnormal movements are the defining feature of dystonia, a larger nonmovement endophenotype can be found in mutation carriers with and without dystonia. Features of this endophenotype include an increased incidence of psychiatric disease,[65–73] abnormalities in sensory gating, motor learning, and sleep physiology. Individuals harboring dystonia-causing mutations also have interrelated abnormalities in neuronal physiology (a failure of central inhibition[12] and abnormal synaptic plasticity[74]), which are potentially clues to an underlying disease mechanism. These broad endophenotypes are valuable clues in determining the pattern of inheritance and are reminders that dystonia is more than just a disorder of movement.

Single-gene defects can produce the full range of dystonia symptoms: focal, segmental, or generalized; primary dystonia, dystonia-plus, paroxysmal dyskinesias, or secondary dystonic syndromes; and can be inherited through dominant, recessive, X-linked, or mitochondrial mechanisms. This diversity of mechanisms, modes of heritability, and other concurrent movement abnormalities makes the diagnosis of dystonia a challenge. However, recognition, subtyping, and management of dystonia are often rewarding, because most patients improve to some degree with therapy. Many patients can be managed with oral agents or botulinum toxin injections. For primary dystonia and dystonia-plus syndromes, DBS of the internal segment of the globus pallidus may lead to marked reduction in dystonia. In secondary dystonias (including monogenic syndromes and idiopathic cerebral palsy), DBS is less efficacious, especially in those patients with basal ganglia lesions on MRI.

Although the last decade has seen substantial increase in identified genes and characterization of the molecular underpinnings of dystonia, careful clinical assessment and detailed family history remain the most valuable tools in diagnosing dystonia. Referral of patients to research studies is essential for identifying the causes and potential novel treatments of dystonia.

REFERENCES

1. Defazio G. The epidemiology of primary dystonia: current evidence and perspectives. Eur J Neurol 2010;17(Suppl 1):9–14.
2. Petrovic I, Klein C, Kostic VS. Delayed-onset dystonia due to perinatal asphyxia: a prospective study. Mov Disord 2007;22(16):2426–9.
3. Brashear A, Dobyns WB, de Carvalho Aguiar P, et al. The phenotypic spectrum of rapid-onset dystonia-parkinsonism (RDP) and mutations in the ATP1A3 gene. Brain 2007;130(Pt 3):828–35.
4. Guerrini R, Mink JW. Paroxysmal disorders associated with PRRT2 mutations shake up expectations on ion channel genes. Neurology 2012;79(21):2086–8.

5. Suls A, Dedeken P, Goffin K, et al. Paroxysmal exercise-induced dyskinesia and epilepsy is due to mutations in SLC2A1, encoding the glucose transporter GLUT1. Brain 2008;131(Pt 7):1831–44.

6. Kagi G, Bhatia KP, Tolosa E. The role of DAT-SPECT in movement disorders. J Neurol Neurosurg Psychiatry 2010;81(1):5–12.

7. Carbon M, Argyelan M, Eidelberg D. Functional imaging in hereditary dystonia. Eur J Neurol 2010;17(Suppl 1):58–64.

8. Blood AJ, Kuster JK, Woodman SC, et al. Evidence for altered basal ganglia-brainstem connections in cervical dystonia. PLoS One 2012;7(2):e31654.

9. Van Gerpen JA, Matsumoto JY, Ahlskog JE, et al. Utility of an EMG mapping study in treating cervical dystonia. Muscle Nerve 2000;23(11):1752–6.

10. Ridding MC, Sheean G, Rothwell JC, et al. Changes in the balance between motor cortical excitation and inhibition in focal, task specific dystonia. J Neurol Neurosurg Psychiatry 1995;59(5):493–8.

11. Quartarone A, Morgante F, Sant'angelo A, et al. Abnormal plasticity of sensorimotor circuits extends beyond the affected body part in focal dystonia. J Neurol Neurosurg Psychiatry 2008;79(9):985–90.

12. Hallett M. Neurophysiology of dystonia: the role of inhibition. Neurobiol Dis 2011; 42(2):177–84.

13. Stamelou M, Edwards MJ, Hallett M, et al. The non-motor syndrome of primary dystonia: clinical and pathophysiological implications. Brain 2012;135(Pt 6): 1668–81.

14. Bradley D, Whelan R, Kimmich O, et al. Temporal discrimination thresholds in adult-onset primary torsion dystonia: an analysis by task type and by dystonia phenotype. J Neurol 2012;259(1):77–82.

15. Carbon M, Argyelan M, Ghilardi MF, et al. Impaired sequence learning in dystonia mutation carriers: a genotypic effect. Brain 2011;134(Pt 5):1416–27.

16. Kurian MA, McNeill A, Lin JP, et al. Childhood disorders of neurodegeneration with brain iron accumulation (NBIA). Dev Med Child Neurol 2011;53(5):394–404.

17. Klein C, Brin MF, Kramer P, et al. Association of a missense change in the D2 dopamine receptor with myoclonus dystonia. Proc Natl Acad Sci U S A 1999; 96(9):5173–6.

18. Dale RC, Merheb V, Pillai S, et al. Antibodies to surface dopamine-2 receptor in autoimmune movement and psychiatric disorders. Brain 2012;135(Pt 11): 3453–68.

19. Placzek MR, Misbahuddin A, Chaudhuri KR, et al. Cervical dystonia is associated with a polymorphism in the dopamine (D5) receptor gene. J Neurol Neurosurg Psychiatry 2001;71(2):262–4.

20. Brancati F, Valente EM, Castori M, et al. Role of the dopamine D5 receptor (DRD5) as a susceptibility gene for cervical dystonia. J Neurol Neurosurg Psychiatry 2003;74(5):665–6.

21. Balcioglu A, Kim MO, Sharma N, et al. Dopamine release is impaired in a mouse model of DYT1 dystonia. J Neurochem 2007;102(3):783–8.

22. Zhao Y, DeCuypere M, LeDoux MS. Abnormal motor function and dopamine neurotransmission in DYT1 DeltaGAG transgenic mice. Exp Neurol 2008; 210(2):719–30.

23. Page ME, Bao L, Andre P, et al. Cell-autonomous alteration of dopaminergic transmission by wild type and mutant (DeltaE) TorsinA in transgenic mice. Neurobiol Dis 2010;39(3):318–26.

24. Song CH, Fan X, Exeter CJ, et al. Functional analysis of dopaminergic systems in a DYT1 knock-in mouse model of dystonia. Neurobiol Dis 2012;48(1):66–78.

25. Ceballos-Picot I, Mockel L, Potier MC, et al. Hypoxanthine-guanine phosphori-bosyl transferase regulates early developmental programming of dopamine neurons: implications for Lesch-Nyhan disease pathogenesis. Hum Mol Genet 2009;18(13):2317–27.
26. Paris I, Perez-Pastene C, Couve E, et al. Copper dopamine complex induces mitochondrial autophagy preceding caspase-independent apoptotic cell death. J Biol Chem 2009;284(20):13306–15.
27. Carbon M, Eidelberg D. Abnormal structure-function relationships in hereditary dystonia. Neuroscience 2009;164(1):220–9.
28. Neychev VK, Fan X, Mitev VI, et al. The basal ganglia and cerebellum interact in the expression of dystonic movement. Brain 2008;131(Pt 9):2499–509.
29. Calderon DP, Fremont R, Kraenzlin F, et al. The neural substrates of rapid-onset dystonia-parkinsonism. Nat Neurosci 2011;14(3):357–65.
30. Raike RS, Pizoli CE, Weisz C, et al. Limited regional cerebellar dysfunction induces focal dystonia in mice. Neurobiol Dis 2012;49C:200–10.
31. Cheng FB, Wan XH, Feng JC, et al. Clinical and genetic evaluation of DYT1 and DYT6 primary dystonia in China. Eur J Neurol 2011;18(3):497–503.
32. Zorzi G, Garavaglia B, Invernizzi F, et al. Frequency of DYT1 mutation in early onset primary dystonia in Italian patients. Mov Disord 2002;17(2):407–8.
33. Bressman SB, Sabatti C, Raymond D, et al. The DYT1 phenotype and guidelines for diagnostic testing. Neurology 2000;54(9):1746–52.
34. Hewett JW, Nery FC, Niland B, et al. siRNA knock-down of mutant torsinA restores processing through secretory pathway in DYT1 dystonia cells. Hum Mol Genet 2008;17(10):1436–45.
35. Nery FC, Zeng J, Niland BP, et al. TorsinA binds the KASH domain of nesprins and participates in linkage between nuclear envelope and cytoskeleton. J Cell Sci 2008;121(Pt 20):3476–86.
36. Kaiser FJ, Osmanoric A, Rakovic A, et al. The dystonia gene DYT1 is repressed by the transcription factor THAP1 (DYT6). Ann Neurol 2010;68(4):554–9.
37. Gavarini S, Cayrol C, Fuchs T, et al. Direct interaction between causative genes of DYT1 and DYT6 primary dystonia. Ann Neurol 2010;68(4):549–53.
38. Bragg DC, Armata IA, Nery FC, et al. Molecular pathways in dystonia. Neurobiol Dis 2011;42(2):136–47.
39. Doheny D, Danisi F, Smith C, et al. Clinical findings of a myoclonus-dystonia family with two distinct mutations. Neurology 2002;59(8):1244–6.
40. Klein C, Liu L, Doheny D, et al. Epsilon-sarcoglycan mutations found in combination with other dystonia gene mutations. Ann Neurol 2002;52(5):675–9.
41. Yokoi F, Yang G, Li J, et al. Earlier onset of motor deficits in mice with double mutations in Dyt1 and Sgce. J Biochem 2010;148(4):459–66.
42. Vidailhet M, Vercueil L, Houeto JL, et al. Bilateral deep-brain stimulation of the globus pallidus in primary generalized dystonia. N Engl J Med 2005;352(5):459–67.
43. Groen JL, Ritz K, Contarino MF, et al. DYT6 dystonia: mutation screening, phenotype, and response to deep brain stimulation. Mov Disord 2010;25(14):2420–7.
44. Panov F, Tagliati M, Ozelius LJ, et al. Pallidal deep brain stimulation for DYT6 dystonia. J Neurol Neurosurg Psychiatry 2012;83(2):182–7.
45. Volkmann J, Wolters A, Kupsch A, et al. Pallidal deep brain stimulation in patients with primary generalised or segmental dystonia: 5-year follow-up of a randomised trial. Lancet Neurol 2012;11(12):1029–38.

46. Beukers RJ, Contarino MF, Speelman JD, et al. Deep brain stimulation of the pallidum is effective and might stabilize striatal D(2) receptor binding in myoclonus-dystonia. Front Neurol 2012;3:22.
47. Cacciola F, Farah JO, Eldridge PR, et al. Bilateral deep brain stimulation for cervical dystonia: long-term outcome in a series of 10 patients. Neurosurgery 2010;67(4):957–63.
48. Skogseid IM, Ramm-Pettersen J, Volkmann J, et al. Good long-term efficacy of pallidal stimulation in cervical dystonia: a prospective, observer-blinded study. Eur J Neurol 2012;19(4):610–5.
49. Foote KD, Sanchez JC, Okun MS. Staged deep brain stimulation for refractory craniofacial dystonia with blepharospasm: case report and physiology. Neurosurgery 2005;56(2):E415 [discussion: E415].
50. Ghang JY, Lee MK, Jun SM, et al. Outcome of pallidal deep brain stimulation in Meige syndrome. J Korean Neurosurg Soc 2010;48(2):134–8.
51. Reese R, Gruber D, Schoenecker T, et al. Long-term clinical outcome in Meige syndrome treated with internal pallidum deep brain stimulation. Mov Disord 2011;26(4):691–8.
52. Borggraefe I, Mehrkens JH, Telegravciska M, et al. Bilateral pallidal stimulation in children and adolescents with primary generalized dystonia–report of six patients and literature-based analysis of predictive outcomes variables. Brain Dev 2010;32(3):223–8.
53. Markun LC, Starr PA, Air EL, et al. Shorter disease duration correlates with improved long-term deep brain stimulation outcomes in young-onset DYT1 dystonia. Neurosurgery 2012;71(2):325–30.
54. Okun MS, Foote KD. Setting realistic expectations for DBS in dystonia. Lancet Neurol 2012;11(12):1014–5.
55. Welter ML, Grabli D, Vidailhet M. Deep brain stimulation for hyperkinetics disorders: dystonia, tardive dyskinesia, and tics. Curr Opin Neurol 2010;23(4):420–5.
56. Gruber D, Trottenberg T, Kivi A, et al. Long-term effects of pallidal deep brain stimulation in tardive dystonia. Neurology 2009;73(1):53–8.
57. Capelle HH, Blahak C, Schrader C, et al. Chronic deep brain stimulation in patients with tardive dystonia without a history of major psychosis. Mov Disord 2010;25(10):1477–81.
58. Chang EF, Schrock LE, Starr PA, et al. Long-term benefit sustained after bilateral pallidal deep brain stimulation in patients with refractory tardive dystonia. Stereotact Funct Neurosurg 2010;88(5):304–10.
59. Alterman RL, Snyder BJ. Deep brain stimulation for torsion dystonia. Acta Neurochir Suppl 2007;97(Pt 2):191–9.
60. Mikati MA, Yehya A, Darwish H, et al. Deep brain stimulation as a mode of treatment of early onset pantothenate kinase-associated neurodegeneration. Eur J Paediatr Neurol 2009;13(1):61–4.
61. Timmermann L, Pauls KA, Wieland K, et al. Dystonia in neurodegeneration with brain iron accumulation: outcome of bilateral pallidal stimulation. Brain 2010;133(Pt 3):701–12.
62. Lim BC, Ki CS, Cho A, et al. Pantothenate kinase-associated neurodegeneration in Korea: recurrent R440P mutation in PANK2 and outcome of deep brain stimulation. Eur J Neurol 2012;19(4):556–61.
63. Fukaya C, Katayama Y, Kano T, et al. Thalamic deep brain stimulation for writer's cramp. J Neurosurg 2007;107(5):977–82.
64. Cho CB, Park HK, Lee KJ, et al. Thalamic deep brain stimulation for writer's cramp. J Korean Neurosurg Soc 2009;46(1):52–5.

65. Heiman GA, Ottman R, Saunders-Pullman RJ, et al. Increased risk for recurrent major depression in DYT1 dystonia mutation carriers. Neurology 2004;63(4): 631–7.

66. Voon V, Butler TR, Ekanayake V, et al. Psychiatric symptoms associated with focal hand dystonia. Mov Disord 2010;25(13):2249–52.

67. Walterfang M, Evans A, Looi JC, et al. The neuropsychiatry of neuroacanthocytosis syndromes. Neurosci Biobehav Rev 2011;35(5):1275–83.

68. Peall KJ, Waite AJ, Blake DJ, et al. Psychiatric disorders, myoclonus dystonia, and the epsilon-sarcoglycan gene: a systematic review. Mov Disord 2011; 26(10):1939–42.

69. Barahona-Correa B, Bugalho P, Guimaraes J, et al. Obsessive-compulsive symptoms in primary focal dystonia: a controlled study. Mov Disord 2011; 26(12):2274–8.

70. van Tricht MJ, Dreissen YE, Cath D, et al. Cognition and psychopathology in myoclonus-dystonia. J Neurol Neurosurg Psychiatry 2012;83(8):814–20.

71. Brashear A, Cook JF, Hill DF, et al. Psychiatric disorders in rapid-onset dystonia-parkinsonism. Neurology 2012;79(11):1168–73.

72. Mula M, Strigaro G, Marotta AE, et al. Obsessive-compulsive-spectrum symptoms in patients with focal dystonia, hemifacial spasm, and healthy subjects. J Neuropsychiatry Clin Neurosci 2012;24(1):81–6.

73. Louis ED, Huey ED, Gerbin M, et al. Apathy in essential tremor, dystonia, and Parkinson's disease: a comparison with normal controls. Mov Disord 2012; 27(3):432–4.

74. Quartarone A, Pisani A. Abnormal plasticity in dystonia: disruption of synaptic homeostasis. Neurobiol Dis 2011;42(2):162–70.

Clinical Neurogenetics
Autosomal Dominant Spinocerebellar Ataxia

Vikram G. Shakkottai, MD, PhD[a],*, Brent L. Fogel, MD, PhD[b],*

KEYWORDS

- Ataxia • Cerebellum • Spinocerebellar • SCA • Autosomal dominant

KEY POINTS

- The spinocerebellar ataxias (SCAs) are a heterogeneous group of dominantly inherited disorders, the most common of which are SCA1, SCA2, SCA3, SCA6, and SCA7, all of which result from glutamine-encoding repeats in the respective genes.
- The polyglutamine ataxias tend to be ataxia-plus disorders with extrapyramidal symptoms, long tract signs, and cranial nerve dysfunction, and have a poorer prognosis. In addition to polyglutamine ataxias, other molecular mechanisms for ataxia include ion-channel dysfunction, disordered signal transduction, and noncoding repeats.
- Advances in DNA sequencing technologies, including whole-exome sequencing, are expected to improve the diagnosis of genetic ataxias.
- Animal models of disease recapitulate many of the key features of the human disease and may be good model systems to test therapies.
- Current management for the SCAs is mostly supportive. However, exercise therapy has been shown to be beneficial in maintaining patient function over time and should be used for all patients.

INTRODUCTION
Definition

The spinocerebellar ataxias (SCAs) are a heterogeneous group of degenerative disorders with symptoms caused by dysfunction of the cerebellum and brainstem, along with their associated pathways and connections, and with an autosomal dominant pattern of inheritance.

This work was supported by the National Institutes of Health (K08NS072158 to V.G.S. and K08MH086297 to B.L.F).
[a] Department of Neurology, University of Michigan, Ann Arbor, MI 48109, USA; [b] Program in Neurogenetics, Department of Neurology, David Geffen School of Medicine, University of California Los Angeles, Los Angeles, CA 90095, USA
* Corresponding author. University of Michigan, 4009 BSRB, 109 Zina Pitcher Place, Ann Arbor, MI 48109-2200; University of California at Los Angeles, 710 Westwood Plaza, Los Angeles, CA 90095.
E-mail addresses: vikramsh@med.umich.edu; bfogel@ucla.edu

Symptoms and Clinical Course

- All patients exhibit cerebellar ataxia (limb, trunk, and/or gait).
- Additional symptoms are variable and disease specific, including extrapyramidal features, long tract signs, peripheral neuropathy, and, in some cases, cognitive impairment and seizures (**Table 1**).
- Clinical course: the polyglutamine ataxias SCA1, SCA2, and SCA3 are progressive disorders with death resulting primarily from brain stem dysfunction.[1] In one series, median survival was in the mid-50s, 21 to 25 years following symptom onset.[2] The other causes of SCA tend to have a more cerebellar dysfunction leading to significant disability but with normal lifespan.

CLINICAL FINDINGS

Ataxia is defined as a disturbance of balance and coordination occurring in the absence of muscle weakness, and can arise from dysfunction of the cerebellum, the vestibular system, or of proprioception, alone or in combination (**Box 1**).[3,4] The cerebellum plays a critical role in this process through the integration of multimodal sensory data with motor output predictions to yield smooth well-timed movement.[5]

Physical Examination

The focus of the physical examination should be on eliciting signs specific for cerebellar dysfunction and extracerebellar findings.

- Disruption of cerebellar function manifests as impairment in coordinated muscle activity, most often observed clinically as dysarthria, dysphagia, ocular dysmetria, altered visual pursuit, direction-changing nystagmus, limb dysmetria, gait disturbance, and/or falls.[3,4]
- In slowly progressive cases, gait impairment is often seen early and is frequently associated with a sense of imbalance or feelings of generalized leg weakness.
- Exacerbation may occur when walking on uneven surfaces or under conditions of reduced sensory input, such as in low lighting. Stance often widens for additional stabilization and patients may require support to walk, especially on turning. When indoors, the practice of navigating from support to support (eg, across items of furniture) can become a common means of ambulation.
- Depending on the cause of the ataxia, associated clinical features may be present and, in some cases, could be helpful to establishing the diagnosis, particularly in the case of genetic ataxias (see **Table 1**).

GENETICS

Despite their similarity in clinical symptoms, an array of diverse genetic causes underlies the SCAs. The genes accounting for autosomal dominant SCA are summarized in **Table 1**.

MOLECULAR PATHOGENESIS

Although distinct genes account for the more than 30 causes of dominant ataxia, groups of disorders may be recognized with shared molecular mechanisms of disease. These groups include the polyglutamine ataxias, ataxias associated with ion-channel dysfunction, mutations in signal transduction molecules, and disease associated with noncoding repeats.

Table 1
Summary of genes, mutations, and clinical features of autosomal dominant SCAs

Name	Locus/Gene	Protein/Mutation[a]	Normal Function[b]	Year[c]	Pathology[d]	Symptoms/Signs[e]
SCA1	6p23/ATXN1	Ataxin 1 CAG repeats 41–81 (normal 25–36)	Gene transcription and RNA splicing	1994	Inferior olivary nuclei Pontine nuclei Purkinje cells	**Pyramidal signs** Amyotrophy Extrapyramidal signs Ophthalmoparesis
SCA2	12q24/ATXN2	Ataxin 2 CAG repeats 35–59 (normal 15–24)	RNA processing	1996	Basis pontis Inferior olivary nuclei Purkinje cells	**Slow saccades** Extrapyramidal signs Dementia (rarely) Ophthalmoplegia Peripheral neuropathy Pyramidal signs
SCA3 (MJD)	14q24.3-q31/ATXN3	Ataxin-3 CAG repeats 62–82 (normal 13–36)	Deubiquitinating enzyme involved in protein quality control	1994	Anterior horn cells Clarke columns Dentate nuclei Dorsal root ganglia Pontine nuclei Purkinje cells Spinocerebellar tracts Substantia nigra Subthalamic nuclei	**Pyramidal signs** Amyotrophy Exophthalmos Extrapyramidal signs Ophthalmoparesis
SCA4	16q22.1/Unknown but distinct from SCA31	Unknown	Unknown	—	Unknown	**Sensory axonal neuropathy** Pyramidal signs
SCA5	11q13/SPTBN2	β III Spectrin	Scaffolding protein important for glutamate signaling	2006	Unknown	**Pure cerebellar ataxia** (late onset) Pyramidal signs (early onset)

(continued on next page)

Table 1
(continued)

Name	Locus/Gene	Protein/Mutation[a]	Normal Function[b]	Year[c]	Pathology[d]	Symptoms/Signs[e]
SCA6	19p13.2/*CACNA1A*	Cav2.1 CAG repeats 21–30 (normal 6–17)	Calcium channel important for regulating Purkinje neuron excitability	1997	Purkinje cells	**Pure cerebellar ataxia** Late onset, usually >50 y
SCA7	3p21.1-p12/*ATXN7*	Ataxin 7 CAG repeats 38–130 (normal 7–17)	Gene transcription	1997	Cone-rod dystrophy Dentate nuclei Inferior olivary nuclei Pontine neurons Purkinje cells Retinal ganglion cells	**Pigmentary macular degeneration** Ophthalmoplegia Pyramidal signs
SCA8	13q21.33/*ATXN8OS* *ATXN8*	Toxic RNA Pure polyglutamine protein CAG/CTG repeats 80–250 (normal 15–50)	Unknown	1999	Purkinje cells Substantia nigra	**Pyramidal signs** Diminished vibratory sense Spastic and ataxic dysarthria
SCA9	Unknown	Unknown	Unknown	—	Unknown	Central demyelination (1 patient) Extrapyramidal signs Ophthalmoplegia Posterior column loss Pyramidal tract signs
SCA10	22q13.31/*ATXN10*	Ataxin 10 Intronic ATTCT repeats 800-4500 (normal 10-32)	Involved in neuron survival, neuron differentiation, and neuritogenesis	2000	Unknown	**Seizures** Cognitive/neuropsychiatric impairment Polyneuropathy Pyramidal signs

	Locus/Gene	Protein	Function	Year		Clinical features
SCA11	15q15.2/*TTBK2*	Tau tubulin kinase-2	Serine-threonine kinase; putatively phosphorylates tau and tubulin proteins; Regulates the genesis of the primary cilium	2007	Unknown	**Pure cerebellar ataxia**
SCA12	5q32/*PPP2R2B*	Protein phosphatase PP2A; CAG repeats in 5'-UTR 51–78 (normal 7–32)	Serine-threonine phosphatase implicated in the negative control of cell growth and division	1999	Unknown	**Upper extremity tremor** Mild or absent gait ataxia; Hyperreflexia
SCA13	19q13.3-13.4/*KCNC3*	Kv3.3	Potassium channel involved in regulating Purkinje neuron excitability	2006	Unknown	**Intellectual disability** (in French pedigree); Pure cerebellar ataxia (in Filipino pedigree)
SCA14	19q13.4/*PRKCG*	Protein kinase C gamma	Neuronal serine/threonine protein kinase activated by calcium and diacylglycerol	2003	Unknown	**Pure cerebellar ataxia** Rarely chorea and cognitive deficits
SCA15/SCA16	3p26.1/*ITPR1*	Inositol 1,4,5-triphosphate receptor	Intracellular calcium channel involved in regulating neuronal excitability	2007	Unknown	**Pure cerebellar ataxia** Rare tremor or cognitive impairment
SCA17/HDL4	6q27/*TBP*	TATA box-binding protein; CAG repeats 46–63 (normal 25–42)	Gene transcription	2001	Neuronal inclusion bodies in brain; Purkinje cells; Reduction in brain weight	**Chorea** Dementia; Extrapyramidal features; Hyperreflexia; Psychiatric symptoms

(continued on next page)

Table 1
(continued)

Name	Locus/Gene	Protein/Mutation[a]	Normal Function[b]	Year[c]	Pathology[d]	Symptoms/Signs[e]
SCA18/SMNA	7q22-q32	Unknown	Unknown	—	Unknown	**Posterior column loss** Amyotrophy Early onset, usually <20 y Hyporeflexia
SCA19/SCA22	1p13.3/KCND3	Kv4.3	Potassium channel involved in regulating neuronal excitability	2012	Unknown	**Pure cerebellar ataxia** Cognitive impairment Myoclonus Postural tremor
SCA20	11p11.2-q13.3	Gene duplication	Unknown	—	Dentate nucleus calcification	**Spasmodic dysphonia or spasmodic coughing** Palatal tremor
SCA21	7p21.3-p15.1	Unknown	Unknown	—	Unknown	Akinesia Cognitive impairment Dysgraphia Early onset Hyporeflexia Postural tremor Resting tremor Rigidity
SCA23	20p13/PDYN	Prodynorphin	Processed to form secreted opioid peptides that serve as ligands for the kappa-type opioid receptor	2010	Cerebellar vermis Cerebellopontine tracts Dentate nuclei Demyelination of posterior and lateral columns (1 patient) Inferior olivary nuclei	**Late onset**, usually >50 y Decreased vibratory sense
SCA25	2p21-p15	Unknown	Unknown	—	Unknown	Areflexia Peripheral sensory neuropathy
SCA26	19p13.3	Unknown	Unknown	—	Unknown	Pure cerebellar ataxia

SCA	Locus/Gene	Protein	Normal function	Year	Pathology	Clinical features
SCA27	13q34/*FGF14*	Fibroblast growth factor 14	Interacts with voltage-gated sodium channels and regulates Purkinje neuron excitability	2003	Unknown	**Orofacial dyskinesias**; Cognitive impairment; Tremor
SCA28	18p11.22-q11.2/ *AFG3L2*	ATPase family gene 3-like 2	Mitochondrial protein synthesis	2010	Unknown	**Early onset, usually <20 y**; Hyperreflexia; Ophthalmoparesis; Ptosis
SCA29	3p26	Unknown	Unknown	—	Unknown	**Congenital**; Nonprogressive
SCA30	4q34.3-q35.1	Unknown	Unknown	—	Unknown	Late onset, usually >50 y; Pure cerebellar ataxia
SCA31	16q22/*BEAN1* and *TK2*	Brain expressed, associated with NEDD4; Thymidine kinase-2; TGGAA repeat in intron shared by both genes	Unknown	2009	Purkinje cells	**Pure cerebellar ataxia**; Late onset, usually >50 y; Sensorineural hearing loss
SCA35	20p13/*TGM6*	Transglutaminase 6	Posttranslational modifications of glutamine residues	2010	Unknown	**Pyramidal signs**; Pseudobulbar palsy
SCA36	20p13/*NOP56*	Nucleolar protein 56; Intronic GGCCTG repeat	Pre-mRNA processing	2011	Dentate nuclei; Hypoglossal nucleus; Motor neurons; Purkinje cells	**Lower motor neuron involvement**; Tongue atrophy
DRPLA	12p13.31/*ATN1*	Atrophin 1; CAG repeats; 49–75 (normal 7–23)	Transcriptional coregulator	1994	Cerebellar white matter; Dentate nuclei; Globus pallidus; Red nucleus; Subthalamic nucleus	**Myoclonic epilepsy**; Choreoathetosis; Dementia

Abbreviations: DRPLA, dentatorubral pallidoluysian atrophy; HDL4 Huntington disease–like 4; MJD, Machado-Joseph disease; SMNA, Sensorimotor Neuropathy with Ataxia; UTR, untranslated region.

[a] Mutation refers to point mutations in the respective genes, unless otherwise specified.

[b] The normal function of all proteins has not been fully established.

[c] Year refers to initial year of publication of the identified gene.

[d] Pathology refers to loss of neurons in the indicated regions.

[e] Not all patients have the symptoms/signs that are mentioned. Bold typeface refers to symptoms either characteristic or unique to the particular SCA and thus helpful to diagnosis.

Box 1
Physical examination findings in a patient with ataxia[a]

- Cerebellar examination
  - Gaze-evoked nystagmus
  - Abnormal eye movements (ocular dysmetria, impaired smooth pursuit)
  - Dysarthria (scanning)
  - Limb dysmetria (finger-to-nose, finger chase, heel-shin testing)
  - Dysdiadochokinesia
  - Loss of check on removal of extremity resistance
  - Truncal ataxia and/or head titubation
  - Wide-based unsteady gait (drunken gait)
  - Inability to tandem walk
- Vestibular examination
  - Spontaneous nystagmus
  - Past-pointing
  - Abnormal head thrust or Dix-Hallpike testing
- Sensory examination
  - Reduced proprioception
  - Reduced vibration sense
  - Abnormal Romberg test

[a] Not comprehensive. Not all patients exhibit all features.

Polyglutamine Ataxias

These include SCA1, SCA2, SCA3, SCA6, SCA7, SCA12, SCA17, and dentatorubral pallidoluysian atrophy (DRPLA), in which expansion within a glutamine-encoding CAG repeat accounts for disease. An additional disorder, SCA8, likely arises from the combined effects of a noncoding CTG repeat expansion and the generation of a pure polyglutamine protein from the corresponding CAG repeat on the opposite strand.[6]

The exact mechanism for how a polyglutamine protein causes ataxia is not understood. Potential mechanisms[7] include:

1. Protein misfolding resulting in altered function
2. Formation of toxic oligomeric complexes
3. Transcriptional dysregulation
4. Mitochondrial dysfunction
5. Impaired axonal transport
6. Aberrant neuronal signaling including excitotoxicity
7. Cellular protein homeostasis impairment
8. RNA toxicity

Ion-channel Mutations/Dysfunction

Either direct ion-channel mutations or secondary ion-channel dysfunction has been implicated in the pathogenesis of SCA5, SCA6, SCA13, SCA15/16, SCA19/22, and SCA27.[8]

1. SCA5: mutations in the structural protein, beta-3 spectrin result in SCA5. In a mouse model of disease, Purkinje neurons exhibit reduced spontaneous firing, smaller sodium currents, and dysregulation of glutamatergic neurotransmission.[9]
2. SCA6: results from a modest polyglutamine expansion in the C-terminus of a neuronal calcium channel, Cav2.1. The exact mechanism for disease pathogenesis may include calcium channel dysfunction and/or polyglutamine protein–associated toxicity.[10]
3. SCA13: mutations in *KCNC3*, the gene encoding the Kv3.3 potassium channel, either suppress currents or alter channel gating in a dominant-negative manner.[11] The SCA13 mutations in Kv3.3 also reduce neuronal excitability in a zebra fish model of disease.[12]
4. SCA15/16: mutations in the inositol 1,4,5-triphosphate receptor, an intracellular ligand-gated calcium channel, underlie this disorder. Decreased modulation of Purkinje neuron intrinsic firing by excitatory synaptic input is described in a mouse model of disease.[13]
5. SCA19/22: loss-of-function mutations in Kv4.3 cause ataxia.[14,15] The physiologic basis for this recently identified cause of SCA is unclear.
6. SCA27: although SCA27 does not result from an ion-channel mutation, the causative FGF14 mutations likely result in perturbed expression of voltage-gated sodium channels in cerebellar neurons.[16]

Signal Transduction

Although alterations in cellular signal transduction likely play a role in most ataxias, mutations in signal transduction molecules are the direct cause of disease in SCA11, SCA12, SCA14, and SCA23.

1. SCA11: results from loss-of-function mutations in TTBK2, a casein kinase 1 family member. Recent work has implicated this kinase as a dedicated regulator of the initiation of ciliogenesis.[17]
2. SCA12: results from a CAG repeat expansion in the 5′-untranslated region of protein phosphatase, PP2A. The mechanism for disease pathogenesis likely shares common features with the other noncoding repeat disorders.
3. SCA14: results from mutations in a serine-threonine family kinase, a protein kinase C isoform that is highly enriched in Purkinje neurons. In a mouse model of disease, mutant PKC gamma reduced long-term depression at parallel fiber–Purkinje cell synapses and increased slow EPSC (excitatory post-synaptic current) amplitude.[18]
4. SCA23: mutations in PDYN, encoding prodynorphin, the precursor protein for the opioid neuropeptides, alpha-neoendorphin, and dynorphins A and B (Dyn A and B) cause SCA23. Cellular models of disease suggest that alterations in Dyn A activities and/or impairment of secretory pathways by mutant PDYN may lead to glutamate neurotoxicity, underlying Purkinje cell degeneration and ataxia.[19]

Noncoding Repeats/RNA Toxicity

This is the likely mechanism of pathogenesis in SCA8, SCA10, SCA31, and SCA36. The putative mechanism of disease includes[20]:

1. Transcriptional alterations and the generation of antisense transcripts
2. Sequestration of mRNA-associated protein complexes that lead to aberrant mRNA splicing and processing
3. Alterations in cellular processes, including activation of abnormal signaling cascades and failure of protein quality control pathways

GENOMICS

1. Anticipation: the polyglutamine ataxias show the phenomenon of anticipation, in which disease onset is seen earlier in successive generations because of germ line CAG repeat instability leading to additional repeat expansion. For example, SCA7 has marked anticipation of approximately 20 years/generation.[21]
2. Association with other neurologic disorders: intermediate-length polyQ expansions (27–33 glutamines) in ATXN2 are significantly associated with amyotrophic lateral sclerosis (ALS).[22] Ataxin 2 acts as a modifier of TDP-43 toxicity, a protein thought to be critical for ALS pathogenesis, in animal and cellular models. ATXN2 and TDP-43 associate in a complex that depends on RNA.

DISEASE MODELS

The autosomal dominant SCA disorders have been studied in cultured cells, animal models, and, most recently, in human inducible pluripotent stem cell–derived neurons.

1. Cultured cells: mutations have been studied in both cultured neurons and non-neuronal cell lines.
2. Animal models: various animal models of these disorders exist and include mouse, zebra fish, and fly models of disease, and these are summarized in **Table 2**.
3. Inducible pluripotent stem cell–derived neurons: patient-derived cells lines have been generated for SCA3.[23]

Evaluation and Management

The evaluation and management of a patient with SCA involves the rapid identification of any treatable causes and, once those are excluded, an efficient and systematic search for a genetic cause, coupled with symptomatic therapies to minimize functional loss.

Clinical Examination and Diagnostic Testing

- A detailed neurologic assessment with careful attention to the examination of co-ordination, sensation (especially proprioception), and vestibular function is essential to the diagnosis of an ataxia (see **Box 1**).[3,4]
- Examination must include a careful evaluation of the movements of the eyes for errors in targeting, errors in tracking, dysmetria, or nystagmus.
- Speech may be dysarthric, typically with a scanning quality.
- Ataxia must be defined as either sporadic or familial. Sporadic cases typically favor an acquired process, which should be prioritized for initial testing (**Fig. 1**) because this has the greatest potential for effective treatment.
- In sporadic cases, once acquired conditions are excluded, genetic and idio-pathic disorders represent the next line of investigation.
- A familial history of ataxia necessitates earlier consideration of genetic causes, but acquired processes must still be adequately explored (see **Fig. 1**).
- The tempo of disease onset and progression can be helpful in the prioritization of acquired causes for subsequent testing (**Table 3**).
- Idiopathic disorders, of which multiple system atrophy is the most likely to pre-sent initially with ataxia,[3,4,24] remain diagnoses of exclusion and should not be made unless a reasonable exploration of acquired and genetic causes has first been pursued.
- For cerebellar ataxia, magnetic resonance imaging (MRI) of the brain is the initial diagnostic test of choice.[3,4,25,26] Imaging is critical to assess for the presence of

Table 2
Animal models of SCA

Name	Type of Model[a]	Phenotype	Pathology	Selected Therapy Trials
SCA1	Transgenic-(Purkinje neuron specific), 82Q[45]	Motor incoordination	Shrinkage and marked loss of Purkinje neurons	shRNA[47]
	Knock-in, 154Q[46]	Cognitive impairment Kyphosis Motor incoordination Premature death Weight loss	Mild loss of Purkinje neurons	Lithium[48] VEGF[49]
SCA2	Transgenic 58Q and 127Q (Purkinje neuron specific)[50]	Motor incoordination	Shrinkage and mild loss of Purkinje neurons	Dantrolene[51] SK channel activator[52]
SCA3 (MJD)	Transgenic (many models including 79Q,[53] 148Q,[54] 71Q,[55] 94Q,[56] 77Q[57])	Motor incoordination Premature death	Variable shrinkage and mild neuronal loss	Sodium butyrate[63]
	Yeast artificial chromosome transgenic[58–60]	Motor incoordination	Mild and late loss of brain stem and cerebellar neurons	Dantrolene[59]
	Rat model lentiviral injection and overexpression of mutant ataxin-3 in the striatum or substantia nigra[61]	Circling behavior following unilateral substantia nigra injection	Fluoro-jade positive neurons and cell shrinkage	shRNA[64]
	Fly eye[62]	Loss of ommatidia		
SCA5	Knockout[9]	Motor incoordination	Shrinkage and mild loss of Purkinje neurons	—
SCA6	Knockin 84Q[65]	Motor incoordination	Very mild Purkinje neuron loss	—
SCA7	Transgenic[66]	Motor incoordination	Mild Purkinje neuron loss	—
SCA8	Klh1 deletion[67]	Motor incoordination	Purkinje neuron shrinkage	—

(continued on next page)

Table 2
(continued)

Name	Type of Model[a]	Phenotype	Pathology	Selected Therapy Trials
SCA10	Transgenic 500 repeats in 3′ UTR[68]	Motor incoordination Seizure susceptibility	Loss of CA3 hippocampal neurons	—
SCA13	Knockout[69] Zebra fish R420H human mutation[12]	Motor incoordination	No neuronal loss No neuronal loss	—
SCA14	Transgenic H501Y[70]	Abnormal clasping	Altered Purkinje neuron morphology	—
SCA15/SCA16	Knockout[13]	Motor incoordination Seizures	No neuronal loss	—
SCA17/HDL4	Transgenic 109Q[71]	Motor incoordination	Loss of Purkinje neurons	—
SCA27	Knockout[72]	Cognitive deficits Motor incoordination	No neuronal loss	—
DRPLA	Transgenic variable repeat length 76Q–129Q[73]	Cognitive deficits Motor incoordination Premature death	Purkinje neuron shrinkage and progressive brain atrophy	—

Abbreviation: VEGF, vascular endothelial growth factor.
  [a] Refers to mouse models unless otherwise specified.

cerebellar atrophy (**Fig. 2**) as well as for the presence of any identifiable evidence of structural or vascular damage (eg, stroke, tumor)[27] and/or other lesions or associated neurodegeneration that could be diagnostically useful (eg, white matter hyperintensities, atrophy of the brainstem or spinal cord, loss of transverse pontine fibers).[4,25,26]

- Subsequent laboratory and diagnostic studies for acquired causes of cerebellar ataxia should be performed in a stepwise fashion and tailored to the presentation of the individual patient (see **Fig. 1**).

Genetic Testing

- Careful attention must be paid to clinical phenotype. In general, the autosomal dominant SCAs show phenotypic heterogeneity[1,3,4]; however, certain clinical features can aid in the prioritization of disorders for genetic testing (eg, seizures in SCA10, parkinsonism in SCA3, or dementia in SCA17; see **Table 1**).
- Ethnicity and geographic origin should also be considered, because several SCAs are more common in specific populations (eg, SCA3 in Brazil or DRPLA in Japan).[1,4,28] Worldwide, the most common SCA is SCA3, which, together with SCA1, SCA2, SCA6, and SCA7, comprises 50% of all dominant ataxias.[1,28,29] In late-onset cases (onset greater than age 50 years), SCA6 and fragile X tremor/ataxia syndrome are the most frequent.[1,3,4]

- Genetic testing should be performed in a stratified fashion based on phenotype (**Fig. 3**). In sporadic cases, it may be reasonable to screen for the most common autosomal dominant SCAs; however, widespread screening should be avoided because the diagnostic yield is disproportionately low relative to the cost of testing.[1,4,30]
- Autosomal recessive disorders, particularly late-onset variants of Friedreich ataxia, become a consideration in sporadic patients from small families,[31,32] complicating diagnostic testing (see **Fig. 3**).

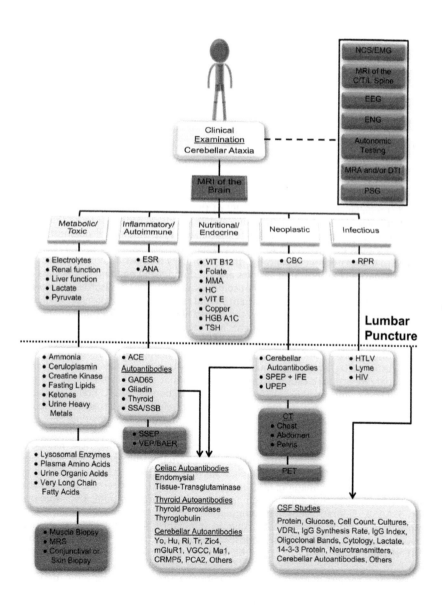

- Newer genome-wide methods of sequencing technology may alleviate most testing problems and become a staple for future testing algorithms (**Box 2**, see **Fig. 3**).[33,34]

Current Management and Therapeutic Options

- Many of the acquired causes of cerebellar ataxia (see **Fig. 1**) can be treated or modified, emphasizing the need for prompt recognition to minimize damage to the cerebellum and its associated pathways.[4]
- Paraneoplastic and other autoimmune mediated ataxias are particularly important to consider because, if left unchecked, rapid and severe damage to the cerebellum can result; current treatments are often not fully effective.[4,35]
- No cures or effective treatments yet exist for genetic or idiopathic ataxias and treatment is therefore wholly symptomatic; however, exercise therapy has been shown to be beneficial in maintaining patient function over time and should be used for all patients.[36,37]

◀──

Fig. 1. Diagnostic evaluation of an acquired cerebellar ataxia. All patients with clinically identified cerebellar ataxia should have MRI of the brain performed to assess for masses, vascular lesions/anomalies, traumatic injury, and/or structural problems in addition to evidence of neurodegeneration and/or white matter changes. Additional diagnostic studies (*gray boxes*) should be performed as warranted based on the clinical examination (*dashed line*). If the MRI does not reveal the cause, then laboratory tests (*white boxes*) should be performed systematically as indicated. Studies are listed under the heading of the class of disorders they most often identify. Note that some tests could identify disorders in more than one class. In a complete evaluation, a patient should receive, at a minimum, all studies listed above the dotted line. Items listed below the dotted line are chosen for more in-depth evaluation of specific causes and not all patients may require all studies. The dotted line represents the threshold for performing a lumbar puncture in a patient undergoing initial work-up. Suggested cerebral spinal fluid studies are indicated (*arrow*). Specific cerebellar (paraneoplastic), celiac, and thyroid autoantibodies are also shown (*arrow*). Note that there are additional rare acquired causes of cerebellar ataxia that are not listed in this figure. ACE, angiotensin-converting enzyme; ANA, antinuclear antibodies; BAER, brainstem auditory evoked response; CBC, complete blood count; C/T/L, cervical, thoracic, and/or lumbar; CSF, cerebral spinal fluid; CT, computed tomography; DTI, diffusion tensor imaging; EEG, electroencephalogram; EMG, electromyogram; ENG, electronystagmogram; ESR, erythrocyte sedimentation rate; GAD, glutamic acid decarboxylase; HC, homocysteine; HGB, hemoglobin; HIV, human immunodeficiency virus; HTLV, human T-lymphotropic virus; IFE, immunofixation electrophoresis; MMA, methylmalonic acid; MRA, magnetic resonance angiography; MRI, magnetic resonance imaging; MRS, magnetic resonance spectroscopy; NCS, nerve conduction study; PET, positron emission tomography; PSG, polysomnogram; RPR, rapid plasma reagin; SSA/SSB, Sjögren syndrome antigen; SPEP, serum protein electrophoresis; SSEP, somatosensory evoked potentials; TSH, thyroid stimulating hormone; UPEP, urine protein electrophoresis; VDRL, venereal disease research laboratory test; VEP, visual evoked potential; VIT, vitamin. (*Reprinted from* Fogel BL, Perlman S. Cerebellar disorders: balancing the approach to cerebellar ataxia. In: Gálvez-Jiménez N, Tuite PJ, editors. Uncommon causes of movement disorders. Cambridge (NY): Cambridge University Press; 2011. p. 198–216; with permission.)

Table 3
Using the tempo of disease onset and progression to aid diagnosis

Symptom Onset/Progression	Causes to Consider[a]
Episodic (minutes to hours)	Genetic Inflammatory Toxic Vascular
Acute (hours to days)	Infection Metabolic Toxic Trauma Vascular
Subacute (weeks to months)	Autoimmune Infection Inflammatory Neoplastic Paraneoplastic
Chronic (months to years)	Autoimmune Degenerative Genetic Inflammatory Metabolic Neoplastic Paraneoplastic
Static (years to decades)	Congenital Cerebellar Injury (any source)

[a] Not a comprehensive list.

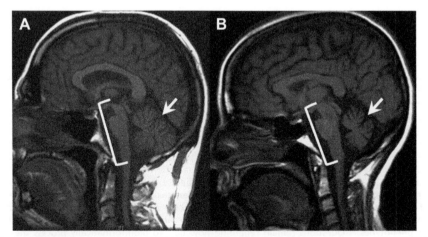

Fig. 2. MRI findings in SCA. Sagittal T1-weighted MRI is shown for a patient with (*A*) SCA3 and (*B*) multiple system atrophy. Cerebellar atrophy (*arrow*) and brainstem atrophy (*bracket*) are noted. Note the similarity in imaging characteristics between these patients; this is common among the different ataxia causes (ie, acquired, hereditary, and idiopathic).

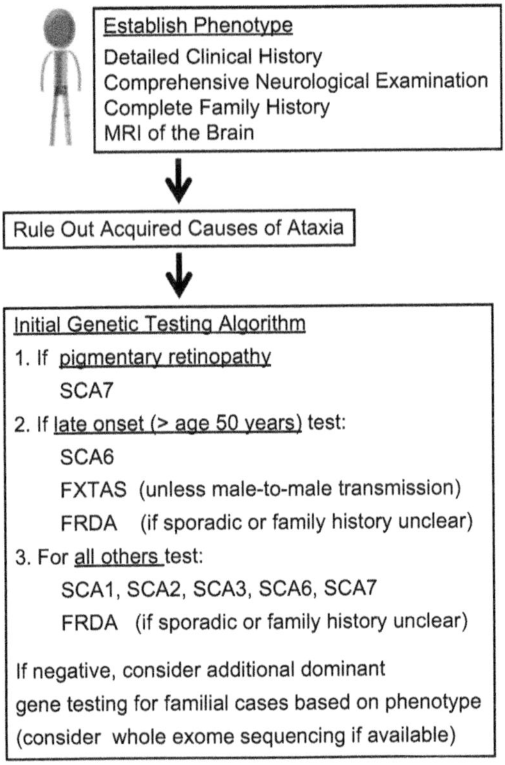

Establish Phenotype
Detailed Clinical History
Comprehensive Neurological Examination
Complete Family History
MRI of the Brain

↓

Rule Out Acquired Causes of Ataxia

↓

Initial Genetic Testing Algorithm
1. If pigmentary retinopathy
    SCA7
2. If late onset (> age 50 years) test:
    SCA6
    FXTAS (unless male-to-male transmission)
    FRDA   (if sporadic or family history unclear)
3. For all others test:
    SCA1, SCA2, SCA3, SCA6, SCA7
    FRDA   (if sporadic or family history unclear)

If negative, consider additional dominant
gene testing for familial cases based on phenotype
(consider whole exome sequencing if available)

Fig. 3. Diagnostic evaluation of a genetic cerebellar ataxia. FRDA, Friedreich ataxia; FXTAS, fragile X tremor/ataxia syndrome.

Box 2
Clinical exome sequencing

Recent advances in DNA sequencing technology have made it possible to rapidly and cheaply sequence large amounts of DNA, including whole genomes.[38,39] Sequencing of the 1% to 2% of the genome expressed as protein (known as the exome) can examine the approximately 20,000 genes in the human genome simultaneously to localize protein-altering sequence variation, and is expected to dramatically affect the evaluation of neurogenetic disease.[33,34,39] Although unable to detect mutations caused by repeat expansion, noncoding variation, or large deletions/duplications,[34] with regard to cerebellar ataxia, there are already key examples of the use of this technology in the identification of new ataxia genes,[40,41] the detection of novel mutations,[42,43] and the diagnosis of patients with clinically heterogeneous spinocerebellar phenotypes.[44] Questions remain regarding how best to bioinformatically process these large amounts of sequence information to identify pathogenic variants in individual patients, particularly those involving novel mutations and genes, but there is little doubt that this technology will see widespread clinical use in the immediate future.[33,34]

SUMMARY

The autosomal dominant SCAs are late-onset progressive degenerative disorders that may be categorized into repeat disorders, disorders of ion-channel dysfunction, and disorders of signal transduction molecules. The identification of additional genes and the development of better cellular and animal model systems of disease pathogenesis continue to advance understanding and suggest new avenues for better diagnosis and potential intervention. Because of the considerable clinical overlap between these disorders and other acquired causes of ataxia, the evaluation of patients with cerebellar ataxia must first include an investigation into potentially treatable causes. If genetic testing is considered, it is best to take a tiered approach, with initial testing including the most common dominant genes, namely SCA1, SCA2, SCA3, SCA6, SCA7, and, in sporadic cases, Friedreich ataxia, the most common recessive cause. Management is mainly supportive, but exercise therapy has been shown to be beneficial in maintaining patient function over time.

REFERENCES

1. Durr A. Autosomal dominant cerebellar ataxias: polyglutamine expansions and beyond. Lancet Neurol 2010;9(9):885–94.
2. Klockgether T, Ludtke R, Kramer B, et al. The natural history of degenerative ataxia: a retrospective study in 466 patients. Brain 1998;121(Pt 4):589–600.
3. Fogel BL, Perlman S. An approach to the patient with late-onset cerebellar ataxia. Nat Clin Pract Neurol 2006;2(11):629–35 [quiz: 1 p following 635].
4. Fogel BL, Perlman S. Cerebellar disorders: balancing the approach to cerebellar ataxia. In: Gálvez-Jiménez N, Tuite PJ, editors. Uncommon causes of movement disorders. Cambridge (NY): Cambridge University Press; 2011. p. 198–216.
5. Manto M, Bower JM, Conforto AB, et al. Consensus paper: roles of the cerebellum in motor control–the diversity of ideas on cerebellar involvement in movement. Cerebellum 2012;11(2):457–87.
6. Ikeda Y, Daughters RS, Ranum LP. Bidirectional expression of the SCA8 expansion mutation: one mutation, two genes. Cerebellum 2008;7(2):150–8.
7. Williams AJ, Paulson HL. Polyglutamine neurodegeneration: protein misfolding revisited. Trends Neurosci 2008;31(10):521–8.
8. Shakkottai VG, Paulson HL. Physiologic alterations in ataxia: channeling changes into novel therapies. Arch Neurol 2009;66(10):1196–201.
9. Perkins EM, Clarkson YL, Sabatier N, et al. Loss of beta-III spectrin leads to Purkinje cell dysfunction recapitulating the behavior and neuropathology of spinocerebellar ataxia type 5 in humans. J Neurosci 2010;30(14):4857–67.
10. Kordasiewicz HB, Gomez CM. Molecular pathogenesis of spinocerebellar ataxia type 6. Neurotherapeutics 2007;4(2):285–94.
11. Waters MF, Minassian NA, Stevanin G, et al. Mutations in voltage-gated potassium channel KCNC3 cause degenerative and developmental central nervous system phenotypes. Nat Genet 2006;38(4):447–51.
12. Issa FA, Mazzochi C, Mock AF, et al. Spinocerebellar ataxia type 13 mutant potassium channel alters neuronal excitability and causes locomotor deficits in zebrafish. J Neurosci 2011;31(18):6831–41.
13. Matsumoto M, Nakagawa T, Inoue T, et al. Ataxia and epileptic seizures in mice lacking type 1 inositol 1,4,5-trisphosphate receptor. Nature 1996;379(6561):168–71.
14. Lee YC, Durr A, Majczenko K, et al. Mutations in KCND3 cause spinocerebellar ataxia type 22. Ann Neurol 2012;72(6):859–69.

15. Duarri A, Jezierska J, Fokkens M, et al. Mutations in potassium channel KCND3 cause spinocerebellar ataxia type 19. Ann Neurol 2012;72(6):870–80.

16. Shakkottai VG, Xiao M, Xu L, et al. FGF14 regulates the intrinsic excitability of cerebellar Purkinje neurons. Neurobiol Dis 2009;33(1):81–8.

17. Goetz SC, Liem KF Jr, Anderson KV. The spinocerebellar ataxia-associated gene tau tubulin kinase 2 controls the initiation of ciliogenesis. Cell 2012; 151(4):847–58.

18. Shuvaev AN, Horiuchi H, Seki T, et al. Mutant PKCgamma in spinocerebellar ataxia type 14 disrupts synapse elimination and long-term depression in Purkinje cells in vivo. J Neurosci 2011;31(40):14324–34.

19. Bakalkin G, Watanabe H, Jezierska J, et al. Prodynorphin mutations cause the neurodegenerative disorder spinocerebellar ataxia type 23. Am J Hum Genet 2010;87(5):593–603.

20. Todd PK, Paulson HL. RNA-mediated neurodegeneration in repeat expansion disorders. Ann Neurol 2010;67(3):291–300.

21. Lebre AS, Brice A. Spinocerebellar ataxia 7 (SCA7). Cytogenet Genome Res 2003;100(1–4):154–63.

22. Elden AC, et al. Ataxin-2 intermediate-length polyglutamine expansions are associated with increased risk for ALS. Nature 2010;466(7310):1069–75.

23. Koch P, Breuer P, Peitz M, et al. Excitation-induced ataxin-3 aggregation in neurons from patients with Machado-Joseph disease. Nature 2011;480(7378): 543–6.

24. Gilman S, Wenning GK, Low PA, et al. Second consensus statement on the diagnosis of multiple system atrophy. Neurology 2008;71(9):670–6.

25. Klockgether T. Sporadic ataxia with adult onset: classification and diagnostic criteria. Lancet Neurol 2010;9(1):94–104.

26. van Gaalen J, van de Warrenburg BP. A practical approach to late-onset cerebellar ataxia: putting the disorder with lack of order into order. Pract Neurol 2012;12(1):14–24.

27. Fogel BL, Salamon N, Perlman S. Progressive spinocerebellar ataxia mimicked by a presumptive cerebellar arteriovenous malformation. Eur J Radiol 2009; 71(1):e1–2.

28. Schols L, Bauer P, Schmidt T, et al. Autosomal dominant cerebellar ataxias: clinical features, genetics, and pathogenesis. Lancet Neurol 2004;3(5):291–304.

29. Finsterer J. Ataxias with autosomal, X-chromosomal or maternal inheritance. Can J Neurol Sci 2009;36(4):409–28.

30. Fogel BL, Lee JY, Lane J, et al. Mutations in rare ataxia genes are uncommon causes of sporadic cerebellar ataxia. Mov Disord 2012;27(3):442–6.

31. Fogel BL. Childhood cerebellar ataxia. J Child Neurol 2012;27(9):1138–45.

32. Fogel BL, Perlman S. Clinical features and molecular genetics of autosomal recessive cerebellar ataxias. Lancet Neurol 2007;6(3):245–57.

33. Coppola G, Geschwind DH. Genomic medicine enters the neurology clinic. Neurology 2012;79(2):112–4.

34. Fogel BL, Geschwind DH. Clinical neurogenetics. In: Daroff R, Fenichel G, Jankovic J, et al, editors. Neurology in clinical practice. 6th edition. Philadelphia: Elsevier/Saunders; 2012. p. 704–34.

35. Panzer J, Dalmau J. Movement disorders in paraneoplastic and autoimmune disease. Curr Opin Neurol 2011;24(4):346–53.

36. Ilg W, Synofzik M, Brotz D, et al. Intensive coordinative training improves motor performance in degenerative cerebellar disease. Neurology 2009;73(22): 1823–30.

37. Ilg W, Brotz D, Burkard S, et al. Long-term effects of coordinative training in degenerative cerebellar disease. Mov Disord 2010;25(13):2239–46.
38. Metzker ML. Sequencing technologies - the next generation. Nat Rev Genet 2010;11(1):31–46.
39. Bras J, Guerreiro R, Hardy J. Use of next-generation sequencing and other whole-genome strategies to dissect neurological disease. Nat Rev Neurosci 2012;13(7):453–64.
40. Doi H, Yoshida K, Yasuda T, et al. Exome sequencing reveals a homozygous SYT14 mutation in adult-onset, autosomal-recessive spinocerebellar ataxia with psychomotor retardation. Am J Hum Genet 2011;89(2):320–7.
41. Wang JL, Yang X, Xia K, et al. TGM6 identified as a novel causative gene of spinocerebellar ataxias using exome sequencing. Brain 2010;133(Pt 12): 3510–8.
42. Dundar H, Ozgul RK, Yalnizoglu D, et al. Identification of a novel Twinkle mutation in a family with infantile onset spinocerebellar ataxia by whole exome sequencing. Pediatr Neurol 2012;46(3):172–7.
43. Li M, Pang S, Song Y, et al. Whole exome sequencing identifies a novel mutation in the transglutaminase 6 gene for spinocerebellar ataxia in a Chinese family. Clin Genet 2013;83(3):269–73.
44. Sailer A, Scholz SW, Gibbs JR, et al. Exome sequencing in an SCA14 family demonstrates its utility in diagnosing heterogeneous diseases. Neurology 2012;79(2):127–31.
45. Burright EN, Clark HB, Servadio A, et al. SCA1 transgenic mice: a model for neurodegeneration caused by an expanded CAG trinucleotide repeat. Cell 1995;82(6):937–48.
46. Watase K, Weeber EJ, Xu B, et al. A long CAG repeat in the mouse Sca1 locus replicates SCA1 features and reveals the impact of protein solubility on selective neurodegeneration. Neuron 2002;34(6):905–19.
47. Xia H, Mao Q, Eliason SL, et al. RNAi suppresses polyglutamine-induced neurodegeneration in a model of spinocerebellar ataxia. Nat Med 2004;10(8): 816–20.
48. Watase K, Gatchel JR, Sun Y, et al. Lithium therapy improves neurological function and hippocampal dendritic arborization in a spinocerebellar ataxia type 1 mouse model. PLoS Med 2007;4(5):e182.
49. Cvetanovic M, Patel JM, Marti HH, et al. Vascular endothelial growth factor ameliorates the ataxic phenotype in a mouse model of spinocerebellar ataxia type 1. Nat Med 2011;17(11):1445–7.
50. Hansen ST, Meera P, Otis TS, et al. Changes in Purkinje cell firing and gene expression precede behavioral pathology in a mouse model of SCA2. Hum Mol Genet 2013; 22(2):271–83.
51. Liu J, Tang TS, Tu H, et al. Deranged calcium signaling and neurodegeneration in spinocerebellar ataxia type 2. J Neurosci 2009;29(29):9148–62.
52. Kasumu AW, Hougaard C, Rode F, et al. Selective positive modulator of calcium-activated potassium channels exerts beneficial effects in a mouse model of spinocerebellar ataxia type 2. Chem Biol 2012;19(10):1340–53.
53. Chou AH, Yeh TH, Ouyang P, et al. Polyglutamine-expanded ataxin-3 causes cerebellar dysfunction of SCA3 transgenic mice by inducing transcriptional dysregulation. Neurobiol Dis 2008;31(1):89–101.
54. Boy J, Schmidt T, Schumann U, et al. A transgenic mouse model of spinocerebellar ataxia type 3 resembling late disease onset and gender-specific instability of CAG repeats. Neurobiol Dis 2010;37(2):284–93.

55. Goti D, Katzen SM, Mez J, et al. A mutant ataxin-3 putative-cleavage fragment in brains of Machado-Joseph disease patients and transgenic mice is cytotoxic above a critical concentration. J Neurosci 2004;24(45):10266–79.

56. Silva-Fernandes A, Costa Mdo C, Duarte-Silva S, et al. Motor uncoordination and neuropathology in a transgenic mouse model of Machado-Joseph disease lacking intranuclear inclusions and ataxin-3 cleavage products. Neurobiol Dis 2010;40(1):163–76.

57. Boy J, Schmidt T, Wolburg H, et al. Reversibility of symptoms in a conditional mouse model of spinocerebellar ataxia type 3. Hum Mol Genet 2009;18(22):4282–95.

58. Cemal CK, Carroll CJ, Lawrence L, et al. YAC transgenic mice carrying pathological alleles of the MJD1 locus exhibit a mild and slowly progressive cerebellar deficit. Hum Mol Genet 2002;11(9):1075–94.

59. Chen X, Tang TS, Tu H, et al. Deranged calcium signaling and neurodegeneration in spinocerebellar ataxia type 3. J Neurosci 2008;28(48):12713–24.

60. Shakkottai VG, do Carmo Costa M, Dell'Orco JM, et al. Early changes in cerebellar physiology accompany motor dysfunction in the polyglutamine disease spinocerebellar ataxia type 3. J Neurosci 2011;31(36):13002–14.

61. Alves S, Regulier E, Nascimento-Ferreira I, et al. Striatal and nigral pathology in a lentiviral rat model of Machado-Joseph disease. Hum Mol Genet 2008;17(14):2071–83.

62. Warrick JM, Paulson HL, Gray-Board GL, et al. Expanded polyglutamine protein forms nuclear inclusions and causes neural degeneration in *Drosophila*. Cell 1998;93(6):939–49.

63. Chou AH, Chen SY, Yeh TH, et al. HDAC inhibitor sodium butyrate reverses transcriptional downregulation and ameliorates ataxic symptoms in a transgenic mouse model of SCA3. Neurobiol Dis 2011;41(2):481–8.

64. Alves S, Nascimento-Ferreira I, Dufour N, et al. Silencing ataxin-3 mitigates degeneration in a rat model of Machado-Joseph disease: no role for wild-type ataxin-3? Hum Mol Genet 2010;19(12):2380–94.

65. Watase K, Barrett CF, Miyazaki T, et al. Spinocerebellar ataxia type 6 knockin mice develop a progressive neuronal dysfunction with age-dependent accumulation of mutant CaV2.1 channels. Proc Natl Acad Sci U S A 2008;105(33):11987–92.

66. Furrer SA, Mohanachandran MS, Waldherr SM, et al. Spinocerebellar ataxia type 7 cerebellar disease requires the coordinated action of mutant ataxin-7 in neurons and glia, and displays non-cell-autonomous Bergmann glia degeneration. J Neurosci 2011;31(45):16269–78.

67. He Y, Zu T, Benzow KA, et al. Targeted deletion of a single Sca8 ataxia locus allele in mice causes abnormal gait, progressive loss of motor coordination, and Purkinje cell dendritic deficits. J Neurosci 2006;26(39):9975–82.

68. White M, Xia G, Gao R, et al. Transgenic mice with SCA10 pentanucleotide repeats show motor phenotype and susceptibility to seizure: a toxic RNA gain-of-function model. J Neurosci Res 2012;90(3):706–14.

69. Hurlock EC, McMahon A, Joho RH. Purkinje-cell-restricted restoration of Kv3.3 function restores complex spikes and rescues motor coordination in Kcnc3 mutants. J Neurosci 2008;28(18):4640–8.

70. Zhang Y, Snider A, Willard L, et al. Loss of Purkinje cells in the PKCgamma H101Y transgenic mouse. Biochem Biophys Res Commun 2009;378(3):524–8.

71. Chang YC, Lin CY, Hsu CM, et al. Neuroprotective effects of granulocyte-colony stimulating factor in a novel transgenic mouse model of SCA17. J Neurochem 2011;118(2):288–303.
72. Wang Q, Bardgett ME, Wong M, et al. Ataxia and paroxysmal dyskinesia in mice lacking axonally transported FGF14. Neuron 2002;35(1):25–38.
73. Sato T, Miura M, Yamada M, et al. Severe neurological phenotypes of Q129 DRPLA transgenic mice serendipitously created by en masse expansion of CAG repeats in Q76 DRPLA mice. Hum Mol Genet 2009;18(4):723–36.

Muscular Dystrophies and Other Genetic Myopathies

Perry B. Shieh, MD, PhD

KEYWORDS

- Muscular dystrophy • Myopathy • Limb-Girdle • FSHD • Myotonic dystrophy
- Congenital • Metabolic

KEY POINTS

- Muscular dystrophy refers to a collection of genetic progressive muscle diseases.
- If relevant, preventive screening for cardiac manifestations and ventilatory insufficiency is an important management consideration.
- Novel therapies tailored to the genetics of the disease are entering clinical trials for some of these diseases.
- Definitive genetic diagnosis is important to optimally manage patients with muscle disease.

INTRODUCTION

Historically, the term, *muscular dystrophy*, was used to describe a progressive genetic myopathy with muscle histologic changes, including fibrosis, muscle fiber size variation, and abnormal internalization of muscle nuclei (**Fig. 1**). Fibrofatty replacement, inflammation, and degenerative fibers are also commonly described histologic features. Hence, the diagnostic evaluation often included a muscle biopsy to demonstrate these histologic features. The most common muscular dystrophies include Duchenne muscular dystrophy (DMD), Becker muscular dystrophy (BMD), facioscapulohumeral muscular dystrophy (FSHD), and myotonic dystrophy. Other conditions were also recognized, but these syndromes were defined clinically.

The classification of many muscular dystrophies has been based on clinical presentation. Specifically, the pattern of weakness has been the means of identifying clinical syndrome. For example, limb-girdle muscular dystrophy (LGMD), distal myopathies, and FSHD are muscular dystrophy syndromes named based on the pattern of weakness.

With improved understanding of the underlying genetics of muscle disease, the list of genetic syndromes associated with muscle disease has expanded dramatically and

Department of Neurology, UCLA Medical Center, 300 Medical Plaza, Suite B-200, Los Angeles, CA 90095, USA
E-mail address: PShieh@mednet.ucla.edu

Neurol Clin 31 (2013) 1009–1029
http://dx.doi.org/10.1016/j.ncl.2013.04.004
0733-8619/13/$ – see front matter © 2013 Elsevier Inc. All rights reserved.

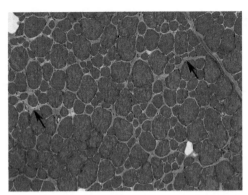

Fig. 1. Cryostat sections of a muscle biopsy from a boy with BMD (original magnification x100). Hematoxylin-eosin preparation shows muscle fibers in cross-section that have significant variability of fiber diameter. Mildly increased fibrosis is also seen in the space between the muscle fibers (endomysial space, examples indicated by *arrows*). Increased internalization of muscle fiber nuclei, however, is not a significant feature of this particular biopsy.

the classification of muscular dystrophy has been revised to incorporate genetic testing. Thus, previously recognized clinical syndromes (eg, DMD) may also be referred to by their genetic locus (eg, dystrophinopathy). Furthermore, conditions that were thought to be different genetic syndromes, such as DMD and BMD, are now recognized as allelic variants of the same genetic locus. Additionally, conditions previously classified as nonprogressive, such as the congenital myopathies, are now loosely categorized as muscular dystrophies based on slow clinical progression and recognition of allelic variability.

The diagnostic criteria for nearly all muscular dystrophies now incorporate genetic testing. Patients with characteristic clinical features and a documented causative mutation may be diagnosed without extensive and invasive diagnostic testing, such as electromyography (EMG) and muscle biopsy, among other tests. In many cases, however, the clinical presentation is not specific and DNA testing may yield sequence variants of unclear clinical significance. Thus, the role of muscle biopsy and other traditional diagnostic tests continues to be helpful although not always essential in the diagnostic evaluation of these patients. With next-generation sequencing and continued improvement in the documentation of causative mutations, it is anticipated that the diagnostic yield of genetic testing will continue to improve in the years to come.

An aggressive effort to identify a definitive diagnosis is recommended because a specific diagnosis affects the management of these patients. For example, many of these conditions are associated with cardiac and pulmonary complications that may require early intervention. Furthermore, potential medical treatments of several of these conditions are available or in the pipeline. An obvious prerequisite for these treatments is for patients to have an accurate genetic diagnosis. This review discusses the clinical and diagnostic features of DMD/BMD, FSHD, and myotonic dystrophy before briefly describing the complex diagnostic landscape of the other muscular dystrophies.

DUCHENNE MUSCULAR DYSTROPHY AND BECKER MUSCULAR DYSTROPHY

DMD affects up to 1 in 3600 boys,[1] making this muscular dystrophy the most common by incidence. Because of the shorter life expectancy, however, DMD ranks second in prevalence among muscular dystrophies. DMD and BMD represent 2 ends of the clinical spectrum associated with mutations in the gene, dystrophin (DMD). The dystrophin gene spans 2.4 million base pairs on chromosome Xp21.2 and codes for a 427-kDa protein through its 79 exons. Dystrophin seems to anchor the actin cytoskeleton to the membrane-bound proteins, thereby protecting the muscle from strain-related damage during muscle exertion. Although many patients inherit the condition through their mother, the size and complexity of the gene provide ample opportunity for sporadic mutations, which are approximately 25% of cases.[2] In most cases, mutations that preserve the reading frame result in the milder Becker phenotype whereas mutations that disrupt the reading frame result in the more severe Duchenne phenotype.[3]

The clinical presentation of boys with DMD includes delayed motor milestones, proximal weakness, hypertrophied calves, and markedly elevated creatine kinase (CK) levels of 20,000 to 40,000. Genetic testing has precluded the need for muscle biopsy in most cases; rarely, however, a muscle biopsy with immunohistochemistry and perhaps cDNA analysis may be necessary because of nondiagnostic DNA testing (eg, intronic mutations).

Standards of care for DMD have been defined[1,4] and include regular monitoring of orthopedic/physical status, nutritional status, cardiac function, and ventilatory function. These measures are aimed at maintaining quality of life and optimal longevity. In particular, 3 medical interventions are thought to improve long-term outcome: (1) corticosteroids, which have been shown to improve muscle strength in DMD patients; (2) angiotensin-converting enzyme inhibitors and angiotensin receptor blockers, which studies have suggested may slow the progression of cardiomyopathy in DMD/BMD patients; and (3) noninvasive ventilator support, which has been shown to significantly improve life-expectancy in DMD patients.

Specific mutations in dystrophin may be amenable to certain treatment strategies.[5,6] Specifically, patients with premature stop codons (nonsense mutations) may be candidates for pharmacologic treatments that suppress stop codons, as suggested by clinical trials with PTC124 (Ataluren).[7] Other patients with large deletions that disrupt the reading frame of the dystrophin gene may be candidates for synthetic antisense oligonucleotide therapy that blocks splice acceptor sites of certain exons (exon skipping), thereby altering the splicing pattern and restoring the reading frame. This strategy has been used by the agents developed by Sarepta Therapeutics (formerly AVI BioPharma) (Eteplirsen [AVI-4658])[8] and by GlaxoSmithKline/Prosensa (PRO051/GSK2402968/Drisapersen)[9] that are designed to cause skipping of exon 51. Clinical trials are ongoing to assess the efficacy of these agents. Agents that are designed to skip other exons are in the pipeline.

FACIOSCAPULOHUMERAL MUSCULAR DYSTROPHY

Classic FSHD is an autosomal dominant muscular dystrophy with variable expressivity. In a recent study, FSHD was found to be the most prevalent muscular dystrophy, with a prevalence of 7 in 100,000.[10] Onset of symptoms is usually during adulthood and the distribution of weakness varies significantly from patient to patient. As the name suggests, the most commonly affected muscles include the facial muscles, scapular stabilizing muscles, and muscles of the upper arm. In some patients, the distal lower extremities may also demonstrate weakness in the early phases of the disease. The deltoid is often spared in these patients, however, resulting in a unique finding of shoulder abduction weakness with preserved deltoid bulk. The pattern of weakness is often asymmetric.[10]

Classic FSHD (FSHD1) is associated with shortening (contraction) of the D4Z4 region in the subtelomeric region of chromosome 4q. The size of the D4Z4 region is assessed based on the size of the EcoR1 fragment on Southern blot and, in phenotypically normal individuals, this fragment is greater than 38 kilobases (kb) in size. In FSHD patients, the EcoR1 fragment of the D4Z4 region is less than 38 kb, and the degree of shortening is correlated with the severity of weakness and with an earlier age of onset of symptoms.

The pathophysiology of classic FSHD involves transcription of the *DUX4* open reading frame, which relies on 2 factors: (1) shortening of the D4Z4 region in the subtelomeric region of chromosome 4q and (2) a polyadenylation-permissive telomeric sequence.

The D4Z4 region comprises tandem repeats of a 3.3-kb fragment and a *DUX4* open reading frame is found in each of these repeats. Phenotypically normal individuals have more than 10 repeats in their D4Z4 region, but FSHD1 patients have fewer than 10 repeats. Recent studies suggest that D4Z4 shortening results in *cis*-hypomethylation, which permits transcription of the *DUX4* open reading frame.[11,12] If this transcription occurs in the setting of a polyadenylation-permissive telomere, the *DUX4* transcript is stable to undergo protein synthesis.

Some normal individuals have contraction of the D4Z4 region but do not demonstrate the FSHD phenotype. This is because, despite the D4Z4 contraction and activation of *DUX4* transcription, these patients do not have the telomere sequences necessary to polyadenylate and stabilize the *DUX4* transcript.

Some phenotypic FSHD patients, however, do not have a D4Z4 contraction but demonstrate hypomethylation, which results in the same endpoint: transcription of the *DUX4* open reading frame. These patients are referred to as FSHD2 patients.[13] Although the D4Z4 region is not contracted in these patients, both alleles of the D4Z4 region are hypomethylated. Recent studies suggest that SMCHD1 plays a role in the hypomethylation seen in FSHD2.[14]

Although the exact function of *DUX4* is still unclear, these recent findings have identified *DUX4* as a potential target for disease-modifying therapeutic agents.[15]

Infantile forms of FSHD have been reported and are associated with shorter D4Z4 fragments,[16] consistent with the inverse relationship that has been established between D4Z4 size and severity of disease.[17] In infantile FSHD, patients develop facial weakness before the age of 5 and shoulder and hip girdle weakness by age 10. Sensorineural hearing loss is common in these patients. A retinal vasculopathy has been reported but is not common.[16] Patients are generally intellectually normal although they may appear cognitively impaired because of hearing loss and facial weakness. Cardiac and respiratory complications are rare as well.

MYOTONIC DYSTROPHY

Myotonic dystrophy is an autosomal dominant condition and is probably the third most common muscular dystrophy with a prevalence of approximately 4.5 per 100,000.[18] In addition to muscle weakness and stiffness, patients develop variable degrees of cognitive impairment, endocrine abnormalities, cataracts, cardiac conduction abnormalities, and cardiomyopathy.[19] Classic myotonic dystrophy is also known as myotonic dystrophy type 1 and is associated with a CTG trinucleotide repeat in the 3' untranslated region of the *DMPK* gene on chromosome 19q.[19] Affected patients have greater than 100 repeats, although subtle or mild symptoms may be seen with 51 to 99 repeats.[19] The pathogenesis of myotonic dystrophy is not related to the function of the *DMPK* gene; rather, the expanded CUG trinucleotide RNA repeat forms hairpin structures that bind to proteins that regulate the splicing machinery, including members of the muscleblind family of RNA-binding proteins.[20] As a result, the splicing of other genes is altered, including that of the insulin receptor (resulting in diabetes) and chloride channel CLCN1 (resulting in clinical myotonia).[20] Presumably the splicing of additional genes is also affected, resulting in the constellation of clinical symptoms seen in myotonic dystrophy.

Children of affected individuals may be more severely affected than their parents; this phenomenon is known as *anticipation* and results from expansion of the trinucle-otide repeat number in subsequent generations. Congenital myotonic dystrophy affects infants of mothers with myotonic dystrophy and is associated with severe expansions of the trinucleotide repeat number, with most cases showing greater than 1000 repeats. The pathogenic mechanism of this dramatic expansion of the trinu-cleotide repeat in mothers of congential myotonic dystrophy patients is still unclear.

Proximal myotonic myopathy (PROMM), or myotonic dystrophy type 2, is a milder disease that has many of the same features as myotonic dystrophy type 1.[19] A CCTG tetranucleotide repeat within an intron of the CNBP (ZNF9) gene has been iden-tified to be responsible for PROMM. As with the CUG trinucleotide repeat in myotonic dystrophy type 1, the CCUG tetranucleotide repeat forms a hairpin structure that binds proteins that regulate the splicing machinery. Patients have such a mild phenotype, however, that many do not present until the sixth or seventh decade. Symptomatic patients with PROMM may have mild proximal muscle weakness and pain/stiffness along with milder degree of cognitive impairment, endocrine abnormalities, cataracts, cardiac conduction abnormalities, and cardiomyopathy.[19]

Management of patients with myotonic dystrophy should focus on monitoring of ventilatory function, development of obstructive sleep apnea, and periodic screening for cardiac conduction abnormalities and cardiomyopathy.[19] Appropriate interven-tions include noninvasive ventilatory support and antiarrhythmic agents. Automatic implantable cardioverter-defibrillator placement has been suggested in patients with significant arrhythmias.[19]

The role of RNA in pathogenesis of the myotonic dystrophies makes antisense oligonucleotide therapy an attractive disease-modifying approach. Specifically, anti-sense DNA with flanking synthetic nucleotides (gapmers) that target DMPK mRNA has been proposed as a potential therapy. The hybridized RNA sequences would be cleaved by endogenous ribonuclease H1, thus destabilizing and/or silencing unde-sired RNA sequences. This strategy was used by Wheeler and colleagues[21] in a trans-genic mouse model of myotonic dystrophy type 1. The results hold promise for a treatment of myotonic dystrophy in humans.

LIMB-GIRDLE MUSCULAR DYSTROPHY

LGMD refers to a large collection of progressive muscle diseases with proximal weak-ness greater than distal weakness. Autosomal dominant conditions are designated as LGMD 1X, where X currently ranges from A to H, and autosomal recessive conditions are LGMD 2X, where X currently ranges from A to Q. The list of LGMDs is long and continues to expand, with new letters in each category appearing on a regular basis. Some of the more common LGMDs are listed in **Table 1**.[22] In particular, lamin A/C (LMNA) is a common cause of LGMD 1, and calpain-3 (CAPN3), dysferlin (DYSF), FKRP, and ANO5 are some of the common causes of LGMD 2. Among children, the sarcoglycan genes should be considered. Some genes that have been associated with the more severe congenital muscular dystrophy (CMD) phenotype have also been shown to have milder variants that present with an LGMD phenotype.

Table 1
Limb-girdle muscular dystrophies

Type	Gene	Features
1A	Myotilin (MYOT)	Adult-onset proximal weakness with myofibrillar changes and rimmed vacuoles on muscle biopsy. CK levels are often normal or mildly elevated. Cardiac arrhythmias and cardiomyopathy should be monitored.
1B	Lamin A/C (LMNA)	Adult-onset proximal weakness, occasionally with contractures. CK levels are usually moderately elevated. Phenotypic variant with contractures more prominent than weakness is also known as autosomal dominant EDMD.[23] Cardiac arrhythmias are a distinguishing feature of laminopathies and require routine surveillance. Early cardiac defibrillator placement may be considered in these patients.[47]
1C	Caveolin-3 (CAV3)	Wide range of phenotypes and severity, often associated with cramps. CKs are usually markedly elevated. Rippling muscle disease has been seen in these patients. Cardiomyopathy has been reported.
2A	Calpain-3 (CAPN3)	Adult-onset proximal weakness and scapular winging. CK levels usually markedly elevated. Muscle biopsy may show inflammation No cardiac involvement has been reported.
2B	Dysferlin (DYSF)	Adult-onset proximal weakness without scapular winging. No cardiac involvement has been reported. CKs are markedly elevated. Muscle biopsy may demonstrate inflammation and decreased staining for dysferlin on immunohistochemistry. LGMD 2B and Miyoshi distal myopathy are phenotypic variants of the same disease and both may appear the same in later stages; calf weakness is usually apparent these patients.
2C 2D 2E 2F	γ-Sarcoglycan (SGCG) α-Sarcoglycan (SGCA) β-Sarcoglycan (SGCB) δ-Sarcoglycan (SGCD)	Onset of weakness usually within the first decade of life. Scapular winging is usually present. Calf hypertrophy is a common finding. CK levels are usually markedly elevated. Cardiac involvement has been reported with mutations in β-sarcoglycan.
2I	FKRP	Adult-onset proximal weakness with scapular winging. Calf hypertrophy is common. Cardiomyopathy and respiratory involvement are features of this condition, although variable severity is commonly seen. CKs are typically significantly elevated. FKRP is a putative glycosyltransferase involved in processing α-dystroglycan, which is implicated in CMDs. Certain FKRP mutations may cause a CMD phenotype.
2L	Anoctamin-5 (ANO5)	Adult-onset proximal weakness with significant variability of phenotype. Calf weakness is a common finding. Presentation may be asymmetric. CKs are typically significantly elevated.

EMERY-DREIFUSS MUSCULAR DYSTROPHY

Emery-Dreifuss muscular dystrophy (EDMD) refers to a phenotype characterized by early contractures that are out of proportion to the degree of weakness. Contractures are most prominently found in the spine, ankles, and elbows; 7 different subtypes have been described (**Table 2**).[23–26]

Table 2
Emery-Dreifuss muscular dystrophies

Type	Gene	Features
1	Emerin (*EMD*)	X-linked with slowly progressive weakness. Contractures are often more debilitating than the weakness. Cardiac arrhythmias and the risk of sudden death require surveillance and possible intervention with defibrillator placement.[23]
2	Lamin A/C (*LMNA*)	Autosomal dominant with a phenotype that is indistinguishable from type 1 (emerin) cases.[23] This form of EDMD seems the most common.
3	Lamin A/C (*LMNA*)	Rare mutations in lamin A/C that are autosomal recessive[23]
4	Nesprin-1 (*SYNE1*)	Autosomal dominant mutations in a nuclear membrane protein that binds emerin and lamin A/C[24]
5	Nesprin-2 (*SYNE2*)	Like Nesprin-1, Nesprin-2 is a nuclear membrane protein that binds emerin and lamin A/C.[24]
6	*FHL1*	X-linked with slowly progressive weakness. A rigid spine may be seen in some cases.[25]
a	*TMEM43*	Recently reported autosomal dominant form of EDMD[26]

[a] Type is not yet officially designated.

DISTAL MYOPATHIES

Although distal weakness is an uncommon phenotype in myopathies, when it is the predominant finding it has a limited differential diagnosis. It may be helpful to divide distal myopathies into (1) early onset (prior to 40 years of age) and (2) late onset (after 40 years of age). Classic distal myopathies known to most specialists who see muscular dystrophy are detailed in **Table 3**.[27–30]

OCULOPHARYNGEAL MUSCULAR DYSTROPHIES

Oculopharyngeal muscular dystrophy (OPMD) is a late-onset muscle disease beginning with ptosis and dysphagia. The age of onset is typically in the fifth decade of life. Patients may eventually develop proximal muscle weakness. Muscle biopsies of affected muscles may show rimmed vacuoles, and electron microscopy reveals 8-nm tubulofilamentous inclusions within the nuclei of the muscle fibers. OPMD is caused by a small expansion of the GCN repeat region of the polyadenylate-binding protein nuclear 1 (*PABN1*) gene, resulting in an expansion of the polyalanine stretch near the N-terminus of the protein. Normal individuals have 10 GCN repeats; autosomal recessive alleles contain 11 GCN repeats; and 12 GCN repeats or more is associated with autosomal dominant disease. The well-described French Canadian founder mutation contains 13 GCN repeats, and alleles with up to 17 repeats have been reported. A point mutation that converts at glycine codon (GGN) to an alanine codon (GCN) has been reported to result in a pseudoexpansion of the GCN repeat that also results in OPMD.[31] The role of the *PABN1* in the pathogenesis of this disease is not known. Ptosis often requires surgical intervention and/or eyelid crutches. Dysphagia eventually becomes so severe that patients may become at risk for malnutrition and aspiration pneumonia.

A similar phenotype is seen in oculopharyngodistal myopathy (OPDM). OPDM is extremely rare and begins with ptosis, mild ophthalmoparesis, weakness of the lower facial muscles, and dysphagia. Onset of symptoms, although variable, is typically in the second or third decade of life. Within 5 years of onset, weakness begins to develop

Table 3
Distal myopathies

Syndrome	Gene (s)	Features
Miyoshi	Dysferlin (*DYSF*)	Autosomal recessive condition that typically presents in the third decade of life with calf weakness and atrophy, an unusual phenotype. CK levels are markedly elevated. Miyoshi myopathy is a phenotypic variant of LGMD 2B.
Miyoshi-like	Anoctamin-5 (*ANO5*)	In addition to the proximal weakness phenotype (also listed in **Table 1** as LGMD 2L), patients with mutations in anoctamin-5 may also present with predominantly calf weakness. The age of onset may be as early as 20, which makes this phenotype a mimicker of Miyoshi myopathy. Weakness is often asymmetric. CKs are usually markedly elevated.
Nonaka/ DMRV/ hIBM	*GNE*	Autosomal recessive condition that presents with dorsiflexion weakness during the twenties. Proximal weakness develops later, although quadriceps muscles are often relative spared. Muscle biopsy shows rimmed vacuoles. CK levels are usually mildly elevated with levels typically under 1000. *GNE* is responsible for the synthesis of sialic acid; clinical trials assessing the efficacy of replacement with sialic acid or *N*-acetylmannosamine (a precursor of sialic acid) are ongoing.
Laing	*MYH7*	Autosomal dominant condition with onset is typically within the first 5 years of life, but may be as late as the second decade. Patients usually present with dorsiflexion and finger extension weakness. Neck flexion and mild facial weakness can be appreciated as well. Cardiac surveillance is suggested.
Welander	*TIA1*	Autosomal dominant condition that is rare outside of Sweden and Finland. The phenotype is that of wrist extensor weakness and foot-drop beginning in the fifth decade of life.[28]
Markesbery-Griggs	*LDB3* (*ZASP*)	Autosomal dominant condition that presents with foot drop typically during the fifth decade of life. Weakness gradually spreads to more proximal muscles. Muscle biopsy may show myofibrillar changes. Monitoring for cardiomyopathy is suggested.
Udd	Titin (*TTN*)	Also known as tibial muscular dystrophy, this autosomal dominant condition affects predominantly the tibialis anterior muscles beginning in fifth decade of life. CKs are usually normal or mildly elevated. Progression to other muscles is typically limited.
Myofibrillar myopathies	Desmin (*DES*) αB crystallin (*CRYAB*) Myotilin (*MYOT*) *LDB3* (*ZASP*) Filamin-C (*FLNC*) *BAG3* *FHL1* *DNAJB6*	Myofibrillar myopathy refers to muscle diseases defined by significant intracellular myofibrillar disruption. Desmin staining on immunohistochemistry is helpful, but electron microscopy is often necessary. The phenotypes vary significantly from gene to gene, and some may have multiple phenotypes. Distal or distal-and-proximal weakness has been described for most of these genes. Cardiac surveillance for cardiomyopathy and cardiac conduction abnormalities is suggested for nearly all of these conditions.[26,27,29,30]

in the limbs, usually predominantly affecting distal muscles.[32] Most of the patients described in the literature follow an autosomal dominant pattern of inheritance. CK levels may be normal or mildly elevated. Muscle biopsy reveals rimmed vacuoles. The genetic locus for this entity has not yet been determined.

CONGENITAL MYOPATHIES

Congenital Myopathies were originally clinically defined by nonprogressive weakness and hypotonia within the first year of life. The specific myopathies were named based on characteristic histologic features: centronuclear myopathy[33,34] nemaline myopathy,[35] and central core myopathy (**Fig. 2**).[36] In many of these cases, type 1 (oxidative/slow) fibers are small (hypotrophic) and constitute the majority of muscle fibers seen (thus, type 1 fiber predominance). When patients with congenital hypotonia and nonprogressive weakness are found to have type 1 hypotrophy and predominance without cores, nemaline bodies, or centralized nuclei, this clinicopathologic entity is known as congenital fiber type disproportion (CFTD).[37] These 4 histologic diagnoses have gradually being replaced with genetic diagnoses (**Table 4**). This has provided a genetic basis for the phenotypic variability that was seen with these pathologically defined entities.

Some patients develop weakness later in life but are found to have central nuclei or nemaline rods. Despite that their weakness was not congenital, by convention, these patients are still categorized as having a congenital myopathy.

CONGENITAL MUSCULAR DYSTROPHIES

In contrast to congenital myopathies, CMDs are defined as (1) progressive, (2) often having brain and other organ abnormalities, and (3) having nonspecific dystrophic changes on muscle histology. The list of genes associated with this class of muscle diseases is expanding but includes the genes shown in **Table 5**.[38] Many of the genes associated with CMDs, including *POMT1, POMT2, ISPD, GTDC2, B3GNT1, B3GNT2, POMGnT1, LARGE, FKRP, FKTN*, collagen VI (*COL6A1, COL6A2, COL6A3*), and laminin α2 (*LAMA2*), all play role in the interaction of α-dystroglycan with the extracellular matrix.

CONGENITAL MYASTHENIC SYNDROMES

Mutations in proteins that form the neuromuscular junction typically cause fluctuating weakness. Although these are often classified separately from myopathies, many of these genes are actually expressed within the muscle and many of these conditions may clinically resemble congenital myopathies and muscular dystrophies. Repetitive nerve stimulation and single-fiber EMG are often helpful in distinguishing these conditions from the other muscle diseases (discussed in this review). In addition, conditions that result in overactive neuromuscular transmission, such as slow channel syndrome and acetylcholinesterase (*COLQ*) deficiency, may demonstrate a repetitive (double-peaked) motor response. Treatment depends on the diagnosis, and response to treatment is variable. For completeness, a brief summary of these genes is provided in **Table 6**.[39,40] Several of these genes, including *DOK7* and *RAPSN*, have been established to result in late-onset weakness. Thus, the term, *congenital*, is used loosely in this article to indicate that the condition is genetic.

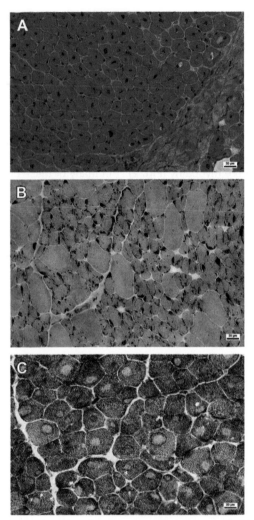

Fig. 2. (*A*) Hematoxylin-eosin stain of cryostat sections of a muscle biopsy from a patient with BIN1-associated centronuclear myopathy (original magnification ×200). Muscle fibers are cut in cross-section and demonstrate centralized in most fibers shown. (*B*) Modified Gomori trichrome stain of cryostat sections of a muscle biopsy from a patient with nemaline myopathy (original magnification ×200). The nemaline rods are mostly seen in the smaller type 1 fibers, which are more numerous than the larger type 2 fibers. Fiber typing demonstrated on myosin ATPase staining (not shown). (*C*) Reduced nicotinamide adenine dinucleotide–tetrazolium reducatase staining of cryostat sections of a muscle biopsy from a patient with RYR1 associated central core myopathy (original magnification ×200). The core structures are the circular regions of decreased staining.

METABOLIC MYOPATHIES

Metabolic myopathies may be divided into lipid metabolic disorders, glycogen metabolic disorders, and mitochondrial disorders.[41] Symptoms may be provoked by exercise or any factor that induces metabolic stress. A patient's dynamic symptoms may be superimposed on a static-progressive clinical course of weakness. Patients often

Table 4		
Congenital myopathies		
Type	**Genes**	**Features**
Centronuclear	*MTM1* *DNM2* *BIN1* *RYR1* *TTN*	Defined by the histologic finding of centrally located nuclei in a large proportion of fibers with radially oriented sarcoplasmic strands and a predominance of type 1 (oxidative) fibers.[33] The X-linked form associated with myotubularin (*MTM1*) is the most severe form that usually presents with severe congenital hypotonia. Ophthalmoplegia is almost always present, along with significant neck weakness. Dynamin-2 (*DNM2*) mutation, responsible for autosomal dominant centronuclear myopathy, is a much milder phenotype that typically presents with mild congenital hypotonia that slowly progresses over many decades. Some patients are so mild that they do not realize they have a myopathy until the fourth decade. Ptosis and mild extraocular weakness are common. *BIN1* is responsible for an autosomal recessive form, where onset of weakness is typically during early childhood with slow progression over the next 2–3 decades. Ophthalmoplegia is common. More recently, mutations in *RYR1*[33] and *TTN* have been described as causing autosomal recessive centronuclear myopathy; there is considerable phenotypic variability, however.
Nemaline	*ACTA1* *TPM3* *CFL2* *NEB* *TPM2* *KBTBD13* *TNNT1*	Associated with mutations in multiple genes.[35] With up to 25% of cases, actin alpha 1 (*ACTA1*) seems the most common cause of nemaline myopathy. The inheritance pattern may be recessive or dominant. Phenotypic variability is seen, ranging from severe congenital hypotonia to childhood onset. Marked facial weakness is common. Less common causes of nemaline rod myopathy include tropomyosin-3 (*TPM3*) (variable phenotypes, dominant or recessive), cofilin 2 (*CFL2*) (congenital, recessive), nebulin (*NEB*) (variable, but often congenital, recessive), β-tropomyosin (*TPM2*) (congenital, dominant), *KBTBD13* (childhood onset, dominant), and troponin T1 (*TNNT1*) (seen in Amish, recessive).
Cores	*RYR1* *SEPN1*	Myopathy that demonstrates cores on NADH staining of the muscle.[36] This condition is most strongly associated with mutations in ryanodine receptor 1 (*RYR1*). Weakness and hypotonia is often evident at birth, and progression is slow. Patients have an increased risk of malignant hyperthermia. Smaller core structures, called minicores, may be seen with mutations in selenoprotein N (*SEPN1*). The cores are not seen with all patients, however. The subtle phenotypic and histologic differences have resulted in *SEPN1* also being associated with CFTD and rigid spine muscular dystrophy (see **Table 5**). Patients with *SEPN1* mutations typically demonstrate weakness and hypotonia in early childhood, but progression is slow and CKs are usually normal. There is often prominent neck weakness and some respiratory insufficiency, however; thus, monitoring for decreased ventilatory capacity is crucial in the management of these patients.
CFTD	*ACTA1* *SEPN1* *TPM3*	Nonprogressive or slowly progressive congenital hypotonia and weakness with only type 1 predominance and hypotrophy on muscle biopsy.[37] Genes associated with CFTD have been associated with genes that are associated with nemaline myopathy (*ACTA1* and *TPM3*) and multiminicore myopathy (*SEPN1*). Thus, CFTD may represent a variant of these other congenital myopathies.

Abbreviation: NADH, Nicotinamide Adenine Dinucleotide-tetrazolium reductase.

Table 5
Congenital muscular dystrophies

Syndrome	Genes	Features
Walker-Warburg syndrome, muscle-eye-brain disease, and Fukuyama CMD	POMT1 POMT2 LARGE FKTN FKRP POMGnT1 ISPD GTDC2 B3GNT1 B3GNT2	Called α-dystroglycanopathies because all of these are believed due to defects in glycosylation of α-dystroglycan. Muscle biopsies show decreased immunohistochemical staining of glycosylated α-dystroglycan. Walker-Warburg syndrome, a severe phenotype of congenital hypotonia and brain malformations, has been associated with mutations in POMT1,[49] POMT2,[50] LARGE,[51] FKTN (Fukutin),[52] and FKRP.[53] ISPD, GTDC2, B3GNT1, and B3GNT2 have recently shown to also cause Walker-Warburg syndrome.[54–58] Muscle-eye-brain disease is a milder disease associated with mutations in POMGnT1.[59] Although all α-dystroglycanopathies may have cerebellar cysts, prominent cysts are a distinguishing feature of muscle-eye-brain disease. Fukuyama CMD[60] is found almost exclusively in Japan and is associated with founder mutation with a retrotransposon insertion in the FKTN gene. Fukuyama patients have typically a milder phenotype than muscle-eye-brain disease patients. Because of similar etiologies, these 3 phenotypes overlap to some extent, and genotype-phenotype correlation is occasionally challenging.[61]
Ullrich CMD/ Bethlem myopathy	Collagen VI (COL6A1, COL6A2, COL6A3)	Ullrich CMD results in congenital weakness that is slowly progressive with contractures that are out of proportion to the degree of weakness. Usually autosomal recessive. Dermatologic abnormalities include keloids and hyperkeratosis pilaris. Ventilatory capacity should be monitored regularly to screen declining function that requires noninvasive ventilation.[62] Bethlem myopathy, a milder form of this disease, presents later in childhood or adolescence.
Merosin deficiency	Laminin α2 (LAMA2)	Laminin is comprised of 3 polypeptides: α, β, and γ. The laminin trimer: α2, β1, γ1 (laminin 211) is known as merosin. Thus, laminin α2 (LAMA2) mutations are often referred to as merosin deficiency.[62] The phenotype is variable, but severely affected patients may present with loss of motor milestones within the first few years of life. Brain MRI demonstrates diffuse white matter hyperintensity and occasionally occipital cortical malformations. Contractures are common. Approximately 40% of patients develop epilepsy. Intelligence is often normal in these patients, however.
Rigid spine muscular dystrophy	SEPN1	These patients are on the spectrum of congenital myopathy and CMD, with mild progressive weakness.[62] SEPN1 patients often have rigid spine and scoliosis. These patients have progressive respiratory weakness that is out of proportion to the degree of limb weakness. Thus, frequent monitoring of ventilatory function is imperative.
L-CMD	Lamin A/C (LMNA)	A rare congenital/severe variant of LGMD 1B/autosomal dominant EDMD.[63] Progression is slow but, as seen with LGMD 1B, patients may have prominent contractures. Neck muscles are often weak. Cardiac conduction abnormalities are often seen in these patients and, thus, surveillance for arrhythmias should be conducted and defibrillator placement should be considered in patients who are deemed to be at risk for sudden death.[48]

Table 6
Congenital myasthenic syndromes

Location	Syndrome	Features	Treatment
Presynaptic	Choline acetyltransferase (*CHAT*)	Catalyzes the synthesis of acetylcholine. Reduced synthesis of acetylcholine results in periods of depletion, which clinically manifests with attacks of apnea. Worsened by cold temperatures.	Portable ventilator and apnea monitor, AchE inhibitors may be helpful.
Synaptic	*COLQ*	Acetylcholinesterase inactivates acetylcholine by cleaving it. *COLQ* is collagen-like subunit that anchors acetylcholinesterase to neuromuscular junction. *COLQ* deficiency prolongs the lifetime of acetylcholine in the synaptic cleft. Nerve conduction studies may demonstrate a repetitive (double peaked) CMAP in some patients. Cholinergic over-activity results in degeneration junctional folds of the neuromuscular junction. Clinical presentation is variable, but patients may have significant axial muscle weakness. Autonomic involvement may result in sluggish pupillary responses.	Albuterol
Postsynaptic	Slow channel (*CHRNA1, CHRNB1, CHRND, CHRNE*)	Autosomal dominant mutations in the acetylcholine receptor subunits (most commonly α) that result in prolongation of the open time. Nerve conduction studies may demonstrate a repetitive (double peaked) CMAP. Prolonged depolarization results in fewer channels that are open for activation.	Fluoxetine, quinine, or quinidine
	Fast channel (*CHRNA1, CHRNB1, CHRND, CHRNE*)	Autosomal recessive mutations in the acetylcholine receptor subunits that result in early closure after activation. Clinical severity is variable.	3,4-DAP and an AchE inhibitor
	AchR deficiency (mostly *CHRNE*)	Autosomal recessive mutations that result in a severe loss of acetylcholine receptor expression. Epsilon subunit mutations are most common because expression of the fetal gamma subunit may partially rescue a deficiency of the epsilon subunit. Deficiency of the other subunits is likely to be lethal.	AchE inhibitor and 3,4-DAP; may consider albuterol
	Rapsyn (*RAPSN*)	Isolated facial weakness is seen with E-box mutation of the promoter seen in the Middle Eastern Jewish patients. Mutations in the coding regions demonstrate a phenotype more typical of autoimmune myasthenia with less extraocular weakness.	AchE inhibitor and 3,4-DAP; may consider albuterol or ephedrine
	DOK7	Variable phenotypes, but limb-girdle weakness is common. Bulbar weakness with vocal cord paralysis, stridor, and swallowing difficulty are also common.	Ephedrine or salbutamol/ alberterol
	GFPT1	Limb-girdle weakness with tubular aggregates on muscle biopsy.	AchE inhibitor and 3,4-DAP

Abbreviations: AchE, acetylcholinesterase; AchR, acetylcholine receptor; CMAP, compound muscle action potential; 3,4-DAP = 3,4-Diaminopyridine.

are to describe what activities worsen or provoke symptoms. This information is useful in determining which diagnostic tests to order. If multiple organ systems seem involved, mitochondrial disorders should be considered.

Plasma carnitine, lactate, pyruvate, and CK levels should be checked. An exaggerated lactate response (relative to the pyruvate response) to exercise may be suggestive of mitochondrial disease because it implies overflow from a congested Krebs cycle. Muscle biopsy is often helpful in showing excessive glycogen (for glycogen disorders), excessive lipid droplets (for glycogen disorders), or ragged red fibers, which represent focal regions of mitochondrial clumping that result from mitochondria proliferation and dysfunction. The muscle tissue is also useful for biochemical testing of specific metabolic pathways. These diagnostic test helps determine which DNA testing can be performed to establish a definitive diagnosis.

A full discussion of metabolic disorders is beyond the scope of this review. **Table 7** highlights some of the more important disorders, including the few common disorders and some of the rare but treatable disorders.

PERIODIC PARALYSIS AND OTHER MUSCLE CHANNELOPATHIES

Mutations in muscle ion channels may manifest with intermittent weakness (periodic paralysis) or delayed relaxation (myotonia). The most well-established muscle channelopathies are detailed in **Table 8**.[42,43]

AUTOPHAGIC VACULOLAR MYOPATHIES

A small but growing number of muscle diseases are associated with defects of lysosomal storage.[44] A defect of myocyte lysosomal function may activate autophagy, a cellular reaction to starvation, [45] resulting in recycling of cellular organelles, resulting in the formation of autophagic vacolues that can be seen in the muscle biopsy.

The best-characterized autophagic vacuolar myopathies are Pompe disease, Danon disease, and X-linked myopathy with excessive autophagy (XMEA). Pompe disease is also considered metabolic myopathy and results from a defect of acid α-glucosidase, a lyososomal enzyme. Both infantile and late-onset forms have been described and treatment with parenteral enzyme replacement is available (see **Table 7**). Danon disease[46] is an X-linked condition that results from mutations in *LAMP2*. Danon patients demonstrate proximal weakness, hypertrophic cardiomyopathy, and delayed cognitive development during childhood. XMEA patients present with weakness during childhood that progresses slowly over decades. Mutations in *VMA21* have been associated with XMEA.[47] No other organs are known to be involved in XMEA.

DIAGNOSTIC APPROACH

Patients who have a textbook phenotype and are seen by an experienced clinician may be diagnosed with a minimal number of diagnostic tests. The remaining cases, however, require a more thorough evaluation with potentially many diagnostic tests.

The significant phenotypic variability seen in muscle disease makes it difficult to develop a robust universal diagnostic algorithm. The clinical history is the most useful starting point for clinicians who are trying to diagnose a genetic myopathy patient. Specifically, the distribution of weakness (proximal vs distal), age of onset (congenital, childhood, and adult onset), and other unique features (contractures, cardiac involvement, and central nervous system involvement) are important clues to establishing a clinical diagnosis. **Table 9** lists some important clinical features to consider in the

Table 7
Selected metabolic disorders associated with muscle disease

Syndrome	Features
CPT2	Carnitine palmitoyl transferase II (CPT2) deficiency is the most common lipid disorder. CPT2 transports acylcarnitine into the mitochondrial matrix for fatty acid metabolism.[41] Patients present with rhabdomyolysis with myoglobinuria after prolonged low-intensity (aerobic) exercise, fasting, or a febrile illness. Onset is usually in the second decade of life. Muscle CPT2 activity is low. The diagnosis can be confirmed with DNA sequencing of the CPT2 gene.
MADD	Multiple acyl–coenzyme A dehydrogenase deficiency (MADD) (or glutaric aciduria II) is a rare, autosomal recessive disorder that affects fatty acid metabolism. A subset of these patients may respond to riboflavin.[64] Riboflavin-responsive MADD may present during childhood or early adulthood with hypoglycemia and progressive weakness. Mutations in electron-transferring flavoprotein (ETFA and ETFB) and electron-transferring flavoprotein dehydrogenase (ETFDH) have also been described to cause MADD. These proteins are responsible for transporting reducing equivalents from the FADH2 to ubiquinone in the electron transport chain. Only milder cases of ETFDH deficiency, however, have been associated with response to riboflavin[65]
Carnitine deficiency	Primary carnitine deficiency is associated with mutations in SLC22A5,[66] which should result in abnormal plasma carnitine levels. Severe deficiency results in a neonatal disorder with multiorgan involvement but mild cases of chronic progressive muscle weakness exist as well. Treatment involves high doses of carnitine.
McArdle disease	The most common glycogen disorder is myophosphorylase (PYGM) deficiency.[41] Myophosphorylase cleavage glucose from glycogen molecules; a partial deficiency results in insufficient ATP generated within the muscle. Glycogen accumulates within the muscle as the patient ages. The patient has clinical episodes of rhabdomyolysis with myoglobinuria are usually elicited by anaerobic (high-intensity) exercise, but CKs are elevated even between episodes. A static-progressive course of muscle weakness develops with time as glycogen accumulates in the muscle tissue. Patients often work around episodes of painful cramps and rhabdomyolysis by consuming more simple sugars before exercise, and waiting for a second wind 10 minutes after beginning exercise,[67] which is the result of increased blood flow to the muscles.
Pompe disease	A deficiency of acid α-glucosidase (GAA), a lysosomal enzyme that cleaves glucose from glycogen. Treatment with parenteral enzyme replacement[68,69] dramatically slows progressive of disease and improves life expectancy.
Chronic progressive external ophthalmoplegia	Chronic progressive external ophthalmoplegia (CPEO)[41] often presents in the fourth or fifth decade of life with progressive ophthalmoplegia and proximal weakness. Large deletions of mitochondrial genome are often seen. In many of these cases, however, the underlying cause seems mutations in one of the nuclear genes (eg, POLG1) that regulate mitochondrial DNA repair. In the pediatric population, the CPEO phenotype is called Kearns-Sayre syndrome and is associated with cardiac conduction defects and pigmentary retinopathy. In contrast to adult CPEO, Kearns-Sayre syndrome patients usually have 2 populations of mitochondrial DNA: a normal-sized mitochondrial genome and a smaller genome with a single, large deletion. This deletion may have developed as a sporadic maternal germline mutation. As patients age, the smaller-sized mitochondrial genome replicates faster than the normal genome, thus accounting for the progressive symptoms seen in these patients.
Mitochondrial DNA point mutations	Mitochondrial point mutations (eg, MELAS and MERRF) may present with episodic symptoms triggered by metabolic stress. Muscle symptoms, however, are often mild compared with symptoms involving other organ systems.

Abbreviations: MELAS, Mitochondrial encephalomyopathy, lactic acidosis, and stroke-like episodes; MERRF, myoclonus epilepsy with ragged red fibers.

Table 8
Muscle channelopathies

Syndrome	Genes	Features
Myotonia congenita	CLCN1	Autosomal dominant or recessive mutations that result in in muscle stiffness. Symptoms improve with exercise. Dominant mutations usually affect upper limbs more than lower limbs, whereas the reverse is true with recessive mutations. Face and eyelids are usually spared in both.
Paramyotonia congenita	SCN4A	Autosomal dominant mutations that result in muscle stiffness that worsens with exercise and cold temperatures. Eyelids and face are often affected.
Sodium channel myotonia	SCN4A	Autosomal dominant mutations that result in muscle stiffness that does not worsen with exercise. Eyelids and face are often affected. Symptoms may worsen with potassium (potassium-aggravated myotonia) and/or respond to acetazolamide.
Hyperkalemic periodic paralysis	SCN4A	Autosomal dominant mutations resulting in fluctuating weakness with occasional episodes of severe paralysis. Weakness is correlated with elevated potassium levels. Patients often begin having symptoms in the first decade of life. Severe attacks usually last 1–4 h and occurring several times a week. Weakness may respond to acetazolamide.
Hypokalemic periodic paralysis	CACNA1S SCN4A	Autosomal dominant mutations resulting in fluctuating weakness with occasional episodes of severe paralysis. Weakness is correlated with low potassium levels. Patients often begin having symptoms in the second decade of life. Severe attacks may last days and occur less frequently than with the hyperkalemic variant. Weakness may also respond to acetazolamide.
Thyrotoxic periodic paralysis	KCNJ18[67]	Seen mostly in Asian men, patients with this condition have episodes of weakness associated with hyperthyroidism and hypokalemia. Patients are treated with potassium during attacks and β-blockers may prevent attacks.
Andersen-Tawil syndrome	KCNJ2	Periodic paralysis episodes are associated with low potassium levels. Patients may have short statures, low-set ears, micrognathia, dental abnormalities, wide-spaced eyes, clinodactyly, and cardiac conduction defects, including long QT.

diagnostic evaluation of genetic myopathy. In any patient with a suspected myopathy, a CK level should always be tested and standard nerve conduction studies and EMG should also be performed to confirm myopathic changes, rule out neurogenic disorders, and evaluate for myotonic discharges. Because congenital myasthenic syndromes can mimic myopathies and muscular dystrophies, repetitive nerve stimulation and/or single-fiber EMG may also be considered if these diagnoses are a possibility. Although the muscle biopsy often does not demonstrate histologic changes that are specific to a particular diagnosis, it should be performed in cases when the diagnosis is not obvious because it often provides some insight that helps navigate the diversity of diagnostic possibilities.

Table 9	
Clinical features to consider in diagnosing genetic muscle diseases	
Clinical Feature	**Consider**
Dynamic or episodic?	Congenital myasthenic syndromes Periodic paralysis Metabolic myopathies
Congenital onset?	Congenital myopathy CMD Congenital myasthenic syndromes
Extraocular weakness	Myotonic dystrophy type 1 Mitochondrial CPEO OPMD/OPDM Centronuclear myopathy Congenital myasthenic syndromes
Contractures	EDMD Bethlem (collagen VI) Merosin deficiency
Distal weakness	Distal myopathies Myotonic dystrophy type 1 FSHD
Proximal weakness	LGMD BMD Myotonic dystrophy type 2 Congenital myasthenic syndromes (*DOK7* and *RAPSN*)
Facial weakness	FSHD Nemaline myopathy Myotonic dystrophy type 1 OPDM

Recently, the use of next-generation sequencing has improved diagnostic yield. Undocumented DNA sequencing variants, however, are common, and thus clinical and pathologic correlation continues to play a vital role in establishing causality in these cases. Clinicians should also be aware that the current implementation of next-generation sequencing is limited by its inability to identify oligonucleotide repeat sizes, large deletions and duplications, intronic mutations, promoter mutations, and low heteroplasmy mitochondrial genome mutations. Awareness of these limitations ensures that appropriate alternative diagnostic testing is considered.

SUMMARY

There has been progress in the field of genetic muscle diseases over the past 20 years. The improved understanding of traditional muscular dystrophies has provided insight into optimal supportive treatment as well as potential novel genetic therapies. In addition, newly recognized genetic syndromes have been established. Although genetic testing has improved the efficiency and accuracy of the diagnostic algorithm for patients with muscular dystrophy, muscle biopsy, EMG, and other traditional diagnostic tests still play a significant role in the diagnostic evaluation of many of these patients.

A definitive genetic diagnosis in patients with muscle disease is imperative because it can help tailor preventive and supportive management of comorbid issues as well as any future treatments that may become available. Ultimately, optimal management will lead to improve longevity and quality of life for patients with genetic muscle diseases.

REFERENCES

1. Bushby K, Finkel R, Birnkrant DJ, et al. Diagnosis and management of Duchenne muscular dystrophy, part 1: diagnosis, and pharmacological and psychosocial management. Lancet Neurol 2010;9:77–93.
2. Barbujani G, Russo A, Danieli GA, et al. Segregation analysis of 1885 DMD families: significant departure from the expected proportion of sporadic cases. Hum Genet 1990;84:522–6.
3. Monaco AP, Bertelson CJ, Liechti-Gallati S, et al. An explanation for the phenotypic differences between patients bearing partial deletions of the DMD locus. Genomics 1988;2:90–5.
4. Bushby K, Finkel R, Birnkrant DJ, et al. Diagnosis and management of Duchenne muscular dystrophy, part 2: implementation of multidisciplinary care. Lancet Neurol 2010;9:177–89.
5. Nelson SF, Crosbie RH, Miceli MC, et al. Emerging genetic therapies to treat Duchenne muscular dystrophy. Curr Opin Neurol 2009;22:532–8.
6. Verhaart IE, Aartsma-Rus A. Gene therapy for Duchenne muscular dystrophy. Curr Opin Neurol 2012;25:588–96.
7. Finkel RS. Read-through strategies for suppression of nonsense mutations in Duchenne/Becker muscular dystrophy: aminoglycosides and ataluren (PTC124). J Child Neurol 2010;25:1158–64.
8. Cirak S, Arechavala-Gomeza V, Guglieri M, et al. Exon skipping and dystrophin restoration in patients with Duchenne muscular dystrophy after systemic phosphorodiamidate morpholino oligomer treatment: an open-label, phase 2, dose-escalation study. Lancet 2011;378:595–605.
9. Goemans NM, Tulinius M, van den Akker JT, et al. Systemic administration of PRO051 in Duchenne's muscular dystrophy. N Engl J Med 2011;364:1513–22.
10. van der Maarel SM, Miller DG, Tawil R, et al. Facioscapulohumeral muscular dystrophy: consequences of chromatin relaxation. Curr Opin Neurol 2012;25:614–20.
11. van Overveld PG, LEmmers RJ, Sandkuijl LA, et al. Hypomethylation of D4Z4 in 4q-linked and non-4q-linked facioscapulohumeral muscular dystrophy. Nat Genet 2003;35:315–7.
12. Lemmers RJ, van der Vliet PJ, Klooster R. A unifying genetic model for facioscapulohumeral muscular dystrophy. Science 2010;329:1650–3.
13. de Greef JC, Lemmers RJ, Camaño P, et al. Clinical features of facioscapulohumeral muscular dystrophy 2. Neurology 2010;75:1548–54.
14. Lemmers RJ, Tawil R, Petek LM, et al. Digenic inheritance of an SMCHD1 mutation and an FSHD-permissive D4Z4 allele causes facioscapulohumeral muscular dystrophy type 2. Nat Genet 2012;44:1370–4.
15. Sahenk Z, Mendell JR. The muscular dystrophies: distinct pathogenic mechanisms invite novel therapeutic approaches. Curr Rheumatol Rep 2011;13:199–207.
16. Klinge L, Eagle M, Haggerty ID, et al. Severe phenotype in infantile facioscapulohumeral muscular dystrophy. Neuromuscul Disord 2006;16:553–8.
17. Tawil R, Figlewicz DA, Griggs RC, et al. Facioscapulohumeral Dystrophy: a distinct regional myopathy with a novel molefular pathogenesis. Ann Neurol 1998;432:279–82.
18. Orphanet Report Series—Prevalence of rare diseases: Bibliographic data—November 2012-Number 1. Available at: http://www.orpha.net/consor/cgi-bin/Education.php?lng=EN.

19. Udd B, Krahe R. The myotonic dystrophies: molecular, clinical, and therapeutic challenges. Lancet Neurol 2012;11:891–905.
20. Wheeler TM, Thornton CA. Myotonic dystrophy: RNA-mediated muscle disease. Curr Opin Neurol 2007;20:572–6.
21. Wheeler TM, Leger AJ, Pandey SK, et al. Targeting nuclear RNA for in vivo correction of myotonic dystrophy. Nature 2012;488:111–5.
22. Bushby K. Diagnosis and management of the limb girdle muscular dystrophies. Pract Neurol 2009;9:314–23.
23. Ellis JA. Emery–Dreifuss muscular dystrophy at the nuclear envelope: 10 years on. Cell Mol Life Sci 2006;63:2702–9.
24. Zhang Q, Bethmann C, Worth NF, et al. Nesprin-1 and -2 are involved in the pathogenesis of Emery–Dreifuss muscular dystrophy and are critical for nuclear envelope integrity. Hum Mol Genet 2007;16:2816–33.
25. Gueneau L, Bertrand AT, Jais JP, et al. Mutations of the FHL1 gene cause Emery–Dreifuss muscular dystrophy. Am J Hum Genet 2009;85(3):338–53.
26. Liang WC, Mitsuhashi H, Keduka E, et al. TMEM43 mutations in Emery-Dreifuss muscular dystrophy-related myopathy. Ann Neurol 2011;69:1005–13.
27. Udd B. Distal myopathies – new genetic entities expand diagnostic challenge. Neuromuscul Disord 2012;22:5–12.
28. Hackman P, Sarparanta J, Lehtinen S, et al. Welander distal myopathy is caused by a mutation in the RNA-binding protein TIA1. Ann Neurol 2013;73:500–9.
29. Selcen D. Myofibrillar myopathies. Neuromuscul Disord 2011;21:161–71.
30. Sarparanta J, Jonson PH, Golzio C, et al. Mutations affecting the cytoplasmic functions of the co-chaperone DNAJB6 cause limb-girdle muscular dystrophy. Nat Genet 2012;44:450–5.
31. Brais B. Oculopharyngeal muscular dystrophy: a polyalanine myopathy. Curr Neurol Neurosci Rep 2009;9:76–82.
32. Durmus H, Laval SH, Deymeer F, et al. Oculopharyngodistal myopathy is a distinct entity: clinical and genetic features of 47 patients. Neurology 2011;76:227–35.
33. Romero NB, Bitoun M. Centronuclear mypoathies. Semin Pediatr Neurol 2011;18:250–6.
34. Ceyhan O, Agrawal PB, Hidalgo C, et al. Recessive truncating titin gene, TTN, mutations presenting as centronuclear myopathy. Neurology 2013;81:1205–14.
35. Wallgren-Pettersson C, Sewry CA, Nowak KJ, et al. Nemaline myopathies. Semin Pediatr Neurol 2011;18:230–8.
36. Jungbluth H, Sewry CA, Muntoni F. Core myopathies. Semin Pediatr Neurol 2011;18:239–49.
37. Clarke NF. Congenital fiber type disproportion. Semin Pediatr Neurol 2011;18:264–71.
38. Mercuri E, Muntoni F. The ever-expanding spectrum of congenital muscular dystrophies. Ann Neurol 2012;72:9–17.
39. Engel AG. Current status of the congenital myasthenic syndromes. Neuromuscul Disord 2012;22:99–111.
40. Chaouch A, Beeson D, Hantaï D, et al. 186th ENMC international workshop: congenital myasthenic syndromes 24-26 June 2011, Naarden, The Netherlands. Neuromuscul Disord 2012;22:566–76.
41. Berardo A, DiMauro S, Hirano M. A diagnostic algorithm for metabolic myopathies. Curr Neurol Neurosci Rep 2010;10:118–26.
42. Raja Rayan DL, Hanna MG. Skeletal muscle channelopathies: nondystrophic myotonias and periodic paralysis. Curr Opin Neurol 2010;23:466–76.

43. Ryan DP, da Silva MR, Soong TW, et al. Mutations in potassium channel Kir2.6 cause susceptibility to thyrotoxic hypokalemic periodic paralysis. Cell 2010;140:88–98.
44. Nishino I. Autophagic vacuolar myopathy. Semin Pediatr Neurol 2006;13:90–5.
45. Mizushima N, Levine B, Cuervo AM, et al. Autophagy fights disease through cellular self digestion. Nature 2008;451:1069–75.
46. Sugie K, Yamamoto A, Murayama K, et al. Clinicopathological features of genetically confirmed Danon disease. Neurology 2002;58:1773–8.
47. Ramachandran N, Munteanu I, Wang P, et al. VMA21 deficiency prevents vacuolar ATPase assembly and cause autophagic vacuolar myopathy. Acta Neuropathol 2013;125:439–57.
48. Sylvius N, Tesson F. Lamin A/C and cardiac diseases. Curr Opin Cardiol 2006;21:159–65.
49. Beltrán-Valero de Bernabé D, Currier S, Steinbrecher A, et al. Mutations in the O-mannosyltransferase gene POMT1 give rise to the severe neuronal migration disorder Walker-Warburg syndrome. Am J Hum Genet 2002;71:1033–43.
50. van Reeuwijk J, Janssen M, van den Elzen C, et al. POMT2 mutations cause alpha-dystroglycan hypoglycosylation and Walker-Warburg syndrome. J Med Genet 2005;42:907–12.
51. van Reeuwijk J, Grewal PK, Salih MA, et al. Intragenic deletion in the LARGE gene causes Walker-Warburg syndrome. Hum Genet 2007;121:685–90.
52. de Bernabé DB, van Bokhoven H, van Beusekom E, et al. A homozygous nonsense mutation in the fukutin gene causes a Walker-Warburg syndrome phenotype. J Med Genet 2003;40:845–8.
53. Beltran-Valero de Bernabé D, Voit T, Longman C, et al. Mutations in the FKRP gene can cause muscle-eye-brain disease and Walker-Warburg syndrome. J Med Genet 2004;41:e61.
54. Willer T, Lee H, Lommel M, et al. ISPD loss-of-function mutations disrupt dystroglycan O-mannosylation and cause Walker-Warburg syndrome. Nat Genet 2012;44:575–80.
55. Roscioli T, Kamsteeg EJ, Buysse K, et al. Mutations in ISPD cause Walker-Warburg syndrome and defective glycosylation of α-dystroglycan. Nat Genet 2012;44:581–5.
56. Manzini MC, Tambunan DE, Hill RS, et al. Exome sequencing and functional validation in zebrafish identify GTDC2 mutations as a cause of Walker–Warburg syndrome. Am J Hum Genet 2012;91:541–7.
57. Buysse K, Riemersma M, Powell G, et al. Missense mutations in β-1,3-N-acetyl-glucosaminyltransferase 1 (B3GNT1) cause Walker-Warburg syndrome. Hum Mol Genet 2013;22:1746–54.
58. Stevens E, Carss KJ, Cirak S, et al. Mutations in b3galnt2 cause congenital muscular dystrophy and hypoglycosylation of α-dystroglycan. Am J Hum Genet 2013;92:354–65.
59. Yoshida A, Kobayashi K, Manya H, et al. Muscular dystrophy and neuronal migration disorder caused by mutations in a glycosyltransferase, POMGnT1. Dev Cell 2001;1:717–24.
60. Kobayashi K, Nakahori Y, Miyake M, et al. An ancient retrotransposal insertion causes Fukuyama-type congenital muscular dystrophy. Nature 1998;394:388–92.
61. Taniguchi K, Kobayashi K, Saito K, et al. Worldwide distribution and broader clinical spectrum of muscle–eye–brain disease. Hum Mol Genet 2003;12:527–34.

62. Collins J, Bönnemann CG. Congenital muscular dystrophies: toward molecular therapeutic interventions. Curr Neurol Neurosci Rep 2010;10:83–91.
63. Mercuri E, Poppe M, Quinlivan R, et al. Extreme variability of phenotype in patients with an identical missense mutation in the lamin A/C gene: from congenital onset with severe phenotype to milder classic Emery-Dreifuss variant. Arch Neurol 2004;61:690–4.
64. Liang WC, Ohkuma A, Hayashi YK, et al. ETFDH mutations, CoQ10 levels, and respiratory chain activities in patients with riboflavin-responsive multiple acyl-CoA dehydrogenase deficiency. Neuromuscul Disord 2009;19:212–6.
65. Wen B, Dai T, Li W, et al. Riboflavin-responsive lipid-storage myopathy caused by ETFDH gene mutations. J Neurol Neurosurg Psychiatry 2010;81:231–6.
66. Vielhaber S, Feistner H, Weis J, et al. Primary carnitine deficiency: adult onset lipid storage myopathy with a mild clinical course. J Clin Neurosci 2004;11:919–24.
67. Braakhekke JP, de Bruin MI, Stegeman DF, et al. The second wind phenomenon in McArdle's disease. Brain 1986;109:1087–101.
68. Kishnani PS, Corzo D, Nicolino M, et al. Recombinant human acid [alpha]-glucosidase: major clinical benefits in infantile onset Pompe disease. Neurology 2007;68:99–109.
69. van der Ploeg AT, Clemens PR, Corzo D, et al. A randomized study of alglucosidase alfa in late-onset pompe's disease. N Engl J Med 2010;362:1396–406.

Clinical Neurogenetics
Neurologic Presentations of Metabolic Disorders

Jennifer M. Kwon, MD[a,b,*], Kristin E. D'Aco, MD[c]

KEYWORDS

- Metabolic genetics • Amino acid disorders • Organic acid disorders
- Urea cycle defect • Small molecule disorder • Inborn error of metabolism

KEY POINTS

- Inherited metabolic disorders are rare causes of neurologic disease, but they should always be considered because many are treatable.
- The characteristics of treatable metabolic disorders are:
  - Although their clinical presentations are often seen early in line with abrupt onset, these can present subacutely during later childhood and adult years
  - Episodic relapses
  - Nonspecific clinical/physical features
- Although many are identified through newborn screening programs, specific screening for inherited metabolic disorders remains useful.

Case

The patient was a previously healthy, successful attorney who developed social withdrawal and difficulty with calculations at age 45 years.[1] Over the subsequent months, he had problems with social interactions and became lost easily. Six months after presentation, he was alert but could not recall items after 5 minutes and had trouble initiating speech. His motor function, sensation, and coordination were normal.

His family history was notable for a brother who had developed progressive leg weakness and numbness with incontinence in his 30s. He had no dementia; he died of complications of frequent urinary tract infections.

The patient and his brother may have had dissimilar presentations but their brain magnetic resonance imaging (MRI) was notable for periventricular, nonenhancing, increased signal

(continued on next page)

---

[a] Division of Child Neurology, Department of Neurology, University of Rochester Medical Center, Rochester, NY, USA; [b] Division of Child Neurology, Department of Pediatrics, University of Rochester Medical Center, Rochester, NY, USA; [c] Division of Medical Genetics, Department of Pediatrics, Golisano Children's Hospital, University of Rochester Medical Center, Rochester, NY, USA
* Corresponding author. Division of Child Neurology, Department of Neurology, University of Rochester Medical Center, 601 Elmwood Avenue, Box 631 (Child Neurology), Rochester, NY 14642.
E-mail address: jennifer_kwon@urmc.rochester.edu

Neurol Clin 31 (2013) 1031–1050
http://dx.doi.org/10.1016/j.ncl.2013.04.005
0733-8619/13/$ – see front matter © 2013 Elsevier Inc. All rights reserved.

(continued)

abnormalities on T2-weighted imaging confluent in the occipital lobes (despite the brother's myelopathic presentation, his spine MRI was normal).

The patient's initial evaluation included cerebrospinal fluid (CSF) showing increased protein (61 mg/dL, normal 15–45 mg/dL), normal CSF immunoglobulin G index, and no oligoclonal bands. Thyroid and cortisol function were normal. Electroencephalogram (EEG) was normal. Hemoglobin; mean corpuscular volume; erythrocyte sedimentation rate; and vitamins E, B_{12}, and folate levels were normal.

Although the patient could have had an acquired condition, the family history suggested an inherited disorder of myelin. In this situation, neurologists should consider disorders arising from defects in metabolism at the organelle level, such as metachromatic leukodystrophy and peroxisomal disorders, or at the small molecule level, such as organic acidemias and urea cycle defects. Although the latter category of disorders are rare in neurologic practice, they are important because they are often treatable.

Additional testing showed plasma homocysteine, 220 μM (normal <20 μM) and methylmalonic acid, 1051 μM (normal <30 μM). These results helped to diagnose this patient with a form of combined methylmalonic aciduria (MMA) and homocystinuria caused by a cobalamin (Cbl) C defect. The patient showed improvement with cobalamin injections, a treatment that might have saved his brother's life.

SMALL MOLECULE DISORDERS: OVERVIEW

The small molecule disorders described later are caused by enzyme defects in pathways of intermediary metabolism (in contrast with the organelle disorders exemplified by lysosomal storage diseases).[2,3] These disorders tend to present early in life, often with abrupt onset with encephalopathy and metabolic crises. Apart from the history of obtundation, vomiting, acidosis, or hyperammonemia, there are few other physical or neurologic findings that are specific for these disorders.

Although they are rare causes of neurologic disease, they remain important because, with prompt identification, there can be effective treatment. For this reason, current newborn screening programs identify many of these conditions.

Disorders of small molecules that are particularly likely to be seen by neurologists include those associated with defects in amino acid metabolism: organic acidemias, aminoacidopathies, and urea cycle defects (**Fig. 1**). The diseases described in this article represent a subset of the biochemical genetic abnormalities likely to be encountered by neurologists. Certain treatable disorders, such as defects of fatty acid oxidation, are not included, despite their frequency in the population. Other disorders of small molecule metabolism will be are discussed as additional examples in which early treatments have the potential for better outcomes.

DEFECTS OF AMINO ACID METABOLISM
Introduction: Clinical Aspects

Disorders of amino acid metabolism tend to be sudden in onset, characterized by episodic relapses and remissions, with nonspecific physical findings. They may respond rapidly to appropriate treatment. If left untreated, many of these disorders develop a more chronic progressive neurologic picture reminiscent of disorders of organelle metabolism. Metabolic screening (**Tables 1** and **2**) in blood and urine may detect many small molecule disorders. In nearly all these cases, the short-term and

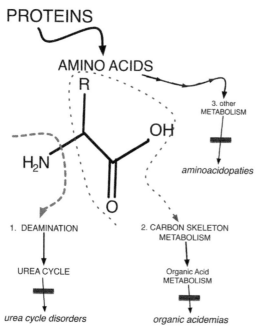

Fig. 1. Metabolism of amino acids proceeds by (1) deamination: removal of the amino group, which is then further metabolized in the urea cycle (eg, urea cycle defects), (2) metabolism of the carbon skeleton of the amino acid (eg, organic acidemias), or (3) transformation into other amino acids or compounds (eg, phenylalanine to tyrosine, in phenylketonuria). These steps are discussed in the text.

Table 1
Biochemical screening tests for identifying treatable disorders of amino acid metabolism

Test	Conditions Screened
Ammonia	Urea cycle defects, organic acidemias
PlAA	Aminoacidopathies, urea cycle disorders, some organic acidemias
UrOA	Organic acidemias, some aminoacidopathies
Plasma acylcarnitine profile	Organic acidemias

Abbreviations: PlAA, plasma amino acids; UrOA, urine organic acids.

Table 2
Clinical findings/presentations and the suggested tests to screen for treatable metabolic diagnoses

Test	Hypogly-cemia	Metabolic Acidosis	Hypoketotic Hypoglycemia	Seizures or Obtundation	Respiratory Alkalosis	Reyes Syndrome or Hepatic Encephalopathy
Ammonia	—	—	—	x	x	x
Plasma amino acids	x	x	—	x	x	x
Plasma acylcarni-tine	x	x	x	x	—	x
Urine organic acids	x	x	x	x	—	x

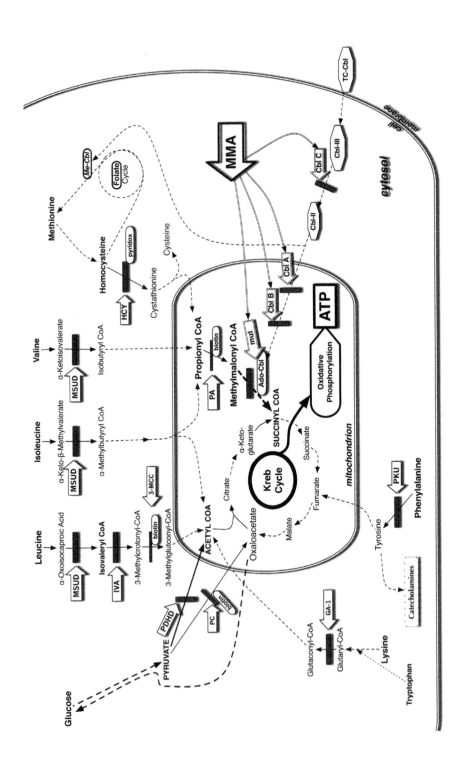

long-term medical and therapeutic management of these patients requires the involvement of specialists with expertise in metabolic disorders.

The tests listed in **Table 1** are often ordered together if a patient presents with a history of sudden deterioration or episodic relapses without other clinical findings or clues on initial screening evaluation. Certain associated findings, such as respiratory alkalosis or hypoglycemia, can narrow the list of screening tests further (see **Table 2**). Consultation with a genetic/metabolic specialist helps any time a metabolic condition is being considered but is essential if a patient is acutely ill or decompensating.

Organic Acidemias

1. Introduction (**Fig. 2, Table 3**)[4–8]
   a. Definition: disorders caused by enzyme deficiencies impairing the metabolism of amino acid carbon skeletons.
   b. Characteristics: symptoms caused by accumulation of organic acids upstream of the enzyme blockage, leading to metabolic acidosis (with anion gap) and hyperammonemia (secondary to impaired urea cycle function).
2. Clinical presentation
   a. Pathogenesis: accumulation of substances proximal to the enzyme block leads to metabolic acidosis and toxicity. Inhibition of N-acetylglutamate (NAG; **Fig. 3**) production occurs (possibly secondary to acetyl coenzyme A [CoA] depletion vs competition from accumulating propionyl CoA), impairing urea cycle reactions and leading to hyperammonemia.[9] Carnitine availability is also affected, restricting mitochondrial transport of fatty acids.
   b. Encephalopathy: caused by acidosis and hyperammonemia. In infants, tachypnea and hyperventilation are common, and seizures may also be seen.
   c. Bone marrow suppression may occur, likely caused by direct toxic effects of organic acids.
   d. Other late effects may include cardiomyopathy, nephritis/renal failure, and pancreatitis.
3. Diagnosis
   a. Abnormalities on urine organic acids (UrOA) testing together with other screening test results can suggest a specific metabolic diagnosis.
   b. For all the disorders of organic acids described later, there are more specific confirmatory diagnostic tests, usually of DNA or enzyme activity.
   c. Confirmation of these metabolic diagnoses requires the assistance of metabolic genetics specialists.

Fig. 2. Intermediary metabolism leads to ATP production. Pathways of intermediary metabolism of glucose and selected amino acids are shown as solid ⟶ (1 enzymatic step) or dashed - - ➔ (multiple enzymatic steps) thin arrows. All pathways lead to the Krebs cycle, which in turn drives oxidative phosphorylation to make ATP. Disorders are labeled in the open arrows ⟹ that point to dark bars ▬ identifying the location of the metabolic defect. Vitamin cofactors are shown as open ovals ⬭. Biotin, pyridox (pyridoxine), folate, Ado-cbl, and Me-cbl (two forms of cobalamin, or vitamin B_{12}). Cobalamin is transported across the cell membrane (transcobalamin [TC-Cbl]) and processed (Cbl-III, Cbl-II) to two active forms: adenosyl-cobalamin (Ado-Cbl) and methylcobalamin (Me-Cbl). Methylmalonic acidemia (MMA) is caused by methylmalonyl-CoA mutase (mut) deficiency. 3-MCC, 3-methyl crotonyl CoA carboxylase deficiency; Cbl A, B, or C: cobalamin processing defects type A, B, or C; GA-1, glutaric aciduria type 1; HCY, homocystinuria; IVA, isovaleric acidemia; MSUD, maple syrup urine disease; PA, propionic acidemia; PC, pyruvate carboxylase deficiency; PDHD, pyruvate dehydrogenase deficiency; PKU, phenylketonuria.

Table 3
Other organic acidemias (see Fig. 2)

Name	Enzyme Defect/Deficiency	Clinical Findings	Findings on Biochemical Screening (see Table 1)	Management
PA	Propionyl CoA carboxylase	1. Infants with classic PA present with encephalopathy, severe metabolic acidosis, hyperammonemia, and neutropenia 2. Imaging may show white matter and basal ganglia abnormalities 3. Later complications include cardiomyopathy, pancreatitis	Increased 3-hydroxypropionate, methylcitrate, tiglylglycine, and propionylglycine in UrOA Increased propionylcarnitine and glycine in blood	Similar to that for MMA. However, in PA, the administration of biotin may be helpful[4]
IVA	Isovaleryl-CoA dehydrogenase	Similar to presentation of MMA and PA, although often more mild. Urine of these infants is said to have a sweaty-feet odor 1. About half of patients have a late-onset, chronic form of the disease 2. Potential for normal outcome if disorder is promptly diagnosed and treated	Isovaleryl-glycine and isovaleric acid, in UrOA	1. Acute management is similar to MMA and PA, requiring parenteral fluids containing glucose and electrolytes 2. Long-term management requires glycine and carnitine supplementation with dietary restriction of leucine, and avoidance of fasting[4]
MCD	Two conditions: Biotinidase deficiency and HS deficiency can impair the 4 biotin-requiring carboxylase enzymes (**Fig 2** shows 3 of the enzymes; also see text)	1. Both forms are associated with hypotonia, seizures, lethargy, irritability, and laryngeal stridor 2. Biotinidase deficiency is a milder disorder that presents later than neonatal MCD caused by HS defects 3. Often there is alopecia and a skin rash similar to atopic dermatitis or seborrheic dermatitis.	3-Hydroxypropionate, 3-hydroxyisovalerate, and 3-methylcrotonylglycine in UrOA	Patients with HS and biotinidase deficiency respond well to high doses of biotin[5]

	4. Urine may have a strong (tomcat) odor 5. Later complications can include ataxia, optic atrophy and hearing loss 6. Without treatment, there may be episodes of metabolic acidosis with increased lactate and hyperammonemia		
GA-1 Glutaryl CoA dehydrogenase	1. Typically presents in infancy, when, after a period of normal development, the infant abruptly develops episodes of metabolic crises associated with hypotonia, dystonia, opisthotonus, and seizures 2. The child may have macrocephaly and involuntary movements 3. Often these episodes are precipitated by infections and illness; although there may be partial recovery, permanent injury may result 4. CNS imaging shows widened sylvian fissures and increased subarachnoid spaces commonly interpreted as cortical atrophy.[6,7] After a metabolic crisis, there may be atrophy of the caudate and putamen	Glutaric acid and 3-hydroxyglutarate in UrOA glutarylcarnitine in plasma acylcarnitines	1. This disorder can have an improved prognosis if the metabolic crises are managed appropriately with hydration, glucose, and carnitine supplementation to reverse the catabolic demands 2. Maintenance therapy consists of a lysine-restricted diet with carnitine (and possibly riboflavin) supplementation[6,7]

Abbreviations: CNS, central nervous system; HS, holocarboxylase synthase; MCD, multiple carboxylase deficiency.

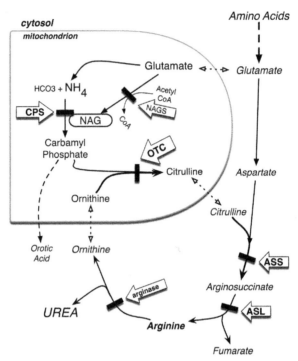

Fig. 3. Urea cycle. Pathways of the urea cycle are shown as solid ⟶ (1 enzymatic step) or dashed ⇢ (multiple enzymatic steps) thin arrows. Double-headed, dotted arrows ◁ ⋯ ▷ show amino acids that are transported between cytosol and mitochondrion. Disorders of the urea cycle are caused by deficiencies of enzymes labeled in open arrows ⇨ pointing to dark bars ▬ identifying the location of the metabolic defect. ASL, arginosuccinate lyase; ASS, arginosuccinate synthetase; CoA, coenzyme A; CPS, carbamoyl phosphate synthetase I; OTC, ornithine transcarbamylase.

4. Genetics: the disorders described here are inherited as autosomal recessive conditions. Carrier parents are unaffected. Siblings are at risk and genetic counseling should be sought.

Example: methylmalonic aciduria[4,8–10]; a common biochemical phenotype associated with early-onset and late-onset neurologic complications.
1. Definition: MMA has an incidence of 1/40,000. Several genetic defects can result in the increased production and excretion of methylmalonic acid, the most common being absent methylmalonyl-CoA mutase activity. Abnormal cobalamin processing (see **Fig. 2**) can present with MMA with or without increased homocysteine; the resulting disorders may respond to cobalamin supplementation.
2. Clinical findings
   a. Classic MMA (absent mutase) presents in neonates with acute encephalopathy including coma, lethargy, hypotonia, vomiting, respiratory distress, and poor feeding.
   b. Laboratory findings: severe metabolic acidosis, hypoglycemia, ketonuria, hyperammonemia, neutropenia, and thrombocytopenia.
   c. Imaging: may show damage to the basal ganglia (globus pallidus or putamen) or strokes. Extrapyramidal symptoms such as dystonia are a long-term problem in these patients.

   d. Later onset forms: when MMA presents after the neonatal period, the initial presentation may be nonspecific (isolated hypotonia or mild developmental delay) requiring additional metabolic screening to identify.

   e. Defects of cobalamin processing can cause neurologic symptoms such as adult-onset myelopathy, dementia, and psychiatric symptoms. The most common form, MMA Cbl C type,[10] has increases of both methylmalonic acid and homocysteine (see **Fig. 2**).

   f. Renal involvement is common in patients with mutase or Cbl B disease; end-stage renal disease may be the cause of demise in patients who survive the neonatal period. Acute or chronic pancreatitis is another common complication in patients with MMA.

3. Diagnosis is suggested by the presence of abnormal compounds (methylmalonic acid, 3-hydroxypropionate, 2-methylcitrate, and tiglylglycine) in UrOA; also, increased plasma methylmalonic acid, propionylcarnitine, and glycine.

4. Management
   a. Acute[4,10]:
     i. Correction of acidosis, hypoglycemia, hyperammonemia, and hypovolemia.
     ii. Carnitine and (for patients with Cbl A, B and C), cobalamin supplementation.
   b. Maintenance treatment includes protein restriction and avoidance of fasting.
   c. Some benefit from liver/kidney transplantation.

Aminoacidopathies

1. Introduction (see **Fig. 2**)
   a. Definition: caused by enzyme defects in amino acid metabolism identifiable on plasma amino acid (PIAA) assays.
   b. Characteristics: early encephalopathy without metabolic acidosis.
   c. Diagnostic tests: screening plasma (and sometimes urine) amino acids

2. Clinical presentation: varies with the enzyme involved.

3. Diagnosis:
   a. PIAA abnormalities can suggest a specific diagnosis.
   b. More specific testing exists for these disorders and should be considered in consultation with a metabolic specialist.

4. Genetics:

Example 1: phenylketonuria[11]

1. Definition: caused by defective phenylalanine hydroxylase (see **Fig. 2**). The most common treatable aminoacidopathy, with an incidence of 1/10,000.

2. Clinical findings
   a. Phenylketonuria (PKU) caused severe mental retardation before the widespread institution of newborn screening in the early 1960s.
   b. The increased phenylalanine (Phe) in PKU acts as a neurotoxin during early development, leading to severe, irreversible mental retardation.
   c. The effects of increased Phe can only be prevented by initiation of a phenylalanine-restricted diet within the first weeks of life. Thanks to newborn screening, prompt identification, and early treatment, children with PKU are able to avoid permanent mental retardation.
   d. An unintended consequence of screening and early treatment of PKU is that infants of mothers with PKU can develop birth defects if the women do not stringently control their Phe levels during pregnancy. The effects of maternal PKU include microcephaly, retardation, and cardiac anomalies.

3. Diagnosis: PKU is suggested by increased plasma phenylalanine.

4. Management: phenylalanine-restricted diet started within the first 10 days of life and maintained for life.

> Note: screening for PKU may also reveal other disorders of phenylalanine and tyrosine metabolism, including abnormalities of the tetrahydrobiopterin and dihydrobiopterin pathways[12] that may result in severe movement disorders and neurologic symptoms. Therefore, a positive screen for PKU prompts additional screening of blood and urine for tetrahydrobiopterin deficiency.

Example 2: homocystinuria[13,14]

1. Definition: caused by cystathionine beta-synthase deficiency. This enzyme requires pyridoxine (vitamin B_6) as a cofactor.
2. Clinical findings: tend to be worse in those who are not pyridoxine responsive. The accumulation of homocystine, a dimer of homocysteine, is associated with childhood onset of mental retardation, skeletal abnormalities including osteoporosis and marfanoid habitus, lens dislocation, marked myopia, and vascular disease with strokes and pulmonary embolism.
3. Diagnosis: suggested by increased homocysteine and homocystine in plasma.
4. Management:
   a. Pyridoxine-responsive patients likely have residual enzyme activity and may benefit from additional folate and cobalamin supplementation (see **Fig. 2**).
   b. Patients who do not respond to pyridoxine are placed on a methionine-restricted, cysteine-supplemented diet and may also receive betaine, a methyl donor that remethylates homocysteine to methionine. These treatments seem to lower the risk of intravascular thrombosis.[14]

Example 3: maple syrup urine disease[15]

1. Definition: caused by defects in the branched-chain α-keto acid dehydrogenase.
2. Clinical findings:
   a. Maple syrup urine disease (MSUD) is a rare disorder with an incidence of approximately 1/250,000.[15]
   b. The most typical time of presentation is in the early neonatal period. Infants develop feeding difficulties and decreased responsiveness in the first 1 to 2 weeks of life, after which there may be the development of stupor, respiratory abnormalities, myoclonus, posturing, and spasms. The characteristic odor of burnt sugar may be detected at this time.
   c. Imaging studies may show cerebral edema and the fontanelle may be full or bulging.
   d. Routine laboratory evaluation may show ketonemia/ketonuria, metabolic acidosis, and hypoglycemia.
   e. Less common presentations of MSUD include neonatal ophthalmoplegia (with or without other cranial nerve palsies) and hypotonia.
   f. Later in infancy, there may be episodic decompensations, including coma and signs of raised intracranial pressure, in the setting of more chronic failure to thrive and slowed development. At this stage, routine laboratory testing often does not show metabolic acidosis, so a high index of suspicion is required to make the diagnosis.
3. Diagnosis: the presence of alloisoleucine on PIAA analysis is pathognomonic and diagnostic for MSUD. There are also increases in leucine, isoleucine, valine, and in PIAA, and also increases in their keto acid derivatives in UrOA.
4. Management:
   a. The acute effects of MSUD require aggressive supportive measures including intravenous fluid hydration and dextrose administration, and branched chain amino acid–free parenteral nutrition solutions.

b. Maintenance treatment with branched chain amino acid–free formulas, low-protein diet, and avoidance of fasting.
c. Thiamine supplementation is beneficial in some cases.
d. Relapses can occur in the setting of illness or increased protein intake.
e. Although individuals with less typical presentations generally have some residual enzyme function, their overall prognosis may be poor if their disorder is unrecognized.

Urea Cycle Defects

The reactions of the urea cycle (**Fig. 3**)[16,17]:

1. Take nitrogen (in the form of ammonia and glutamate) and convert toxic ammonia (NH_4) into excretable urea.
2. Produce arginine, which is necessary for creatine and nitric oxide production.

Fig. 3 and **Table 4** show some of the clinically relevant urea cycle reactions. The initial steps of the urea cycle are intramitochondrial, and the rest occur in the cytosol. Glutamate is converted to N-acetylglutamate (NAG) by N-acetylglutamate synthase (NAGS). NAG activates carbamoyl phosphate synthetase I (CPS) to make carbamoyl phosphate from ammonia. Carbamoyl phosphate joined with ornithine via ornithine transcarbamylase (OTC) makes citrulline. Citrulline moves out of the mitochondria to the cytosol where arginosuccinate synthetase (ASS) condenses it with aspartate to form arginosuccinate, which is cleaved by arginosuccinate lyase (ASL) to form arginine and fumarate. As the final step in the cycle, arginine is cleaved by arginase to urea, which is excreted, and ornithine, which is transported from the cytosol to the mitochondria to restart the cycle.

Table 4 shows the clinical and distinguishing biochemical characteristics of selected urea cycle enzyme deficiencies of relevance to neurologists. CPS, OTC, ASS, and ASL deficiencies have similar clinical presentations in the neonatal period. Neonates with urea cycle defects (UCDs) generally appear normal for their first 24 hours of life and afterward become lethargic, with difficulty feeding. Vomiting, hypothermia, and hyperventilation develop. This presentation may seem similar to the organic acidemias or MSUD but, in the UCDs, there is no metabolic acidosis; these infants have respiratory alkalosis. They may also develop a bulging fontanelle and cerebral edema on cranial imaging. Routine laboratories studies are often unremarkable or may only show low blood urea nitrogen (as low as 1 mg/dL). Arginase deficiency is distinct in that it is characterized by a progressive spastic quadriparesis with mental retardation with less apparent hyperammonemia.

OTHER SMALL MOLECULE DISORDERS

Example 1: pyruvate dehydrogenase complex deficiency (see **Fig. 2**)[18,19]
1. Definition: caused by impaired function of one of the 3 components of the PDHC, which converts pyruvate into acetyl CoA, a crucial initial step of the tricarboxylic acid (TCA) cycle (**Table 5**). In pyruvate dehydrogenase complex (PDHC) deficiency, energy production from carbohydrate metabolism is severely reduced, and excess pyruvate is converted to lactate. The most common defect is in the alpha subunit of the E1 PDHC component, encoded on the X chromosome.
2. Clinical findings of PDHE1α deficiency:
   a. Male patients present with a spectrum of clinical phenotypes, depending on mutation:
      i. Severe neonatal lactic acidosis, often associated with brain malformations such as agenesis of the corpus callosum

Table 4
Urea cycle disorders: Biochemical findings and selected clinical characteristics

Enzyme Deficiency	Mode of Inheritance	Urine Orotic Acid	Plasma Citrulline	Clinical Characteristics and Treatment
CPS (also applies to NAGS)	AR	Low	Low	Within 24–72 h after birth infant becomes lethargic, needs stimulation to feed, and has vomiting, increasing lethargy, hypothermia, and hyperventilation; treat with intravenous arginine and Ammonul (sodium phenylacetate/sodium benzoate) during hyperammonemic crisis, may require dialysis to reduce ammonia. Routine management includes high-carbohydrate, low-protein diet; citrulline; nitrogen scavenging with sodium phenylacetate and/or sodium benzoate
OTC	X-linked	High	Low	Most common UCD; often lethal in boys; girls who present in the neonatal period may do poorly as well; girls may present later with episodic ataxia/intoxication syndrome, especially with illness or high protein load; later onset in men with liver failure and hyperammonemia has also been described; treat with intravenous arginine and Ammonul (sodium phenylacetate/sodium benzoate) during hyperammonemic crisis, may require dialysis to reduce ammonia. Routine management includes high-carbohydrate, low-protein diet; citrulline; nitrogen scavenging with sodium phenylacetate and/or sodium benzoate

ASS, usually called citrullinemia	AR	High	Very high	Episodic hyperammonemia, vomiting, lethargy, ataxia, seizures, eventual coma: treat with intravenous arginine and Ammonul (sodium phenylacetate/sodium benzoate) during hyperammonemic crisis. Routine management includes arginine administration to enhance citrulline excretion, and a nitrogen scavenging agent such as sodium benzoate
ASL	AR	High	High, with high arginosuccinate	Episodic hyperammonemia with a unique set of symptoms including hypertension, liver fibrosis, and developmental delay. Nitric oxide synthesis impaired. Increased plasma and cerebral spinal fluid argininosuccinate: treat with arginine and sodium benzoate
Arginase	AR	High	Normal	Very rare UCD: progressive spastic quadriplegia and mental retardation; ammonia and arginine high in cerebral spinal fluid and serum; arginine, lysine, and ornithine high in urine. Treatment includes diet of essential amino acids excluding arginine, and a low-protein diet

Abbreviations: AR, autosomal recessive; ASL, arginosuccinate lyase; ASS, arginosuccinate synthetase; CPS, carbamoyl phosphate synthetase I; NAGS, *N*-acetylglutamate synthase; UCD, urea cycle defect.

Table 5
Other treatable small molecule disorders

Name	Genetic Cause (Recessive Disorder, Unless Otherwise Noted)	Clinical Findings	Diagnosis	Management
Pyruvate carboxylase deficiency (see **Fig. 2**)	Caused by deficiency of the pyruvate carboxylase enzyme (*PC* gene), which converts pyruvate and CO_2 into oxaloacetate, essential for the Krebs cycle and gluconeogenesis	1. Infantile form (type A): primary lactic acidosis with developmental delay, failure to thrive, hypotonia, seizures, pyramidal tract signs, ataxia, nystagmus. Intellectual disability in survivors. Brain MRI may show symmetric cystic lesions and gliosis, hypomyelination, or hyperintensity of subcortical white matter 2. Neonatal form (type B): primary lactic acidosis with hepatomegaly, seizures, stupor, hypotonia, pyramidal tract signs, tremor or dyskinesia, and abnormal ocular behavior. Most die in infancy. Brain MRI may show ventricular dilatation, brain atrophy, or periventricular cysts 3. Intermittent form (type C): mildly delayed neurologic development and episodic metabolic acidosis	1. Lactate, pyruvate, ammonia, PIAA (increased alanine, citrulline, lysine, low aspartic acid and glutamine) 2. UrOA: ketone metabolites 3. CSF LP increased, CSF amino acids show increased glutamic acid and proline, low glutamine 4. Molecular testing of *PC* gene	1. Biotin supplementation (cofactor for PC enzyme) 2. Citrate and aspartic acid supplementation as Krebs cycle intermediates 3. Treatment of persistent acidosis with chronic bicarbonate therapy 4. Avoidance of ketogenic diet and fasting[20]

Pyridoxine-dependent seizures	Antiquitin (ALDH7A1)[21]	1. The classic presentation is an infant with severe neonatal seizures refractory to anticonvulsant therapy whose seizures respond both clinically and electrographically to large daily doses of pyridoxine (vitamin B_6) 2. Atypical cases include late-onset seizures (up to 2 y of age); seizures that initially respond to anticonvulsants and then become intractable; seizures during early life that do not respond to pyridoxine but are later controlled with pyridoxine 3. Mental retardation is common	1. 100–500 mg of intravenous pyridoxine stops both clinical and EEG seizures 2. Confirmed by finding increases in plasma and urine alpha-aminoadipic semialdehyde 3. Molecular testing of ALDH7A1 gene	1. Seizures are treated with high doses of daily pyridoxine 2. A related disorder of pyridoxine metabolism (PNPO deficiency) causing neonatal encephalopathy is treated with pyridoxal phosphate rather than pyridoxine[22,23]
Glucose transporter type 1 deficiency syndrome	Caused by impaired transport of glucose across the blood-brain-barrier caused by a mutation of a solute carrier family 2 gene (SLC2A1). Most affected have dominant (new) mutations	1. Children often present in early infancy with seizures and later develop hypotonia with a complex movement disorder. They have global developmental delay that may be nonprogressive 2. The clinical phenotype seems to be broad and should be considered whenever there is mental retardation with fluctuating ataxia, dystonia, motor incoordination, or altered consciousness	1. Low CSF glucose in the setting of normal blood glucose levels 2. CSF lactate is low. (distinguishes from mitochondrial disorders in which CSF lactate is high) 3. Molecular testing of SLC2A1 gene	Management: treatment with the ketogenic diet provides a consistent alternative fuel source, and has been shown to stop the seizures and may prevent other neurologic sequelae[24,25]

(continued on next page)

Table 5
(continued)

Name	Genetic Cause (Recessive Disorder, Unless Otherwise Noted)	Clinical Findings	Diagnosis	Management
Menkes disease	X-linked disorder of copper transport caused by mutations in a copper-transporting ATPase gene (*ATP7A*)	1. Boys with classic Menkes disease initially appear healthy but develop loss of developmental milestones, hypotonia, seizures, and failure to thrive at 2–3 mo of age 2. Characteristic facial features (sagging cheeks) and distinctive hair that is short, sparse, and twisted 3. Imaging of the brain may show atrophy of the hemispheres and tortuosity of blood vessels. Temperature instability and hypoglycemia may be present in the neonatal period 4. Death usually occurs by age 3 y 5. Another syndrome caused by *ATP7A* mutations that is distinct from Menkes is occipital horn syndrome, characterized by occipital horns (calcifications on the occipital bone), and lax skin and joints. Intellect is normal or slightly reduced	1. Low concentrations of copper and ceruloplasmin 2. 3-Hydroxypropionate, 3-hydroxyisovalerate, and 3-methylcrotonylglycine in UrOA 3. Molecular testing of *ATP7A* gene	1. There is no treatment of symptomatic affected infants 2. However, infant boys who are presymptomatically diagnosed and started on copper injections before 10 d of life may show improvement and even normal development[26,27]

Wilson disease (hepatolenticular degeneration)	Autosomal recessive disorder of copper transport caused by mutations in a copper-transporting ATPase gene (*ATP7B*)	1. Gradual copper accumulation in the liver, brain, kidney and cornea, presenting first with either: 2. Hepatic (childhood) presentation: acute hepatitis, jaundice, liver failure progressing ultimately to cirrhosis. Transaminases not as high as with viral or autoimmune hepatitis 3. Neurologic (adult) presentation: psychiatric symptoms, deterioration of handwriting, dysarthria, tremors, rigidity, swallowing dysfunction	1. Low serum ceruloplasmin and copper, increased urinary copper, increased liver copper 2. Molecular testing of *ATP7B* gene	1. Copper chelation with penicillamine or trientine, zinc to interfere with copper absorption, avoidance of high copper–containing foods 2. Liver transplant for those who cannot tolerate medical therapy[28]
Creatine deficiency syndromes (3 forms)	Caused by defects in (1) creatine biosynthesis (AGAT deficiency or GAMT deficiency), or (2) creatine transport (*SLC6A8*), an X-linked disorder	1. All 3 forms lead to a nonspecific syndrome of mental retardation, global delays, and epilepsy 2. In GAMT deficiency, the epilepsy may be intractable and patients may also develop a movement disorder with basal ganglia abnormalities on MRI	1. Magnetic resonance spectroscopy shows deficient creatine peak 2. Measurement of guanidinoacetate, creatine, and creatinine in urine and plasma 3. Molecular testing of causative genes	The creatine depletion and clinical effects of GAMT and AGAT deficiency (but not the transporter defect) may be partially reversed with creatine supplementation[29]

Abbreviations: AGAT, arginine:glycine amidinotransferase; *ALDH7A1*, aldehyde dehydrogenase 7 family member A1; GAMT, guanidinoacetate methyltransferase; LP, lactate and pyruvate; PNPO, pyridoxine-5'-phosphate oxidase.

　　　　ii. Leigh encephalopathy, presenting in the first few years of life with apnea; intermittent weakness/ataxia; absent reflexes; lower limb dystonia; progressive, severe developmental delay; and characteristic brain MRI findings

　　　　iii. Intermittent ataxia, worse after carbohydrate-rich meals, progressing slowly into a milder Leigh encephalopathy

　　b. Female patients typically have seizures (infantile spasms and myoclonic seizures are common), microcephaly, spasticity, mental retardation, and dysmorphic facial features. Abnormal brain MRI findings are common. Severity may be based on distribution of X-inactivation.

3. Diagnosis:

　　a. Increased blood and CSF lactate and pyruvate (LP). LP ratio is usually normal. LP increases in the setting of carbohydrate loading.

　　b. Alanine increased in PIAA. UrOA may show increased LP.

　　c. Enzyme can be measured in skin biopsy fibroblasts or leukocytes; may be inconclusive in affected female patients

　　d. PDHE1α mutational analysis may be especially helpful in diagnosing female patients

4. Management: ketogenic diet and thiamine supplementation may lead to clinical improvement and longer survival.

SUMMARY

The treatable disorders of metabolism described earlier are collectively rare in neurology practice. Patients with epilepsy, intellectual disability, and movement disorders are more likely to have specific genetic diagnoses made using the newer and much-heralded next-generation sequencing techniques. However, the disorders described earlier, whose screening (see **Tables 1** and **2**) is rapid, straightforward, and inexpensive, all have treatments that can radically alter the course of their conditions, which is in contrast with other genetic diagnoses that promise information but little in the way of diagnosis-specific therapies.

　　In the United States and in many other countries, there are newborn screening programs to identify this same group of disorders, namely those that present early in life, are serious, and are treatable. However, these screening efforts are new, and they do not include all of the treatable conditions mentioned earlier. Newborn screening programs in the United States are state managed, leading to regional variations in clinical follow-up and care. Furthermore, as the case discussed earlier shows, some patients present as adults who were born before the era of widespread screening for metabolic disorders. For these reasons, it is preferable to repeat metabolic screening tests, even if the newborn screen was known to be normal, if testing seems clinically indicated.

REFERENCES

1. This case of two brothers was adapted from a case report Powers JM, Rosenblatt DS, Schmidt RE, et al. Neurological and neuropathologic heterogeneity in two brothers with cobalamin C deficiency. Ann Neurol 2001;49:396–400.

2. For this review, as in their clinical practices, the authors relied on the excellent and current disease-specific reviews (eg, organic acidurias, homocystinuria, pyridoxine-dependent epilepsy) in GeneReviews. Available at: www.ncbi.nlm. nih.gov/sites/GeneTests/review. Accessed January 2, 2013.

3. Fernandes J, Saudubray JM, van den Berghe G, et al, editors. Inborn metabolic diseases: diagnosis and treatment. 4th edition. Heidelberg (Germany): Springer Medizin Verlag; 2006.

4. Knerr I, Weinhold N, Vockley J, et al. Advances and challenges in the treatment of branched-chain amino/keto acid metabolic defects. J Inherit Metab Dis 2012;35: 29–40.
5. Wolf B. Clinical issues and frequent questions about biotinidase deficiency. Mol Genet Metab 2010;100:6–13.
6. Kolker S, Christensen E, Leonard JV, et al. Diagnosis and management of glutaric aciduria type I – revised recommendations. J Inherit Metab Dis 2011;34:677–94.
7. Hedlund GL, Longo N, Pasquali M. Glutaric acidemia type 1. Am J Med Genet C Semin Med Genet 2006;142C:86–94.
8. Vockley J, Zschocke J, Knerr I, et al. Branched chain organic acidurias. In: Valle D, Beaudet AL, Vogelstein B, et al, editors. Scriver's online metabolic and molecular bases of inherited disease. 2006. Available at: http://dx.doi.org/10.1036/ommbid.172. Accessed January 2, 2013.
9. Stewart PM, Walser M. Failure of the normal ureagenic response to amino acids in organic acid-loaded rats: proposed mechanism for the hyperammonemia of propionic and methylmalonic acidemia. J Clin Invest 1980;66:484–92.
10. Carrillo-Carrasco N, Chandler RJ, Venditti CP. Combined methylmalonic acidemia and homocystinuria, cblC type. I. Clinical presentations, diagnosis and management. J Inherit Metab Dis 2012;35:95–102.
11. Blau N, van Spronsen FJ, Levy HL. Phenylketonuria. Lancet 2010;376:1417–27.
12. Blau N, Hennermann JB, Langenbeck U, et al. Diagnosis, classification, and genetics of phenylketonuria and tetrahydrobiopterin (BH4) deficiencies. Mol Genet Metab 2011;104:S2–9.
13. Picker JD, Levy HL. Homocystinuria caused by cystathionine beta-synthase deficiency. 2004 Jan 15 [Updated 2011 Apr 26]. In: Pagon RA, Bird TD, Dolan CR, et al, editors. GeneReviews. Seattle (WA): University of Washington; 1993 [Internet]. Available at: http://www.ncbi.nlm.nih.gov/books/NBK1524/. Accessed January 2, 2013.
14. Yap S. Classical homocystinuria: vascular risk and its prevention. J Inherit Metab Dis 2003;26:259–65.
15. Strauss KA, Puffenberger EG, Morton DH. Maple syrup urine disease. 2006 Jan 30 [Updated 2009 Dec 15]. In: Pagon RA, Bird TD, Dolan CR, et al, editors. GeneReviews. Seattle (WA): University of Washington; 1993 [Internet]. Available at: http://www.ncbi.nlm.nih.gov/books/NBK1319/. Accessed January 2, 2013.
16. Nassogne MC, Heron B, Touati G, et al. Urea cycle defects: management and outcome. J Inherit Metab Dis 2005;28:407–14.
17. Lanpher BC, Gropman A, Chapman KA, et al. Urea cycle disorders overview. 2003 Apr 29 [Updated 2011 Sep 1]. In: Pagon RA, Bird TD, Dolan CR, et al, editors. GeneReviews. Seattle (WA): University of Washington; 1993 [Internet]. Available at: http://www.ncbi.nlm.nih.gov/books/NBK1217/. Accessed January 2, 2013.
18. Patel KP, O'Brien TW, Subramony SH, et al. The spectrum of pyruvate dehydrogenase complex deficiency: clinical, biochemical and genetic features in 371 patients. Mol Genet Metab 2012;105:34–43.
19. Prasad C, Rupar T, Prasad AN. Pyruvate dehydrogenase deficiency and epilepsy. Brain Dev 2011;33:856–65.
20. Wang D, De Vivo D. Pyruvate carboxylase deficiency. 2009 Jun 2 [Updated 2011 Jul 21]. In: Pagon RA, Bird TD, Dolan CR, et al, editors. GeneReviews. Seattle (WA): University of Washington; 1993 [Internet]. Available at: http://www.ncbi.nlm.nih.gov/books/NBK6852/. Accessed January 2, 2013.
21. Mills PB, Struys E, Jakobs C, et al. Mutations in antiquitin in individuals with pyridoxine-dependent seizures. Nat Med 2006;12:307–9.

22. Gospe SM. Pyridoxine-dependent seizures: new genetic and biochemical clues to help with diagnosis and treatment. Curr Opin Neurol 2006;19:148–53.

23. Mills PB, Surtees RA, Champion MP, et al. Neonatal epileptic encephalopathy caused by mutations in the PNPO gene encoding pyridox(am)ine 50-phosphate oxidase. Hum Mol Genet 2005;14:1077–86.

24. Klepper J. Impaired glucose transport into the brain: the expanding spectrum of glucose transporter type 1 deficiency syndrome. Curr Opin Neurol 2004;17:193–6.

25. Klepper J. GLUT1 deficiency in clinical practice. Epilepsy Res 2012;100:272–7.

26. Kaler SG, Holmes CS, Goldstein DS, et al. Neonatal diagnosis and treatment of Menkes disease. N Engl J Med 2008;358:605–14.

27. Kaler SG. ATP7A-related copper transport disorders. 2003 May 9 [Updated 2010 Oct 14]. In: Pagon RA, Bird TD, Dolan CR, et al, editors. GeneReviews. Seattle (WA): University of Washington; 1993 [Internet]. Available at: http://www.ncbi. nlm.nih.gov/books/NBK1413/. Accessed January 2, 2013.

28. Lorincz MT. Neurologic Wilson's disease. Ann N Y Acad Sci 2010;1184:173–87.

29. Almeida LS, Verhoeven NM, Roos B, et al. Creatine and guanidinoacetate: diagnostic markers of inborn errors in creatine biosynthesis and transport. Mol Genet Metab 2004;82:214–9.

Clinical Neurogenetics
Neuropathic Lysosomal Storage Disorders

Gregory M. Pastores, MD[a,b,*], Gustavo H.B. Maegawa, MD, PhD[c]

KEYWORDS

- Lysosomal storage disorders • Stroke • Myopathy • Leukodystrophy

KEY POINTS

- Patients with a lysosomal storage disorder may present with neurologic problems, such as developmental delay, myoclonic seizures, ataxia, or stroke, and the absence of features (eg, hepatosplenomegaly) suggestive of an underlying storage disorder may lead to misdiagnosis.
- Diagnosis can be readily confirmed by blood tests, although testing may be limited to specialized laboratories.
- Carrier testing and preimplantation or prenatal diagnosis are available options for carrier couples at risk of having an affected child.
- Treatment is available for certain subtypes and early diagnosis and intervention is critical in enabling optimal outcomes. Although ultimate neurologic prognosis may not be fully modified, available therapies can improve quality of life.
- Elucidation of pathophysiology is shedding light on disease mechanisms that may be broadly applicable to the understanding of more common disorders, such as Parkinson disease and other neurodegenerative disorders.
- Several novel therapeutic strategies, such as substrate reduction therapy, use of pharmacologic chaperones, and gene therapy, are being pursued to expand the number of potentially treatable conditions.

INTRODUCTION
Definition

The lysosome is a subcellular organelle with an acidified milieu, wherein metabolites that are generated as a byproduct of cellular turnover are directed for degradation.[1] Deficiency of a particular enzyme or its cofactor results in the accumulation of various

[a] Departments of Neurology and Pediatrics, New York University School of Medicine, NYU at Rivergate, 403 East 34th Street, 2nd Floor, New York, NY 10016, USA; [b] Neurogenetics Laboratory, New York University School of Medicine, NYU at Rivergate, 403 East 34th Street, 2nd Floor, New York, NY 10016, USA; [c] Department of Pediatrics, McKusick-Nathans Institute of Genetic Medicine, The Johns Hopkins University School of Medicine, 733 North Broadway, Room 409, Baltimore, MD 21205, USA
* Corresponding author. Department of Neurology, New York University School of Medicine, NYU at Rivergate, 403 East 34th Street, 2nd Floor, New York, NY 10016.
E-mail address: gregory.pastores@nyumc.org

Neurol Clin 31 (2013) 1051–1071
http://dx.doi.org/10.1016/j.ncl.2013.04.007
0733-8619/13/$ – see front matter © 2013 Elsevier Inc. All rights reserved.

substrates within the lysosome, which initiate a cascade of cellular events including aberrant inflammatory and apoptotic responses. Affected individuals may present with clinical signs of tissue storage, such as hepatosplenomegaly or cardiomyopathy, although these may not be evident in those with predominant neuropathic involvement, in whom developmental delay and subsequent regression develop.[2,3] Neuronopathic subtypes, particularly those without overt visceral signs, are often associated with delayed or missed diagnoses, particularly in adult-onset cases and in the absence of a family history. **Tables 1** and **2** list the various lysosomal storage disorders (LSDs), the underlying gene affected, and its respective locus.

Symptoms and Clinical Course

The LSDs are mainly chronic conditions, and clinical problems may evolve over years to decades. In contrast to other inborn errors of metabolism due to defects in intermediate metabolism (such as amino acidopathies, organic acidurias, and fatty acid oxidation defects), the onset of symptoms in LSDs has no temporal relationship to diet or the fasting state.

Age of onset can be broad, with nonimmune hydrops evident at birth, ataxia or spasticity in childhood, and stroke in a young adult without any antecedent risk factors (eg, hypertension, atherosclerosis). Clinical signs, such as the cherry red spot (**Table 3**) or leukodystrophy evident on brain magnetic resonance imaging (MRI), serve as clues to particular clinical forms. Deafness can be a feature of LSDs and can be conductive, sensorineural, or a combination, with involvement of cochlea and central nervous system dysfunction.

Extraneurologic findings can also be instructive (eg, cardiomyopathy in an infant with hypotonia [Pompe disease] or young adult with Fabry disease). **Table 4** lists several clinical features associated with particular LSDs. As noted, there often is multisystemic disease, following a pattern often reflecting the tissue sites of substrate storage.

Late-onset forms of G_{M2}-gangliosidosis and metachromatic leukodystrophy (MLD) may present with impaired intellectual function, emotional lability, hallucinations, and delusions that may initially be attributed to a psychiatric diagnosis.[4,5]

Nature of Disease

Although individually infrequent to rare, collectively the LSDs have a combined prevalence of approximately 1 in 2000.[6,7] Certain entities are overrepresented in particular populations, such as the Ashkenazi Jews (of Central and Eastern European descent) and those of Finnish ancestry, as a consequence of founder effect (**Table 5**).[8]

CLINICAL FINDINGS
Physical Examination

Nonimmune hydrops fetalis may be evident at birth in several conditions (**Box 1**).[9] Dysmorphic features may develop in childhood, primarily in the mucopolysaccharidoses (MPS) and oligosaccharidoses, although these can be subtle in attenuated cases.[10] However, most conditions, particularly those with predominant neurologic involvement, are not associated with distinctive facies. In these cases, affected children may display developmental delay, speech problems, and ataxia. Peripheral neuropathy can also be a problem, and tissue infiltration in the MPS and oligosaccharidoses can lead to carpal tunnel syndrome or a radiculopathy.[11,12] In patients with certain later onset LSDs, psychiatric features may be a presenting complaint.[13]

Table 1
Enzyme-deficiency LSDs, classified according to primary substrate storage

Disease	Defective Protein	Main Storage Materials	Gene and Locus	OMIM
Sphingolipidoses				
Fabry	α-Galactosidase A	Globotriasylceramide	GLA Xq22	301500
Farber	Acid ceramidase	Ceramide	ASAH1 8p22	228000
Gangliosidosis G$_{M1}$ (types I, II, III)	G$_{M1}$-β-galactosidase	G$_{M1}$ ganglioside, Keratan sulfate, oligos, glycolipids	PSAP 10q22.1	230500 230600 230650
Gangliosidosis G$_{M2}$, Tay-Sachs variant	β-Hexosaminidase A	G$_{M2}$ ganglioside, oligos, glycolipids	HEXA 15q23	272800
Gangliosidosis G$_{M2}$, Sandhoff variant	β-Hexosaminidase A+ B	G$_{M2}$ ganglioside, oligos, glycolipids	HEXB 5q13	268800
Gaucher (types I, II, III)	Glucosylceramidase	Glucosylceramide	GBA 1q21	230800 230900 231000
Krabbe	β-Galactosylceramidase	Galactosylceramide	GALC 14q31.3	245200
Metachromatic leukodystrophy	Arylsulphatase A	Sulphatides	ARSA 22q13.33	250100
Niemann-Pick (type A, type B)	Sphingomyelinase	Sphingomyelin	SMPD1 11p15.4	257200 607616

(continued on next page)

Table 1
(continued)

Disease	Defective Protein	Main Storage Materials	Gene and Locus	OMIM
Mucopolysaccharidoses (MPSs)				
MPS I (Hurler, Scheie, Hurler/Scheie)	α-Iduronidase	Dermatan sulfate, heparan sulfate	IDUA 4p16.3	607014 607015 607016
MPS II (Hunter)	Iduronate sulphatase	Dermatan sulfate, heparan sulfate	IDS Xq28	309900
MPS III A (Sanfilippo A)	Heparan sulphamidase	Heparan sulfate	SGSH 17q25.3	252900
MPS III B (Sanfilippo B)	Acetyl α-glucosaminidase	Heparan sulfate	NAGLU 17q21.2	252920
MPS III C (Sanfilippo C)	Acetyl CoA: α-glucosaminide N-acetyltransferase	Heparan sulfate	HGSNAT 8p11.21	252930
MPS III D (Sanfilippo D)	N-acetyl glucosamine-6-sulphatase	Heparan sulfate	GNS 12q14.3	252940
MPS IVA (Morquio A)	Acetyl galactosamine-6-sulphatase	Keratan sulfate, chondroitin 6-sulfate	GALNS 16q24.3	253000
MPS IV B (Morquio B)	β-Galactosidase	Keratan sulfate	GLB1 3p22.3	253010
MPS VI (Maroteaux-Lamy)	Acetyl galactosamine 4-sulphatase (arylsulphatase B)	Dermatan sulfate	ARSB 5q14.1	253200
MPS VII (Sly)	β-Glucuronidase	Dermatan sulfate, heparan sulfate, chondroitin 6-sulfate	GUSB 7q11.21	253220
MPS IX (Natowicz)	Hyaluronidase	Hyluronan	HYAL1 3p21.31	601492

Olygosaccharidoses (glycoproteinoses)

Disorder	Enzyme	Substrate	Gene/Locus	OMIM
Aspartylglicosaminuria	Glycosylasparaginase	Aspartylglucosamine	*AGA* 4q34.3	208400
Fucosidosis	α-Fucosidase	Glycoproteins, glycolipids, Fucoside-rich oligos	*FUCA1* 1p36.11	230000
α-Mannosidosis	α-Mannosidase	Mannose-rich oligos	*MANSA* 19p13.2	248500
β-Mannosidosis	β-Mannosidase	Man(β1 → 4)GlnNAc	*MANBA* 4q24	248510
Schindler	N-acetylgalactosaminidase	Sialylated/asialaglycopeptides, glycolipids	*NAGA* 22q13.2	609241
Sialidosis	Neuraminidase	Oligos, glycopeptides	*NEU1* 6p21.33	256550

Glycogenoses

Disorder	Enzyme	Substrate	Gene/Locus	OMIM
Glycogenosis II/Pompe	α1,4-Glucosidase (acid maltase)	Glycogen	*GAA* 17q25.3	232300

Lipidoses

Disorder	Enzyme	Substrate	Gene/Locus	OMIM
Wolman/CESD	Acid lipase	Cholesterol esters	*LIPA* 10q23.31	278000

Table 2
Other LSDs, classified according to underlying molecular defect disease

Disease	Defective Protein	Main Storage Materials	Gene and Locus	OMIM
Nonenzymatic lysosomal protein defects				
Gangliosidosis G_{M2}, activator defect	G_{M2} activator protein	G_{M2} ganglioside, oligos	GMA2A 5q13.3	272750
Metachromatic leukodystrophy	Saposin B	Sulphatides	PSAP 10q22.1	249900
Krabbe	Saposin A	Galactosylceramide	PSAP 10q22.1	611722
Gaucher	Saposin C	Glucosylceramide	PSAP 10q22.1	610539
Transmembrane protein defects				
Sialic acid storage disease; infantile form (ISSD) and adult form (Salla)	Sialin	Sialic acid	SLC17A5 6q13	269920 604369
Cystinosis	Cystinosin	Cystine	CTNS 17p13.2	219800
Niemann-Pick type C1	Niemann-Pick type 1 (NPC1)	Cholesterol and sphingolipids	NPC1 18q11.2	257220
Niemann-Pick type C2	Niemann-Pick type 2 (NPC2)	Cholesterol and sphingolipids	NPC2 14q24.3	607625
Structural proteins				
Danon	Lysosome-associated membrane protein 2	Cytoplasmatic debris and glycogen	LAMP2A Xq24	300257
Mucolipidosis IV	Mucolipin	Sulphatides, glycolipids, GAGs	TRMPL1 19p13.2	252650

Lysosomal enzyme protection defect

Galactosialidosis	Protective protein cathepsin A	Sialyloligosaccharides	*CTSA* 20q13.12	256540

Posttranslational processing defect

Multiple sulphatase deficiency	Multiple sulphatase	Sulphatides, glycolipids, GAGs	*SUMF1* 3p26.1	272200

Trafficking defect in lysosomal enzymes

Mucolipidosis IIα/β, IIIα/β	GlcNAc-1-P transferase	Oligos, GAGs, lipids	*GNPTAB* 12q23.2	252500 252600
Mucolipidosis IIIγ	GlcNAc-1-P transferase	Oligos, GAGs, lipids		232605

Polypeptide degradation defect

Pycnodysostosis	Cathepsin K	Type I collagen (major component of long bone), and type II collagen (major component of cartilage)	*CTSK* 1q21.3	265800

Neuronal ceroid lipofuscinoses (NCLs)

NCL 1	Palmitoyl protein thioesterase (PPT1)	Saponins A and D (++), oligosaccharyl diphosphodolichol (oligo-PP-dol) (+), subunit c of mitochondrial ATP synthase	*PPT1* 1p34.2	256730
NCL 2	Tripeptidyl peptidase 1	Oligosaccharyl diphosphodolichol (oligo-PP-dol) (++), subunit c of mitochondrial ATP synthase	*CLN2* 11p15.4	204500

(continued on next page)

Table 2
(continued)

Disease	Defective Protein	Main Storage Materials	Gene and Locus	OMIM
NCL 3	Battenin	Oligo-PP-dol (++), subunit c of mitochondrial ATP synthase	*CLN3* 16p11.2	204200
NCL 4B, Parry type	DnaJ homolog subfamily C member 5	Oligo-PP-dol, subunit c of ATP synthase	*DNAJC5* 20q13.33	162350
NCL 5	Ceroid-lipofuscinosis neuronal protein 6	Oligo-PP-dol, subunit c of ATP synthase	*CLN5* 13q22.3	256731
NCL 6	Ceroid-lipofuscinosis neuronal protein 6	Oligo-PP-dol, subunit c of ATP synthase	*CLN6* 15q23	601780
NCL 7	Major facilitator superfamily domain-containing protein 8	Oligo-PP-dol, subunit c of ATP synthase	*MFSD8* 4q28.2	610951
NCL 8	CLN8, transmembrane protein of endoplasmic reticulum	Oligo-PP-dol, subunit c of ATP synthase	*CLN8* 8p23.3	600143
NCL 10	Cathepsin D	Oligo-PP-dol, subunit c of ATP synthase	*CTSD* 11p15.5	610127

Abbreviations: CLN8, neuronal ceroid lipofuscinosis type 8; GAGs, glycosaminoglycans.

Table 3
LSDs associated with cherry red spot and their typical features

Galactosialidosis	Cerebellar ataxia, myoclonus, visual failure; onset in late childhood or adolescence
G_{M1}-gangliosidosis	Coarse facial features, corneal clouding, hepatomegaly, skeletal dysplasia, learning disability, myoclonus
Infantile free sialic acid storage disease (ISSD)	Coarse facies, fair complexion, hepatosplenomegaly, and severe psychomotor retardation, nephrotic syndrome
Mucolipidosis II (I-cell disease)	Coarse facies, short stature, kyphoscolosis, umbilical and inguinal hernias
Mucopolysaccharidosis types IV (MPS IV) and VII (MPS VII)	Short stature, skeletal dysplasia
Neuronal ceroid lipofuscinosis (NCL)	Cerebellar ataxia; myoclonus; visual failure; onset by late childhood or adolescence
Niemann-Pick disease type A	Hepatosplenomegaly, spasticity
Sialidosis type 1	Juvenile or adult onset; intention and action myoclonus
Sandhoff disease	Exaggerated acousticomotor reflex, splenomegaly
Tay-Sachs disease	Exaggerated acousticomotor reflex, megalencephaly

Imaging

Leukodystrophy is predominantly seen in arylsulfatase A deficiency (MLD) and Krabbe disease (globoid cell leukodystrophy, GLD) (**Fig. 1**). Interest in understanding the natural history of disease and investigations of potential therapies have prompted the development of brain disease MRI severity scoring systems for both MLD (Eichler and colleagues[14]) and GLD (Loes and colleagues[15]). These scoring systems were based on the evolution and severity of brain MRI findings observed in X-linked adrenoleukodystrophy (peroxisomal disorder).[16] In 9 infants with GLD, correlations have been shown between neurodevelopmental features (ie, mental development, gross and fine motor dysfunction) and total Loes score.[15]

Other Diagnostic Modalities

Skeletal radiographs of the thoracolumbar spine and long bones reveal a constellation of findings (dysotosis multiplex) in patients with MPS and oligosaccharidosis (**Fig. 2**). Odontoid hypoplasia can also be a feature in these disorders.[3] Hepatosplenomegaly, detectable by ultrasound or palpation, is seen in Gaucher and Niemann-Pick A, B, and C diseases.[10] Cardiomyopathy, detectable by echocardiography, is encountered in infantile Pompe, Fabry, and Danon diseases.[17–19]

Disease Pathology

Until recently, the LSDs were classified according to the nature of the substrate accumulation (ie, glycosphingolipid, glycosaminoglycans), which could be measured in samples obtained during the diagnostic workup (eg, liver or bone marrow tissue, serum, urine). Characterization of the underlying gene defects and molecular basis has enabled the introduction of a molecular classification (eg, enzyme deficiency, transport defect).

Table 4
Neurologic clinical manifestations reported in patients with an LSD

Optic Atrophy, Visual Loss
- Galactosialidosis
- G_{M1}-gangliosidosis
- Infantile free sialic acid storage disease (ISSD)
- Mucolipidosis II (I-cell disease)
- Mucopolysaccharidosis types IV (MPS IV) and VII (MPS VII)
- Neuronal ceroid lipofuscinosis
- Niemann-Pick disease type A
- Sialidosis type 1
- Sandhoff disease
- Tay-Sachs disease

Retinitis pigmentosa
- Neuronal ceroid lipofuscinosis

Corneal opacities (clouding)
- I-cell disease (ML II)
- Mucolipidosis IV
- MPS I, IV, VI
- Oligosaccharidosis (late-onset α-mannosidosis)
- Fabry disease

Lenticular opacities (cataracts)
- Oligosaccharidosis (sialidosis, α-mannosidosis)
- Fabry disease

Ophthalmoplegia (Abnormal eye movements), nystagmus
- Gaucher disease 3
- Niemann-Pick C

Leukodystrophy
- Krabbe disease
- MLD
- Fabry disease[a]

Myoclonic seizures
- Galactosialidosis
- Gaucher disease III
- G_{M2}-gangliosidosis
- Neuronal ceroid lipofuscinosis
- Niemann-Pick C
- Oligosaccharidosis (α-N-acetyl-galactosaminidase deficiency, fucosidosis, Sialidosis type 1)

Deafness
- Fabry disease
- Galactosialidosis
- Gaucher disease type 2
- I-cell disease
- MPS I, II, IV
- Oligosaccharidosis (α-mannosidosis and β-mannosidosis)
- Metachromatic leukodystrophy
- Infantile Pompe disease

Macrocephaly
- Tay-Sachs disease
- Sandhoff disease
- Krabbe disease

Peripheral neuropathy
- Krabbe disease
- MLD (spastic paraplegia)
- Multiple sulfatase deficiency

Cortical atrophy
- Late stage of G_{M1}-gangliosidosis and G_{M2}-gangliosidosis (cerebellar atrophy)
- MLD
- I-cell disease
- Neuronal ceroid lipofuscinosis
- Cerebrovascular or strokelike episodes and other vascular events (eg, Raynaud phenomenon)
- Fabry disease

Ataxia
- Galactosialidosis
- Gaucher disease III
- G_{M1}-gangliosidosis
- Late-onset G_{M2}-gangliosidosis (cerebellar hypoplasia)
- Krabbe disease
- Mucolipidosis IV
- MLD
- Neuronal ceroid lipofucinosis
- Niemann-Pick C
- Salla disease
- Sialidosis I

Extrapyramidal signs
- Gaucher disease 3
- G_{M1}-gangliosidosis (adult form)
- Late-onset G_{M2}-gangliosidosis
- Krabbe disease
- Niemann-Pick C
- Oligosaccharidosis

Dementia, psychosis
- Fabry disease
- Gaucher disease 3
- G_{M1}-gangliosidosis
- Late-onset G_{M2}-gangliosidosis
- Krabbe disease
- MLD
- MPS III (Sanfilippo disease)
- Neuronal ceroid lipofuscinosis
- Niemann-Pick C

a Signal abnormalities consistent with leukoariosis.

Table 5	
LSDs prevalent in 2 communities	
Ashkenazi Jews	**Finns**
• GM2 gangliosidosis (Tay-Sachs disease) • Gaucher disease type 1 • Niemann-Pick A and B disease • Mucolipidosis IV	• Aspartylglucosaminuria • Infantile neuronal ceroid lipofuscinosis

GENETICS
Genetic Basis of Disease

The primary defect can arise in a gene that encodes a hydrolytic enzyme or its cofactor/activator (**Fig. 3**). Alternatively, the mutated gene may encode a transmembrane protein involved with substrate transport or vesicle fusion.[1] Occasionally, the defect may involve a protein required for posttranslational modification of a lysosomal enzyme/protein; consequently, the target protein may be nonfunctional (eg, SUMF-1, a formylglycine-generating enzyme, critical for the introduction of formylglycine residue in sulfatases), prematurely degraded (neuraminidase, which is part of a multiunit complex including protective protein or cathepsin A), or mistargeted (eg, GNPTAB in I-cell disease, resulting in a defect of posttranslation modification/glycosylation, required as most lysosomal enzymes rely on mannose-6-phosphate residues for lysosomal targeting or delivery).

The LSDs are transmitted as autosomal-recessive traits, except for 3 X-linked disorders: Fabry, Danon, and Hunter syndrome (MPS-II). Hunter syndrome only affects male carriers, except for unusual female carriers who either also have Turner syndrome (45,X) or an X-autosome translocation wherein the functional X-chromosome happens to bear a mutation of the *IDS* gene encoding iduronate-2-sulfatase.[20] Male and female patients with a mutation of either the *GLA* gene, which encodes α-galactosidase (deficient in Fabry disease) or the *LAMP2* gene, which encodes the lysosomal-associated membrane protein-2 (defective in Danon disease), show characteristic clinical features encountered in affected male patients. However, age of symptom onset and disease severity can be highly variable among female patients.

Box 1
LSDs associated with nonimmune hydrops fetalis
• Farber disease
• Galactosialidosis
• Gaucher disease type 2
• GM1-gangliosidosis
• I-cell disease
• MPS types IV and VII
• Niemann-Pick types A and C
• Sialidosis type II
• Salla disease and infantile free sialic acid storage disease
• Wolman disease

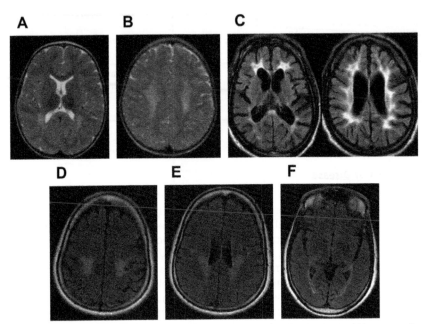

Fig. 1. Leukodystrophic LSDs, brain MRI. In MLD and GLD, there is progressive central nervous system demyelination. (*A, B*) A 22-month-old girl diagnosed with MLD who presented with global psychomotor delay and fronto-occipital periventricular demyelination on imaging. (*C*) A 26-year-old man with late-onset MLD who presented with behavioral disturbances, initially diagnosed with schizophrenia. Diffuse periventricular T2 hyperintensity extending into U-fibers was noted, associated with cerebral atrophy. (*D–F*) A 61-year-old man diagnosed with GLD who presented with late-onset gait problems evolving to spastic paraparesis. Brain MRI showed typical parietal occipital T2 hyperintensity bilaterally with extension to temporal white matter and basal ganglia.

Molecular Pathogenesis

Deleterious alleles cause the complete obliteration of enzyme or protein function, which leads to early onset cases associated with rapid progression and death in infancy or early childhood. Alleles generating a protein with residual function enable a subacute or chronic disease course. In these latter cases, life spans can extend into decades.[10] However, genotype-phenotype correlations are often imperfect, particularly in insidious cases, and there remains incomplete understanding of factors that modify clinical course. In terms of lysosomal hydrolases, in general, a specific critical threshold, below which symptoms have been observed, has been determined (varying between 10% and 25%).[21,22]

Previously, loss of enzyme function was largely attributed to mutations that inactivated the catalytic site or resulted in a gene product subjected to nonsense mediated decay or a highly unstable or truncated nonfunctional protein. However, several studies have shown that certain mutations can result in misfolding of the nascent protein that is subsequently diverted away from the lysosome by its premature elimination via endoplasmic reticulum (ER)-associated degradation (ERAD). This pathway diverts misfolded and unstable proteins in the course of their ER synthesis toward the ubiquitin-proteasome system (UPS) in the cytoplasm.[23] These observations are of particular interest in relation to potential therapeutic approaches, such as the use of pharmacologic chaperones and agents that influence proteostasis regulation (see discussion below).

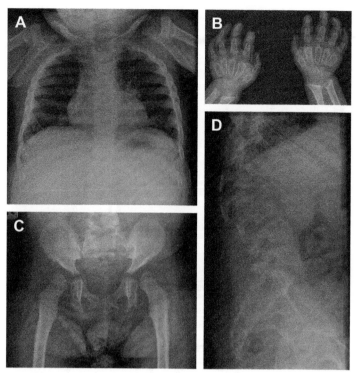

Fig. 2. Multiplex dysostosis associated with MPS. (*A*) Broadened clavicles and ribs. (*B*) Short and thin metacarpals with proximal tapering and distal erosions of middle and distal phalanges. (*C*) Shallow and wider acetabuli, which may result in subluxation or dislocation of the femoral heads. (*D*) Gibbus deformity, with anterior wedging, retrolisthesis of the apex vertebrae at the thoracolumbar transition.

Although substrate accumulation and the resultant altered trafficking and recycling of various metabolites may represent the initial insult to cells, several studies have shown a cascade of pathologic events (**Box 2**).[24–26] It is likely an interplay of factors contribute to disease expression, but the mechanistic links between underlying gene defect and clinical manifestations have not been fully elucidated. For a subset of the sphingolipidosis, the deacylated (psychosine) forms of the primary accumulating substrate might mediate cellular toxicity. For instance, in Fabry disease studies have shown the presence of globotriaosylsphingosine (LysoGb3), which may have a role in the development of increased carotid intima-media thickness and altered brachial flow-mediated dilation. In addition, altered vascular reactivity and a prothrombotic state may contribute to the increased risk for stroke in these patients.

Of various mechanisms, recent interest has focused on the inhibition of autophagy; in particular, its role in Pompe disease, which is an LSD caused by α-glucosidase (GAA) deficiency and characterized by an accumulation of autophagosomes in muscles and tissue wasting. Interestingly, in late onset cases (acid maltase myopathy), a correlation has been demonstrated among autophagy impairment (assessed by monitoring expression of p62-containing protein aggregates), the degree of muscle fiber atrophy, and disease progression.[28] Defects of autophagy seem to also compromise the uptake and delivery to the lysosome of recombinant GAA, which might

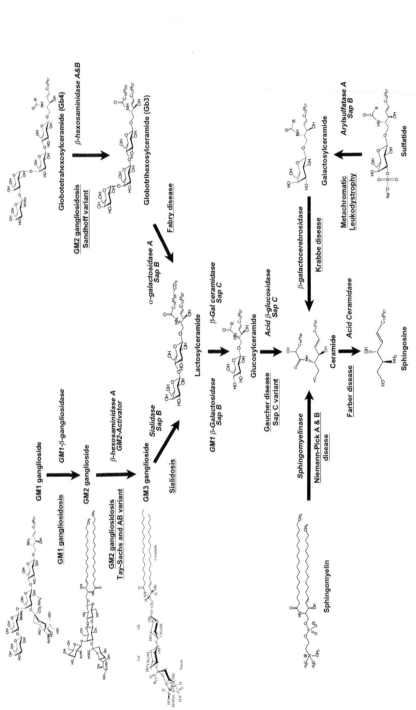

Fig. 3. Sphingolipid molecular structures and their degradation pathway. The sphingolipids consist of a ceramide molecule attached to a long-chain sphingoid base (sphingosine), which is bound to a long-chain fatty acid. The degradation of specific sphingolipids requires specific enzymes, which are depicted here in each step of the pathway. The correspondent lysosomal storage disease (*underlined*) associated with each enzyme (*italic*) is also shown. Some of the lysosomal enzymes need cofactors, called sphingolipid activator proteins, for the catalysis of their specific substrates. Examples of these cofactors are a group of proteins called saponins (Sap), here described as Sap A, B, C, and D.

Box 2
Pathologic events in LSDs[a]

- Accumulation of primary substrates and secondary metabolites
- Increased lysosomal membrane permeability
- Altered lysosomal pH
- Endoplasmic reticulum stress and unfolded protein response activation
- Oxidative stress
- Altered calcium homeostasis
- Autophagy impairment[b]
- Inflammation, microglial activation
- Apoptosis

[a] Reviewed in ref.[24]
[b] Autophagy is a highly conserved homeostatic process for lysosome-mediated degradation of cytoplasmic components, including damaged organelles and toxic protein aggregates.[27]

---

adversely influence therapeutic outcome.[29] Reactivation of autophagy in vitro contributes to GAA maturation in both healthy and diseased myotubes.

A gene-expression array analysis of brain tissue obtained from the MPS VII knockout mouse (gus^{mps}/gus^{mps}) revealed several alterations including up-regulation of key components of the immune system along with those related to inflammatory response.[30] In the MPS-IIIB mouse model, there was down-regulation of major oligodendrocyte-related genes, indicating defects in myelination and perturbations in multiple developmental genes.[31–33] The variation in gene dysregulation observed between brain regions in these mouse models indicates that different neuropathologic mechanisms may predominate within specific regions of a diseased brain, which may translate to differentiating neurologic symptoms and signs.[30]

Relevant Disease Models

Several animal models, including spontaneously occurring and those generated by recombinant genetic techniques, have been described. These models have been invaluable in understanding underlying disease mechanisms, particularly presymptomatic changes. For instance, during myelination, galactosylation of sphingosine produces psychosine, which is catalyzed by uridine diphosphate-galactose:ceramide galactosyltransferase (ie, the Cleland-Kennedy pathway).[34] Physiologically, the low level of psychosine produced is rapidly degraded by GALC.[35] In the setting of GALC deficiency (Krabbe disease), psychosine levels are elevated in the brain.[36] At high levels, psychosine becomes cytotoxic, particularly to oligodendrocytes (myelin-forming neural cells), resulting in apoptosis and extensive demyelination observed in brain imaging studies of Krabbe disease patients.[35] In the *Twitcher,* naturally occurring Krabbe disease mouse model, psychosine has been shown to induce the dephosphorylation of neurofilaments by deregulation of 2 serine/threonine phosphatases (PP1 and PP2A).[37] Studies involving several mouse models of distinct LSDs affecting the sphingolipid metabolism (ie, sphingolipidoses, such as G_{M1}-gangliosidosis and G_{M2}-gangliosidosis) have revealed elevated levels of proinflammatory cytokines (tumor necrosis-α, interleukin-1β).[38]

Moreover, proof of therapeutic potential has been shown in preclinical studies involving several animal models before drug introduction in human clinical trials. However, results of studies in animal models should be interpreted with caution, as occasionally, a particular mouse model may not mimic disease in humans even when biochemical or histologic changes may be present, because of an alternative metabolic pathway or incompletely understood reasons.[39]

EVALUATION AND MANAGEMENT
Strategies for Diagnosis

In suspected cases, diagnosis of a specific LSD can be readily confirmed by a biochemical and/or molecular assay, using cells derived from peripheral blood. Testing is available through specialized laboratories (listed in Genetests; http://www.ncbi.nlm.nih.gov/sites/GeneTests/). ARSA pseudo-deficiency is found in 10% to 15% of individuals in the general population, which can lead to diagnostic errors; rare cases of Saposin deficiency may be missed and usually requires screening for elevated levels of the substrate in body fluids and molecular analysis. Characterization of the putative gene defect as the cause of a particular LSD is increasingly available and molecular confirmation of the diagnosis is ideally undertaken before any therapeutic intervention.

Newborn screening aimed at the identification of inborn errors of metabolism has largely focused on the amino acidopathies and organic acidurias, including fatty acid oxidation defects. The availability of treatment has led to the development of guidelines for managing patients with selected LSDs, potentially including screening of newborns and high-risk populations.

Current Management and Therapeutic Options

Genetic counseling is central to management of affected individuals and their relatives. Geneticists/counselors often facilitate the multidisciplinary care required by patients and can arrange carrier/prenatal testing for individuals/couples at risk.

Symptomatic treatment remains the only option for most LSDs. For certain disorders, such as the MPS, physical and occupational therapy are components of a comprehensive program to facilitate performance of activities of daily living. Special precautions are necessary in children with MPS who need anesthesia, because of risks associated with cardiopulmonary disease and cervical manipulation in cases with odontoid hypoplasia.[40,41] Pulmonary assistance (BiPAP or CPAP) provides significant relief for patients with MPS and sleep apnea, and for those with both infantile and late onset Pompe disease who suffer from intercostal and diaphragmatic muscle weakness.[42,43] Adjunctive therapies to control seizures and behavioral and sleep problems, which can be challenging concerns help improve patient quality of life. Antiplatelet agents and lipid-lowering drugs, in conjunction with enzyme replacement therapy (ERT) in Fabry disease, may reduce the risk for cerebrovascular events.[44]

Disorders caused by a deficiency of an enzyme or soluble protein may be modifiable by cellular (ie, hematopoietic stem cells transplantation [HSCT]) or protein/recombinant enzyme replacement therapy. Microglia derived from donor stem cells can penetrate the blood-brain barrier (BBB) and secrete functional enzyme. In MPS-I (Hurler syndrome), HSCT results in stabilization or improvement of cognitive function[45,46]; in patients with infantile Krabbe disease, HSCT prolongs survival when undertaken in the first weeks of life.[47] However, follow-up studies indicate greater than 80% of transplanted Krabbe disease infants who survive beyond age 2 years experience some degree of motor difficulty.[48] Skeletal dysplasia in the MPS is not fully corrected by HSCT, although there are indications of a positive effect on odontoid hypoplasia.[45] To obtain maximal enzyme activity following HSCT, donor cells should be derived from noncarriers.[46]

ERT has been shown to modify disease course in various LSDs, but not alter ultimate neurologic prognosis in severe subtypes (eg, Hunter syndrome, neuropathic Gaucher disease).[49] In patients with infantile Pompe disease, ERT enables the resolution of cardiomyopathy and increased survival, except for those with high antibody titers in whom prognosis remained guarded to poor.[50] Among survivors, cognitive development at school age ranged between normal and mildly delayed.[51] In a study including 38 adult patients with late onset Pompe disease receiving alglucosidase alfa for 36 months, ERT led to improvement in physical endurance (as measured by the 6-min walk test) and stabilization of forced vital capacity.[52]

In a proportion of ERT-treated patients, antibodies can develop against recombinant enzymes that might neutralize the activity of the infused protein or interfere with its cellular uptake. Long-term studies are required to establish the full efficacy of ERT and its impact on health-related quality of life.[50,53]

Substrate reduction therapy is available for certain glycosphingolipidoses, wherein the use of a small molecular agent (miglustat in Gaucher disease and Niemann-Pick disease type C) has been shown to inhibit precursor synthesis, reduce tissue substrate burden, and alter the rate of disease progression.[54] Other approaches, such as the use of pharmacologic chaperones (migalastat in Fabry disease), or agents that influence proteostasis regulation and gene therapy are under investigation.[55]

Investigations of misfolding mutant protein suggest potential rescue by pharmacologic chaperones, which mimic the natural substrate and act as templates to facilitate proper enzyme folding and its subsequent transit to the lysosome, wherein the higher affinity of the substrate displaces the drug, partially restoring intralysosomal enzyme activity.[56–58] In addition, a potentially complementary approach involves the use of drugs that influence proteostasis regulation.[59] Significant increases of glucocerebrosidase activity were obtained with the use small molecule inhibitors of histone deacetylase that cross the BBB. Gene therapy is the subject of investigations.[60]

Future Directions in Therapy and Diagnosis

Newborn screening aimed at the identification of inborn errors of metabolism has largely focused on conditions that are largely modifiable by dietary modification and/or vitamin/cofactor supplementation. These therapeutic options are not applicable to LSDs, but the increasing availability of approaches such as ERT has led to advocacy for incorporating some these disorders in an expanded newborn screening program. In the State of New York, screening for Krabbe disease was introduced in 2006, which has enabled consideration of HSCT for affected infants and prenatal diagnosis for future pregnancies in couples at risk.[61]

A major challenge in the development of treatment for neuropathic LSD is drug delivery across the BBB, and additionally the likelihood that there are disease mechanisms not modifiable by administration of exogenous enzyme or protein. In this setting, small molecule pharmacological agents are more likely to penetrate the BBB and allow the manipulation of specific upstream (eg, reduction of substrate synthesis) and downstream (eg, autophagy disturbances) pathways and potentially influence disease outcome. Deleterious cellular events precede the onset of clinical symptomatology, and thus early diagnosis and intervention will be a key to achieving an optimal outcome.

Therapeutic approaches under consideration include HSCT with autologous cells that have been genetically modified to constitutively express supraphysiologic enzyme levels. In addition, trials with recombinant enzyme administered intravenously and intrathecally have been undertaken or are on-going.[62] Gene therapy with oligodendroglial, neural progenitor, embryonic, and microencapsulated recombinant cells is also under investigation.

SUMMARY

The LSDs are chronic disorders that can have a significant impact on quality of life and lead to shortened life spans, particularly in the subtypes associated with neuropathic involvement. A high index of suspicion should be maintained, even when signs (eg, hepatosplenomegaly) suggestive of a storage disorder are not evident. Developmental delay and behavioral and/or psychiatric problems may be presenting symptoms. Diagnosis can be confirmed in all LSDs, by biochemical and/or molecular testing, which is essential for appropriate genetic counseling and management. Treatment is available for several, and studies are on-going to expand the therapeutic options for disease control.

ACKNOWLEDGMENTS

Gregory M. Pastores, MD is supported by the NYU-HHC Clinical and Translational Science Institute, which is supported in part by grant UL1 TR000038 from the National Center for Advancing Translational Sciences of the National Institutes of Health. Dr Pastores also receives research funds for clinical trials involving LSDs from Amicus-GSK, Biomarin Pharmaceuticals, Genzyme-Sanofi, Protalix and Shire HGT.

Gustavo Maegawa MD, PhD is currently supported by NIH-NIMH 1R03MH098689 and NIH-NINDS 1R01NS079655 grants. Dr Maegawa also receives research grants from National MPS Society and received research grants from the National Tay-Sachs Disease and Allied Diseases Association (NTSAD). Dr Maegawa receives research funds for clinical and educational studies from Genzyme-Sanofi, Biomarin Pharmaceuticals, Protalix and Shire HGT.

REFERENCES

1. Saftig P, Klumperman J. Lysosome biogenesis and lysosomal membrane proteins: trafficking meets function. Nat Rev Mol Cell Biol 2009;10(9):623–35.
2. Vellodi A, Bembi B, de Villemeur TB, et al. Management of neuronopathic Gaucher disease: a European consensus. J Inherit Metab Dis 2001;24(3): 319–27.
3. Wraith JE. The clinical presentation of lysosomal storage disorders. Acta Neurol Taiwan 2004;13(3):101–6.
4. Maegawa GH, Stockley T, Tropak M, et al. The natural history of juvenile or subacute GM2 gangliosidosis: 21 new cases and literature review of 134 previously reported. Pediatrics 2006;118(5):e1550–62.
5. Zaroff CM, Neudorfer O, Morrison C, et al. Neuropsychological assessment of patients with late onset GM2 gangliosidosis. Neurology 2004;62(12):2283–6.
6. Mechtler TP, Stary S, Metz TF, et al. Neonatal screening for lysosomal storage disorders: feasibility and incidence from a nationwide study in Austria. Lancet 2012;379(9813):335–41.
7. Spada M, Pagliardini S, Yasuda M, et al. High incidence of later-onset fabry disease revealed by newborn screening. Am J Hum Genet 2006;79(1):31–40.
8. Zlotogora J. High frequencies of human genetic diseases: founder effect with genetic drift or selection? Am J Med Genet 1994;49(1):10–3.
9. Wraith JE. Lysosomal disorders. Semin Neonatol 2002;7(1):75–83.
10. Vellodi A. Lysosomal storage disorders. Br J Haematol 2005;128(4):413–31.
11. Muenzer J, Beck M, Eng CM, et al. Multidisciplinary management of Hunter syndrome. Pediatrics 2009;124(6):e1228–39.

12. Muenzer J, Wraith JE, Clarke LA. Mucopolysaccharidosis I: management and treatment guidelines. Pediatrics 2009;123(1):19–29.
13. Staretz-Chacham O, Choi JH, Wakabayashi K, et al. Psychiatric and behavioral manifestations of lysosomal storage disorders. Am J Med Genet B Neuropsychiatr Genet 2010;153B(7):1253–65.
14. Eichler F, Grodd W, Grant E, et al. Metachromatic leukodystrophy: a scoring system for brain MR imaging observations. AJNR Am J Neuroradiol 2009; 30(10):1893–7.
15. Loes DJ, Peters C, Krivit W. Globoid cell leukodystrophy: distinguishing early-onset from late-onset disease using a brain MR imaging scoring method. AJNR Am J Neuroradiol 1999;20(2):316–23.
16. Loes DJ, Stillman AE, Hite S, et al. Childhood cerebral form of adrenoleukodystrophy: short-term effect of bone marrow transplantation on brain MR observations. AJNR Am J Neuroradiol 1994;15(9):1767–71.
17. Byrne BJ, Kishnani PS, Case LE, et al. Pompe disease: design, methodology, and early findings from the Pompe Registry. Mol Genet Metab 2011;103(1): 1–11.
18. Mehta A, Clarke JT, Giugliani R, et al. Natural course of Fabry disease: changing pattern of causes of death in FOS - Fabry Outcome Survey. J Med Genet 2009; 46(8):548–52.
19. Nucifora G, Miani D, Piccoli G, et al. Cardiac magnetic resonance imaging in Danon disease. Cardiology 2012;121(1):27–30.
20. Tuschl K, Gal A, Paschke E, et al. Mucopolysaccharidosis type II in females: case report and review of literature. Pediatr Neurol 2005;32(4):270–2.
21. Conzelmann E, Kytzia HJ, Navon R, et al. Ganglioside GM2 N-acetyl-beta-D-galactosaminidase activity in cultured fibroblasts of late-infantile and adult GM2 gangliosidosis patients and of healthy probands with low hexosaminidase level. Am J Hum Genet 1983;35(5):900–13.
22. Leinekugel P, Michel S, Conzelmann E, et al. Quantitative correlation between the residual activity of beta-hexosaminidase A and arylsulfatase A and the severity of the resulting lysosomal storage disease. Hum Genet 1992;88(5): 513–23.
23. Wiseman RL, Powers ET, Buxbaum JN, et al. An adaptable standard for protein export from the endoplasmic reticulum. Cell 2007;131(4):809–21.
24. Vitner EB, Platt FM, Futerman AH. Common and uncommon pathogenic cascades in lysosomal storage diseases. J Biol Chem 2010;285(27):20423–7.
25. Walkley SU. Pathogenic cascades in lysosomal disease-Why so complex? J Inherit Metab Dis 2009;32(2):181–9.
26. Boya P, Andreau K, Poncet D, et al. Lysosomal membrane permeabilization induces cell death in a mitochondrion-dependent fashion. J Exp Med 2003; 197(10):1323–34.
27. Cuervo AM. Autophagy and aging: keeping that old broom working. Trends Genet 2008;24(12):604–12.
28. Raben N, Roberts A, Plotz PH. Role of autophagy in the pathogenesis of Pompe disease. Acta Myol 2007;26(1):45–8.
29. Raben N, Schreiner C, Baum R, et al. Suppression of autophagy permits successful enzyme replacement therapy in a lysosomal storage disorder–murine Pompe disease. Autophagy 2010;6(8):1078–89.
30. Parente MK, Rozen R, Cearley CN, et al. Dysregulation of gene expression in a lysosomal storage disease varies between brain regions implicating unexpected mechanisms of neuropathology. PLoS One 2012;7(3):e32419.

31. DiRosario J, Divers E, Wang C, et al. Innate and adaptive immune activation in the brain of MPS IIIB mouse model. J Neurosci Res 2009;87(4):978–90.

32. Ausseil J, Desmaris N, Bigou S, et al. Early neurodegeneration progresses independently of microglial activation by heparan sulfate in the brain of mucopolysaccharidosis IIIB mice. PLoS One 2008;3(5):e2296.

33. Killedar S, Dirosario J, Divers E, et al. Mucopolysaccharidosis IIIB, a lysosomal storage disease, triggers a pathogenic CNS autoimmune response. J Neuroinflammation 2010;7:39.

34. Cleland WW, Kennedy EP. The enzymatic synthesis of psychosine. J Biol Chem 1960;235:45–51.

35. Suzuki K. Twenty five years of the "psychosine hypothesis": a personal perspective of its history and present status. Neurochem Res 1998;23(3):251–9.

36. Svennerholm L, Vanier MT, Mansson JE. Krabbe disease: a galactosylsphingosine (psychosine) lipidosis. J Lipid Res 1980;21(1):53–64.

37. Cantuti-Castelvetri L, Zhu H, Givogri MI, et al. Psychosine induces the dephosphorylation of neurofilaments by deregulation of PP1 and PP2A phosphatases. Neurobiol Dis 2012;46(2):325–35.

38. Lee J, Kim HR, Quinley C, et al. Autophagy suppresses interleukin-1beta (IL-1beta) signaling by activation of p62 degradation via lysosomal and proteasomal pathways. J Biol Chem 2012;287(6):4033–40.

39. Haskins ME. Animal models for mucopolysaccharidosis disorders and their clinical relevance. Acta Paediatr Suppl 2007;96(455):56–62.

40. Kirkpatrick K, Ellwood J, Walker RW. Mucopolysaccharidosis type I (Hurler syndrome) and anesthesia: the impact of bone marrow transplantation, enzyme replacement therapy, and fiberoptic intubation on airway management. Paediatr Anaesth 2012;22(8):745–51.

41. Ard JL Jr, Bekker A, Frempong-Boadu AK. Anesthesia for an adult with mucopolysaccharidosis I. J Clin Anesth 2005;17(8):624–6.

42. Jones HN, Moss T, Edwards L, et al. Increased inspiratory and expiratory muscle strength following respiratory muscle strength training (RMST) in two patients with late-onset Pompe disease. Mol Genet Metab 2011;104(3):417–20.

43. Kishnani PS, Corzo D, Leslie ND, et al. Early treatment with alglucosidase alpha prolongs long-term survival of infants with Pompe disease. Pediatr Res 2009;66(3):329–35.

44. Mehta A, Beck M, Eyskens F, et al. Fabry disease: a review of current management strategies. QJM 2010;103(9):641–59.

45. Prasad VK, Kurtzberg J. Transplant outcomes in mucopolysaccharidoses. Semin Hematol 2010;47(1):59–69.

46. Prasad VK, Kurtzberg J. Cord blood and bone marrow transplantation in inherited metabolic diseases: scientific basis, current status and future directions. Br J Haematol 2010;148(3):356–72.

47. Escolar ML, Poe MD, Provenzale JM, et al. Transplantation of umbilical-cord blood in babies with infantile Krabbe's disease. N Engl J Med 2005;352(20):2069–81.

48. Duffner PK, Caviness VS Jr, Erbe RW, et al. The long-term outcomes of presymptomatic infants transplanted for Krabbe disease: report of the workshop held on July 11 and 12, 2008, Holiday Valley, New York. Genet Med 2009;11(6):450–4.

49. Grabowski GA, Hopkin RJ. Enzyme therapy for lysosomal storage disease: principles, practice, and prospects. Annu Rev Genomics Hum Genet 2003;4:403–36.

50. Patel TT, Banugaria SG, Case LE, et al. The impact of antibodies in late-onset Pompe disease: a case series and literature review. Mol Genet Metab 2012; 106(3):301–9.

51. Kishnani PS, Corzo D, Nicolino M, et al. Recombinant human acid {alpha}-glucosidase: major clinical benefits in infantile-onset Pompe disease. Neurology 2011;77(17):1604.

52. van der Ploeg AT, Clemens PR, Corzo D, et al. A randomized study of alglucosidase alfa in late-onset Pompe's disease. N Engl J Med 2010;362(15): 1396–406.

53. Banugaria SG, Patel TT, Kishnani PS. Immune modulation in Pompe disease treated with enzyme replacement therapy. Expert Rev Clin Immunol 2012;8(6): 497–9.

54. Cox TM, Aerts JM, Andria G, et al. The role of the iminosugar N-butyldeoxynojirimycin (miglustat) in the management of type I (non-neuronopathic) Gaucher disease: a position statement. J Inherit Metab Dis 2003;26(6):513–26.

55. Alfonso P, Pampin S, Estrada J, et al. Miglustat (NB-DNJ) works as a chaperone for mutated acid beta-glucosidase in cells transfected with several Gaucher disease mutations. Blood Cells Mol Dis 2005;35(2):268–76.

56. Fan JQ. Pharmacological chaperone therapy for lysosomal storage disorders - leveraging aspects of the folding pathway to maximize activity of misfolded mutant proteins. FEBS J 2007;274(19):4943.

57. Tropak MB, Mahuran D. Lending a helping hand, screening chemical libraries for compounds that enhance beta-hexosaminidase A activity in GM2 gangliosidosis cells. FEBS J 2007;274(19):4951–61.

58. Maegawa GH, Tropak M, Buttner J, et al. Pyrimethamine as a potential pharmacological chaperone for late-onset forms of GM2 gangliosidosis. J Biol Chem 2007;282(12):9150–61.

59. Mu TW, Ong DS, Wang YJ, et al. Chemical and biological approaches synergize to ameliorate protein-folding diseases. Cell 2008;134(5):769–81.

60. Cachon-Gonzalez MB, Wang SZ, Lynch A, et al. Effective gene therapy in an authentic model of Tay-Sachs-related diseases. Proc Natl Acad Sci U S A 2006;103(27):10373–8.

61. Duffner PK, Caggana M, Orsini JJ, et al. Newborn screening for Krabbe disease: the New York State model. Pediatr Neurol 2009;40(4):245–52 [discussion: 53–5].

62. Auclair D, Finnie J, Walkley SU, et al. Intrathecal recombinant human 4-sulfatase reduces accumulation of glycosaminoglycans in dura of mucopolysaccharidosis VI cats. Pediatr Res 2012;71(1):39–45.

Clinical Neurogenetics
Fragile X–Associated Tremor/Ataxia Syndrome

Deborah A. Hall, MD, PhD[a],*, Joan A. O'Keefe, PT, PhD[b]

KEYWORDS

- Fragile X syndrome • *Fragile X mental retardation 1* gene • Ataxia

KEY POINTS

- Fragile X–associated tremor ataxia syndrome (FXTAS) is a progressive neurodegenerative disorder characterized by kinetic tremor and cerebellar ataxia.
- FXTAS is seen in individuals with 55 to 200 CGG repeats in the *fragile X mental retardation 1* gene and shows age-dependent penetrance, with symptoms typically manifesting in individuals older than 55 years.
- Affected individuals also have executive dysfunction, parkinsonism, peripheral neuropathy, and characteristic findings on neuroimaging and pathology.
- The disorder is postulated to be secondary to RNA toxicity.
- Treatment is typically symptomatic, and no medications or disease-modifying treatments of the disorder have been approved by the US Food and Drug Administration.

INTRODUCTION
Definition

The fragile X–associated tremor/ataxia syndrome (FXTAS, pronounced *fax-tas*) is a progressive neurodegenerative disorder characterized by cerebellar gait ataxia and kinetic tremor. The disorder, first reported in 2001, occurs in individuals older than 55 years who are carriers of a premutation size expansion of 55 to 200 repeats in the *fragile X mental retardation 1 (FMR1)* gene.[1,2] Diagnostic criteria for FXTAS, established in 2003, also include minor signs of parkinsonism and cognitive deficits, in addition to radiographic findings (**Box 1**).[3]

Symptoms and Clinical Course

The initial presenting motor symptom of FXTAS was originally described to be predominantly tremor.[4] Patients describe tremor in the hands when performing tasks,

Funding Sources: Dr D.A. Hall, NIH, Pfizer, Ceregene, Phytopharm; Dr J.A. O'Keefe, none.
Conflict of Interest: None.
[a] Department of Neurological Sciences, Rush University, 1725 West Harrison, Suite 755, Chicago, IL 60612, USA; [b] Department of Anatomy and Cell Biology, Rush University, 600 South Paulina Street, Suite 505B AcFac, Chicago, IL 60612-3244, USA
* Corresponding author.
E-mail address: Deborah_A_Hall@rush.edu

Box 1
Diagnostic criteria for FXTAS

Molecular	FMR1 CGG Repeat Size 55–200
Clinical	
Major signs	Intention tremor
	Gait ataxia
Minor signs	Parkinsonism
	Moderate to severe short-term memory deficits
	Executive function deficits
Radiologic	
Major signs	MRI white matter lesions in the middle cerebellar peduncle (MCP sign)
Minor signs	MRI white matter lesions in cerebral white matter
	Moderate to severe generalized atrophy
Diagnostic Categories	
Definite	Presence of 1 major radiologic sign plus 1 major clinical symptom
Probable	Presence of either 1 major radiologic sign plus 1 minor clinical symptom or has 2 major clinical symptoms
Possible	Presence of 1 minor radiologic sign plus 1 major clinical symptom

Adapted from Jacquemont S, Hagerman RJ, Leehey M, et al. Fragile X premutation tremor/ataxia syndrome: molecular, clinical, and neuroimaging correlates. Am J Hum Genet 2003;72(4):869; with permission.
Abbreviation: MRI, magnetic resonance imaging.

which slowly worsens over time. At around 9 years after tremor onset, the tremor interferes with activities of daily living, and writing becomes illegible within 15 years.[4] Gait difficulties start within a few years of tremor onset, with falls commencing by 6 years.[4] Dependence on a walking aid or need for a wheelchair occurs after a decade of disease, with death occurring after approximately 2 decades.[4]

More recently, self-reports of patients with FXTAS show that only 62% (31/50) endorse motor symptoms, despite 92% (46/50) having tremor, ataxia, or both on examination.[5] Those individuals presenting with both tremor and ataxia were most likely to also have cognitive impairment at presentation (69%) compared with those presenting with tremor only (38%).[5] There is now recognized clinical heterogeneity in the disorder, and this may account for the fact that frequently patients with FXTAS are initially diagnosed with other disorders, such as Parkinson disease (PD), tremor, ataxia, dementia, or cerebrovascular disease.[6] The age of onset to FXTAS, typically older than 60 years, is similar to the average age of PD or multiple system atrophy. However, this age is older than is expected in many of the autosomal-dominant spinocerebellar ataxias (SCAs).

Nature of Disease

The FMR1 premutation occurs in 1 of 151 females and 1/468 males.[7] Once FXTAS was described, many researchers screened banked DNA or tested patients sequentially to identify premutation carriers in their clinic populations, focusing on phenotypes reported in the original case series: tremor, ataxia, and parkinsonism. The prevalence of premutation range expansions is highest in populations with ataxia, with the following summarizing epidemiology estimates in movement disorder populations.[8]

- Ataxia populations: adult-onset ataxia (2.2%), patients with ataxia with negative SCA gene testing (4%), and male patients with ataxia with negative SCA testing (5%)[8]
- Parkinsonism populations: multiple system atrophy (0%–4%) and PD (0%–1%)[8]
- Essential tremor (0%)[8]

Given the prevalence of the *FMR1* premutation in the population, it is unclear why FXTAS is only infrequently diagnosed. Reasons for this situation include lack of referral to neurologists for specialty care, misdiagnosis,[6] and potentially decreased penetrance of the disorder.

Clinical Findings

On examination, patients with FXTAS show movement disorders and varying degrees of cognitive dysfunction. Kinetic tremor, especially with intention, is common but has variable severity, with at least 50% of male premutation carriers having at least mild tremor and 17% having moderate tremor.[4] Cerebellar gait ataxia, the other key feature for diagnosis, starts with difficulties on tandem gait on testing before progressing to need for a walking aid or falls within 5 to 10 years. Early in the disease, some patients may not recognize balance difficulties, despite an abnormal neurologic examination or quantitative testing.[5] Parkinsonism is also a common feature, but manifests predominantly with mild bradykinesia in 57% and rigidity in 71%.[4]

The pattern of cognitive dysfunction in FXTAS is frontal-subcortical and develops after the onset of the movement disorder.[9,10] The dysexecutive syndrome is characterized by deficits in control of attention, working memory, and behavioral self-regulation.[11] Significant dementia occurs in a portion of individuals,[3] with some becoming bed-ridden and indistinguishable from late-stage Alzheimer disease. Psychological and psychiatric symptoms can develop with or without cognitive dysfunction. These symptoms include apathy, anxiety, mood lability or disorders, social phobias, and reclusive behaviors.[11,12] This constellation of symptoms may make it less likely that affected patients with FXTAS seek medical care, even from a primary care physician.[6]

Peripheral neuropathy occurs in approximately 60% of patients with FXTAS. The neuropathy is typically axonal, with motor and sensory conduction changes associated with premutation molecular measures.[13] Longer CGG repeat number was associated with slowing of tibial nerve conduction velocity ($P = .04$), and increased messenger RNA levels were associated with a reduction of the tibial compound muscle action potential velocity ($P = .01$).[13] Although women with FXTAS seem to have a length-dependent polyneuropathy, men have a more variable presentation.[14]

Most men with FXTAS have autonomic symptoms, including impotence (80%), bowel and bladder dysfunction (30%–50%), and orthostatic hypotension (15%).[5] Two patients who presented with postprandial hypotension rather than movement disorders but met clinical or autopsy criteria for FXTAS have been reported.[15,16] Other features that have been reported in FXTAS are hearing loss and dysphagia.[2,4]

Although most of the original phenotypic studies in FXTAS focused on men, women with FXTAS have now been reported. Initial case-control studies did not show an association of tremor and ataxia in female premutation carriers, likely because of a lower manifestation of signs from X inactivation effects.[17] A case series was subsequently published describing female *FMR1* premutation carriers with tremor and ataxia, but only 1 had the MCP sign (see description in later discussion) on magnetic resonance imaging (MRI).[1] More recent studies have reported women with FXTAS and spasmodic dysphonia,[18] with FXTAS and multiple sclerosis,[19] and with FXTAS and AD,[20] suggesting that the FXTAS phenotype may be synergistic with other neurologic disorders in female premutation carriers.

Imaging

The classic neuroimaging abnormality reported in FXTAS is the MCP sign, which manifests as hyperintensity on T2-weighted MRI in the middle cerebellar peduncles (**Fig. 1**).[21] The MCP sign is considered a major radiologic feature of FXTAS and is

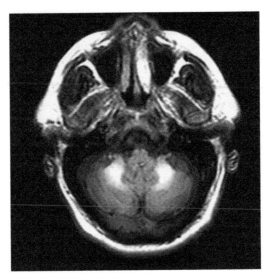

Fig. 1. Axial fluid-attenuated inversion recovery MRI in a patient with FXTAS. Hyperintensity in the middle cerebellar peduncle. (*Courtesy of* RJ Hagerman, University of California Davis, MIND Institute.)

seen in 60% of men with FXTAS, but has been reported in several other diseases, including multiple system atrophy, recessive ataxia, and acquired hepatocerebral degeneration.[22–24] Affected individuals also have moderate to severe generalized brain atrophy, with ventricular enlargement, more severe atrophy in cerebellar regions, and subcortical or pontocerebellar white matter lesions.[3,21]

Other Diagnostic Modalities

Tremor recordings, not typically performed for clinical care, were recently reported in patients with FXTAS and show that there are 3 electroclinical patterns: essential-tremor–like (35%) with small amplitude tremor, cerebellar (29%) with bilateral proximodistal tremor, and parkinsonian (12%) with a unilateral rest tremor.[14]

Disease Pathology

In patients with FXTAS, eosinophilic ubiquitin-positive intranuclear inclusions are found in both neurons and astrocytes in multiple areas: dentate nuclei, inferior olive, basal ganglia, thalamus, and throughout the cerebrum (**Fig. 2**).[25] The spinal cord, autonomic ganglia, and cranial nerve nuclear XII also show inclusions, but widespread disease, including inclusions, have now been reported outside the nervous system, in the endocrine organs, gastrointestinal tract, heart, and kidney.[2,26,27] In addition, there is patchy loss of axons, myelin, and glia, with some cases showing spongiosus.[27] Cerebral white matter disease ranges from microscopic white matter pallor to severe white matter degeneration, especially in the subcortex.[27]

GENETICS
Genetic Basis of Disease

Expansions in the 5′ noncoding region of the *FMR1* gene give rise to several distinct clinical phenotypes, depending on the size (**Fig. 3**). Larger expansions (>200 CGG repeats or full mutation) result in fragile X syndrome, which is the most common cause

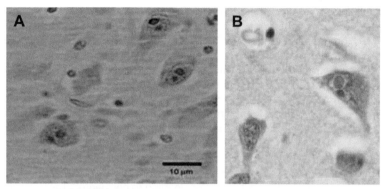

Fig. 2. FXTAS pathology. (*A*) Eosinophilic neuronal intranuclear inclusions. (*B*) Intranuclear inclusions stained with antiubiquitin antibodies.

of inherited intellectual disability in males. Premutation expansions (55–200 CGG repeats) may manifest premature ovarian insufficiency,[28] in addition to FXTAS. Recently, gray zone expansions (41 or 45–54 CGG repeats) have been reported to have parkinsonism or other neurologic signs, but these phenotypes need to be studied in more detail.[29–31]

FXTAS shows age-dependent penetrance, when the disease is defined as the fraction of carriers with intention tremor and gait instability.[32] Manifestation of symptoms occurs in 17% of male *FMR1* premutation carriers aged 50 to 59 years and increases to 75% of carriers aged 80 years or older manifesting symptoms.[32,33] In addition, there is a correlation between increasing CGG repeat size and motor impairment in men, which is more robust for tremor and ataxia.[33] Although a meta-analysis[34] showed that most *FMR1* premutation carriers with ataxia had CGG repeat sizes greater than 70, reports of individuals with FXTAS phenotypes with expansions even in the gray zone have been reported.[35]

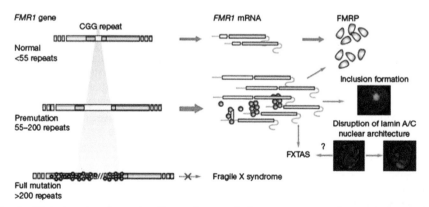

Fig. 3. Clinical and pathogenic effects of expanded CGG repeats in the *FMR1* gene. The repeat expansion ranges are located in the left portion of the figure. In individuals with the premutation, there is an increase in *FMR1* mRNA, which leads to inclusion formation and FXTAS. In individuals with a full mutation, the promoter and CGG repeat is methylated, the gene is silenced, and fragile X syndrome occurs. (*From* Hagerman PJ, Hagerman RJ. Fragile X-associated tremor/ataxia syndrome–an older face of the fragile X gene. Nat Clin Pract Neurol 2007;3(2):107–12; with permission.)

In the full *FMR1* mutation, the gene is methylated and transcriptional silencing occurs, resulting in a lack of fragile X mental retardation protein (FMRP). In individuals in the *FMR1* premutation range, there is only a slight depletion in FMRP levels, but a 2-fold to 10-fold increase of *FMR1* mRNA.[36] The increased transcriptional activity seems to be positively correlated with CGG repeat size.[36] However, X inactivation needs to be accounted for in women. Studies have shown that the relationship of mRNA levels and CGG repeat size is nonlinear in women, with a positive correlation less than 100 CGG.[37] When correcting for the X inactivation ratio, mRNA levels increase as the number of CGG repeats increase and is significant higher than 100 CGG.

Molecular Pathogenesis

It is hypothesized that FXTAS is caused by a toxic RNA gain of function, which may dysregulate neuronal and astrocyte function, leading to cell death.[2] There are multiple isoforms of *FMR1* mRNA that are associated with alternative transcriptional start sites and different polyadenylation sites.[38] Premutation size CGG repeat mRNAs form large intranuclear aggregates that sequester several RNA-binding proteins, including several important in splicing and regulatory function.[39–41] Recently, increased histone acetylation and chromatin remodeling has been shown to occur at the *FMR1* locus and is correlated with *FMR1* mRNA levels in premutation cell lines.[42]

FMRP is an RNA-binding protein containing 2 KH domains and an RGG box and is generally cytoplasmic. FMRP associates with polyribosomes in an RNA-dependent manner and suppresses translation in vitro and in vivo.[43] The lack of FMRP, seen in full-mutation carriers, leads to a persistent abnormal dendritic spine structure in humans.[44] Reduced dendritic branching and abnormal synaptic size compared with controls are also seen in premutation carriers.[45] In addition, embryonic premutation mice show migration defects in the neocortex and altered expression of neuronal lineage markers,[46] which may suggest a role for FMRP in neurodevelopment.

Direct RNA toxicity has been shown in animal and cell models of FXTAS. Pur α and hn RNP A2/B1 are present in the inclusions of FXTAS fly models, and overexpression of these rescues the phenotype.[39] Disrupted lamin A/C expression and organization have been seen in skin fibroblasts from males with FXTAS and may account for peripheral nervous system abnormalities.[47] The fibroblasts also showed increased mRNA of 3 stress response genes: *heat shock protein (HSP) 27, HSP70,* and *αβ-crystallin (CRYAB)*. Although they were not associated with an increase in protein in the fibroblasts, the mRNA was found in the nervous system intranuclear inclusions in individuals with FXTAS.[47] Reduced nuclear export of stress response mRNAs has also been found to contribute to neuronal degeneration in cultured premutation neurons.[48] Mitochondrial dysfunction may account for some of the pathophysiology of the disorder. Lower oxidative phosphorylation capacity with disrupted processing and import of mitochondrial proteins is seen in premutation carrier fibroblasts.[49,50]

Relevant Disease Models

The initial transgenic mouse models with 81 CGG repeats in *FMR1* showed stable transmission from generation to generation, unlike the dynamic mutations seen in families with fragile X. More recently, 2 mouse models have been created that better recapitulate the human condition. A knockin mouse with 98 human CGG repeats has been generated that shows instability on transmission, in addition to a lack of methylation.[51] A similar knockin mouse with 118 CGG repeats has also been developed.[52] The mouse models showed increased *FMR1* mRNA and reduced FMRP expression. The mice also have ubiquitin-positive intranuclear inclusions, declining motor performance on the rotarod, and deficits in learning and memory in the Morris water maze.[53]

A *Drosophila* model for the fragile X premutation has been created with 90 rCGG repeats, which lead to neurodegeneration.[54] The *Drosophila* have neuronal inclusion bodies that are Hsp70 and ubiquitin positive.

EVALUATION AND MANAGEMENT
Strategies for Diagnosis

Epidemiologic studies suggest that patients, especially men, with cerebellar gait ataxia have the highest likelihood of having FXTAS. The presence of kinetic tremor, cognitive deficits, or other features seen in the disorder may increase the yield of testing. Most individuals with FXTAS were originally ascertained through testing individuals in families with a fragile X syndrome proband. However, this situation is changing given that the disease was discovered more than a decade ago. Testing is accomplished easily through clinical laboratories, but coverage for testing varies depending on insurance.

Genetic counseling is vital in families with fragile X–associated disorders. All female offspring of male *FMR1* premutation carriers are at risk for primary ovarian insufficiency, infertility, and having children affected with fragile X syndrome. Cascade testing, as frequently performed when a fragile X syndrome child is identified, can also be offered to families with members affected with FXTAS (see **Box 1**).[55]

Current Management and Therapeutic Options

There are no disease-modifying medical treatments for FXTAS. Like most neurodegenerative diseases, treatment is focused on alleviating symptoms. There are no proven symptomatic agents, but medications used for similar diseases are typically used and may be beneficial (**Table 1**).[56] Kinetic tremor can be treated with β-blockers, primidone, or topiramate, although with less effectiveness than that seen in essential tremor.[56] Benzodiazepines may also be helpful in patients with coexisting anxiety disorders.[57] Levetiracetam was reported to be beneficial in 1 patient with FXTAS.[58]

Table 1
Suggested medications for symptomatic treatment of FXTAS

Sign	Medication
Kinetic tremor	Propranolol
	Primidone
	Topiramate[a]
	Levetiracetam
Gait ataxia	Amantadine
	Varenicline[b]
	Riluzole
	Memantine
	Physical therapy
Parkinsonism	Levodopa
Anxiety	Benzodiazepines
Cognitive decline	Donepezil
	Memantine
Depression	Venlafaxine

[a] May worsen cognitive function.
[b] May worsen tremor.
From Hall D, Berry-Kravis E, Hagerman R, et al. Symptomatic treatment of the fragile X–associated tremor/ataxia syndrome. Mov Disord 2006;21:1743; with permission.

Isolated patients have shown improvement in gait ataxia on ataxia rating scales with amantadine, varenicline, riluzole, and memantine.[17,59,60] Parkinsonism, including problems with balance, may be responsive to levodopa or other dopaminergic agents.[56] Although not specifically studied, physical therapy or exercise is likely to be beneficial in patients with FXTAS who have cerebellar gait ataxia, given the multitude of positive studies in other ataxias.[61] More complex balance protocols, using computerized dynamic posturography with biofeedback retraining devices (available at select centers), might be most beneficial for patients with FXTAS with balance disorders.[62]

Slowing of cognitive decline by anticholinesterase inhibitors has been reported by caregivers of patients with FXTAS.[56] Case reports of venlafaxine alone and in combination with donepezil or memantine have shown improvement in cognitive and psychiatric manifestations in the disease.[63–65]

Future Directions in Therapy and Diagnosis

Recent advances have led to a novel single-tube CGG repeat primed *FMR1* polymerase chain reaction test that quickly detects expanded *FMR1* repeats, with 100% accuracy.[66] In addition, the method also shows AGG interruptor sequences, which may influence expansion in children of some carriers. This method minimizes the number of samples that require Southern blot analysis and quickens diagnosis for patients. Because FXTAS has only recently been discovered, there is only 1 ongoing clinical trial of the disorder. Based on the pathophysiology, which shows that increased histone acetylation occurs in premutation carriers, histone acetyltransferase inhibitors have been used to reduce *FMR1* mRNA to normal levels and suppress CGG repeat neurotoxicity, extending life span in a *Drosophila* model of FXTAS.[42] This finding suggests that the first disease-modifying studies in the disorder may come from these types of agents.

SUMMARY

FXTAS is a progressive neurodegenerative disorder characterized by kinetic tremor and cerebellar ataxia. FXTAS is seen in individuals with 55 to 200 CGG repeats in the *FMR1* gene and shows age-dependent penetrance, with symptoms typically manifesting in patients older than 55 years. Affected individuals also have executive dysfunction, parkinsonism, peripheral neuropathy, and characteristic findings on neuroimaging and pathology. The disorder is postulated to be secondary to RNA toxicity. Treatment is typically symptomatic, and no medications or disease-modifying treatments of the disorder have been approved by the US Food and Drug Administration.

REFERENCES

1. Hagerman RJ, Leavitt BR, Farzin F, et al. Fragile-X–associated tremor/ataxia syndrome (FXTAS) in females with the FMR1 premutation. Am J Hum Genet 2004;74(5):1051–6.
2. Hagerman RJ, Leehey M, Heinrichs W, et al. Intention tremor, parkinsonism, and generalized brain atrophy in male carriers of fragile X. Neurology 2001;57(1): 127–30.
3. Jacquemont S, Hagerman RJ, Leehey M, et al. Fragile X premutation tremor/ ataxia syndrome: molecular, clinical, and neuroimaging correlates. Am J Hum Genet 2003;72(4):869.
4. Leehey MA, Berry-Kravis E, Min SJ, et al. Progression of tremor and ataxia in male carriers of the FMR1 premutation. Mov Disord 2007;22(2):203–6.

5. Juncos JL, Lazarus JT, Graves-Allen E, et al. New clinical findings in the fragile X-associated tremor ataxia syndrome (FXTAS). Neurogenetics 2011;12(2): 123–35.
6. Hall DA, Berry-Kravis E, Jacquemont S, et al. Prior diagnoses given to persons with the fragile X-associated tremor/ataxia syndrome. Neurology 2005;65: 299–301.
7. Seltzer MM, Baker MW, Hong J, et al. Prevalence of CGG expansions of the FMR1 gene in a US population-based sample. Am J Med Genet B Neuropsychiatr Genet 2012;159B(5):589–97.
8. Hall DA, Hagerman RJ, Hagerman PJ, et al. Prevalence of FMR1 repeat expansions in movement disorders. A systematic review. Neuroepidemiology 2006; 26(3):151–5.
9. Bacalman S, Farzin F, Bourgeois JA, et al. Psychiatric phenotype of the fragile X-associated tremor/ataxia syndrome (FXTAS) in males: newly described fronto-subcortical dementia. J Clin Psychiatry 2006;67(1):87–94.
10. Grigsby J, Brega AG, Jacquemont S, et al. Impairment in the cognitive functioning of men with fragile X-associated tremor/ataxia syndrome (FXTAS). J Neurol Sci 2006;248(1–2):227–33.
11. Grigsby J, Brega AG, Engle K, et al. Cognitive profile of fragile X premutation carriers with and without fragile X-associated tremor/ataxia syndrome. Neuropsychology 2008;22(1):48–60.
12. Bourgeois JA, Seritan AL, Casillas EM, et al. Lifetime prevalence of mood and anxiety disorders in fragile X premutation carriers. J Clin Psychiatry 2011; 72(2):175–82.
13. Soontarapornchai K, Maselli R, Fenton-Farrell G, et al. Abnormal nerve conduction features in fragile X premutation carriers. Arch Neurol 2008;65(4): 495–8.
14. Apartis E, Blancher A, Meissner WG, et al. FXTAS: new insights and the need for revised diagnostic criteria. Neurology 2012;79(18):1898–907.
15. Pugliese P, Annesi G, Cutuli N, et al. The fragile X premutation presenting as postprandial hypotension. Neurology 2004;63(11):2188–9.
16. Louis E, Moskowitz C, Friez M, et al. Parkinsonism, dysautonomia, and intranuclear inclusions in a fragile X carrier: a clinical-pathological study. Mov Disord 2006;21(3):420–5.
17. Jacquemont S, Farzin F, Hall D, et al. Aging in individuals with the FMR1 mutation. Am J Ment Retard 2004;109(2):154–64.
18. Horvath J, Burkhard PR, Morris M, et al. Expanding the phenotype of fragile X-associated tremor/ataxia syndrome: a new female case. Mov Disord 2007; 22(11):1677–8.
19. Zhang L, Coffey S, Lua LL, et al. FMR1 premutation in females diagnosed with multiple sclerosis. J Neurol Neurosurg Psychiatr 2009;80(7):812–4.
20. Tassone F, Greco CM, Hunsaker MR, et al. Neuropathological, clinical and molecular pathology in female fragile X premutation carriers with and without FXTAS. Genes Brain Behav 2012;11(5):577–85.
21. Brunberg JA, Jacquemont S, Hagerman RJ, et al. Fragile X premutation carriers: characteristic MR imaging findings of adult male patients with progressive cerebellar and cognitive dysfunction. AJNR Am J Neuroradiol 2002;23(10): 1757–66.
22. Schrag A, Kingsley D, Phatouros C, et al. Clinical usefulness of magnetic resonance imaging in multiple system atrophy. J Neurol Neurosurg Psychiatr 1998; 65(1):65–71.

23. Storey E, Knight MA, Forrest SM, et al. Spinocerebellar ataxia type 20. Cerebellum 2005;4(1):55–7.
24. Lee J, Lacomis D, Comu S, et al. Acquired hepatocerebral degeneration: MR and pathologic findings. AJNR Am J Neuroradiol 1998;19(3):485–7.
25. Greco CM, Hagerman RJ, Tassone F, et al. Neuronal intranuclear inclusions in a new cerebellar tremor/ataxia syndrome among fragile X carriers. Brain 2002; 125:1760–71.
26. Hunsaker MR, Greco CM, Spath MA, et al. Widespread non-central nervous system organ pathology in fragile X premutation carriers with fragile X-associated tremor/ataxia syndrome and CGG knock-in mice. Acta Neuropathol 2011; 122(4):467–79.
27. Greco CM, Berman RF, Martin RM, et al. Neuropathology of fragile X-associated tremor/ataxia syndrome (FXTAS). Brain 2006;129(Pt 1):243–55.
28. Sullivan AK, Marcus M, Epstein MP, et al. Association of FMR1 repeat size with ovarian dysfunction. Hum Reprod 2005;20(2):402–12.
29. Hall D, Berry-Kravis E, Zhang W, et al. FMR1 gray-zone alleles: association with Parkinson's disease in women? Mov Disord 2011. http://dx.doi.org/10.1002/mds.23755.
30. Loesch DZ, Khaniani MS, Slater HR, et al. Small CGG repeat expansion alleles of FMR1 gene are associated with parkinsonism. Clin Genet 2009;76:471–6.
31. Crawford DC, Meadows KL, Newman JL, et al. Prevalence and phenotype consequence of FRAXA and FRAXE alleles in a large, ethnically diverse, special education-needs population. Am J Hum Genet 1999;64:495–507.
32. Jacquemont S, Hagerman RJ, Leehey MA, et al. Penetrance of the fragile X-associated tremor/ataxia syndrome in a premutation carrier population. JAMA 2004;291(4):460.
33. Leehey M, Berry-Kravis E, Goetz C, et al. FMR1 CGG repeat length predicts motor dysfunction in premutation carriers. Neurology 2008;70(16):139–42.
34. Jacquemont S, Leehey MA, Hagerman RJ, et al. Size bias of fragile X premutation alleles in late-onset movement disorders. J Med Genet 2006;43(10): 804–9.
35. Hall D, Tassone F, Klepitskaya O, et al. Fragile X-associated tremor ataxia syndrome in FMR1 gray zone allele carriers. Mov Disord 2011;27(2):296–300.
36. Tassone F, Hagerman RJ, Taylor AK, et al. Elevated levels of FMR1 mRNA in carrier males: a new mechanism of involvement in the fragile X syndrome. Am J Hum Genet 2000;66:6–15.
37. Garcia-Alegria E, Ibanez B, Minguez M, et al. Analysis of FMR1 gene expression in female premutation carriers using robust segmented linear regression models. RNA 2007;13(5):756–62.
38. Tassone F, De Rubeis S, Carosi C, et al. Differential usage of transcriptional start sites and polyadenylation sites in FMR1 premutation alleles. Nucleic Acids Res 2011;39(14):6172–85.
39. Jin P, Duan R, Qurashi A, et al. Pur alpha binds to rCGG repeats and modulates repeat-mediated neurodegeneration in a Drosophila model of fragile X tremor/ataxia syndrome. Neuron 2007;55(4):556–64.
40. Sellier C, Rau F, Liu Y, et al. Sam68 sequestration and partial loss of function are associated with splicing alterations in FXTAS patients. EMBO J 2010;29(7): 1248–61.
41. Sofola OA, Jin P, Qin Y, et al. RNA-binding proteins hnRNP A2/B1 and CUGBP1 suppress fragile X CGG premutation repeat-induced neurodegeneration in a Drosophila model of FXTAS. Neuron 2007;55(4):565–71.

42. Todd PK, Oh SY, Krans A, et al. Histone deacetylases suppress CGG repeat-induced neurodegeneration via transcriptional silencing in models of fragile X tremor ataxia syndrome. PLoS Genet 2010;6(12):e1001240.

43. Gatchel JR, Zoghbi HY. Diseases of unstable repeat expansion: mechanisms and common principles. Nat Rev Genet 2005;6(10):743–55.

44. Irwin SA, Galvez R, Greenough WT. Dendritic spine structural anomalies in fragile-X mental retardation syndrome. Cereb Cortex 2000;10(10):1038–44.

45. Chen Y, Tassone F, Berman RF, et al. Murine hippocampal neurons expressing Fmr1 gene premutations show early developmental deficits and late degeneration. Hum Mol Genet 2010;19(1):196–208.

46. Cunningham CL, Martinez Cerdeno V, Navarro Porras E, et al. Premutation CGG-repeat expansion of the Fmr1 gene impairs mouse neocortical development. Hum Mol Genet 2011;20(1):64–79.

47. Garcia-Arocena D, Yang JE, Brouwer JR, et al. Fibroblast phenotype in male carriers of FMR1 premutation alleles. Hum Mol Genet 2010;19(2):299–312.

48. Qurashi A, Li W, Zhou JY, et al. Nuclear accumulation of stress response mRNAs contributes to the neurodegeneration caused by fragile x premutation rCGG repeats. PLoS Genet 2011;7(6):e1002102.

49. Napoli E, Ross-Inta C, Wong S, et al. Altered zinc transport disrupts mitochondrial protein processing/import in fragile X-associated tremor/ataxia syndrome. Hum Mol Genet 2011;20(15):3079–92.

50. Ross-Inta C, Omanska-Klusek A, Wong S, et al. Evidence of mitochondrial dysfunction in fragile X-associated tremor/ataxia syndrome. Biochem J 2010; 429(3):545–52.

51. Brouwer JR, Mientjes EJ, Bakker CE, et al. Elevated Fmr1 mRNA levels and reduced protein expression in a mouse model with an unmethylated fragile X full mutation. Exp Cell Res 2007;313(2):244–53.

52. Entezam A, Biacsi R, Orrison B, et al. Regional FMRP deficits and large repeat expansions into the full mutation range in a new fragile X premutation mouse model. Gene 2007;395(1–2):125–34.

53. Berman RF, Willemsen R. Mouse models of fragile X-associated tremor ataxia. J Investig Med 2009;57(8):837–41.

54. Jin P, Zarnescu DC, Zhang F, et al. RNA-mediated neurodegeneration caused by the fragile X premutation rCGG repeats in *Drosophila*. Neuron 2003;39(5): 739–47.

55. McConkie-Rosell A, Abrams L, Finucane B, et al. Recommendations from multidisciplinary focus groups on cascade testing and genetic counseling for fragile X-associated disorders. J Genet Couns 2007;16(5):593–606.

56. Hall D, Berry-Kravis E, Hagerman R, et al. Symptomatic treatment of the fragile X-associated tremor/ataxia syndrome. Mov Disord 2006;21:1741–4.

57. Leehey MA. Fragile X-associated tremor/ataxia syndrome: clinical phenotype, diagnosis, and treatment. J Investig Med 2009;57(8):830–6.

58. Saponara R, Greco S, Proto G, et al. Levetiracetam improves intention tremor in fragile X-associated tremor/ataxia syndrome. Clin Neuropharmacol 2009;32(1): 53–4.

59. Zesiewicz TA, Sullivan KL, Freeman A, et al. Treatment of imbalance with varenicline Chantix(R): report of a patient with fragile X tremor/ataxia syndrome. Acta Neurol Scand 2009;119(2):135–8.

60. Ristori G, Romano S, Visconti A, et al. Riluzole in cerebellar ataxia: a randomized, double-blind, placebo-controlled pilot trial. Neurology 2010;74(10): 839–45.

61. Landers M, Adams M, Acosta K, et al. Challenge-oriented gait and balance training in sporadic olivopontocerebellar atrophy: a case study. J Neurol Phys Ther 2009;33(3):160–8.
62. Cohen HS, Kimball KT. Decreased ataxia and improved balance after vestibular rehabilitation. Otolaryngol Head Neck Surg 2004;130(4):418–25.
63. Bourgeois JA, Farzin F, Brunberg JA, et al. Dementia with mood symptoms in a fragile X premutation carrier with the fragile X-associated tremor/ataxia syndrome: clinical intervention with donepezil and venlafaxine. J Neuropsychiatry Clin Neurosci 2006;18(2):171–7.
64. Hagerman RJ, Hall DA, Coffey S, et al. Treatment of fragile X-associated tremor ataxia syndrome (FXTAS) and related neurological problems. Clin Interv Aging 2008;3(2):251–62.
65. Ortigas MC, Bourgeois JA, Schneider A, et al. Improving fragile X-associated tremor/ataxia syndrome symptoms with memantine and venlafaxine. J Clin Psychopharmacol 2010;30(5):642–4.
66. Chen L, Hadd A, Sah S, et al. An information-rich CGG repeat primed PCR that detects the full range of fragile X expanded alleles and minimizes the need for southern blot analysis. J Mol Diagn 2010;12(5):589–600.

Clinical Neurogenetics
Huntington Disease

Yvette M. Bordelon, MD, PhD

KEYWORDS

- Huntingtin • CAG repeat disorder • Striatum • Presymptomatic genetic testing
- Preimplantation genetic diagnosis • Tetrabenazine

KEY POINTS

- Huntington disease (HD) is an autosomal dominant disorder caused by a CAG repeat expansion in the huntingtin gene.
- HD is typically manifest in adulthood and characterized by progressive deterioration in motor, cognitive, and behavioral functions, with chorea as the primary motor manifestation of disease.
- The pathologic hallmark of HD is striatal atrophy, but widespread cell loss, gliosis, and huntingtin-positive neuronal inclusions are demonstrated in cortical and extrastriatal structures.
- HD serves as a model for presymptomatic genetic testing and preimplantation genetic diagnosis for multiple other disorders whose genetic causes are being identified.
- Current treatment approaches are symptomatic, but disease-modifying interventions including medications and gene-based and stem cell–based therapies are under investigation.

INTRODUCTION

Huntington disease (HD) results from an abnormal expansion of a CAG repeat in the huntingtin gene that is dominantly inherited. It is typically an adult-onset disorder that causes the following:

- Abnormal movements
  - Chorea
  - Dystonia
  - Rigidity
  - Bradykinesia

Disclosures: Member of Speakers Bureaus for Lundbeck, Inc, Teva Neuroscience and Medical Education Speakers Network.
Department of Neurology, David Geffen School of Medicine at UCLA, 710 Westwood Plaza, Los Angeles, CA 90210, USA
E-mail address: ybordelon@mednet.ucla.edu

Neurol Clin 31 (2013) 1085–1094
http://dx.doi.org/10.1016/j.ncl.2013.05.004
0733-8619/13/$ – see front matter © 2013 Elsevier Inc. All rights reserved.

neurologic.theclinics.com

- Behavioral manifestations
  - Depression
  - Anxiety
  - Obsessive-compulsive symptoms
  - Irritability/aggression
  - Apathy
  - Psychosis
- Cognitive impairment
  - Impaired attention and concentration
  - Poor organization and planning
  - Memory loss
  - Visuospatial dysfunction

These symptoms appear gradually in any combination varying among individuals and families and progress inexorably leaving the person with HD ultimately mute and akinetic.

CLINICAL FINDINGS

HD was first described by the physician George Huntington in 1872 in his paper entitled "On Chorea," where he reported on the families living in Long Island, New York, affected by "that disorder" who were cared for by him as well as his grandfather and father before him.[1] This paper described the core features of the illness including the typical adult onset, progressive nature of the disease, prominent chorea, and associated psychiatric illness with a tendency to suicide. He also characterized the inheritance pattern remarking that if a person in an affected family was spared the disease, no one descending from that individual would develop it; in other words, an autosomal dominant pattern.

At present, the prevalence of HD is estimated to be 7 to 10 per 100,000 in the United States, and a similar range has also been reported in the United Kingdom, although a debate continues as to whether these are underestimates.[2,3] The typical age of onset is in the fourth decade of life, and progression to death occurs over a 20- to 25-year period. In less than 10% of cases, the onset occurs before age 20 years and is accompanied by more severe motor symptoms of disease, sometimes accompanied by seizures and faster progression over a 10- to 15-year period (Westphal variant).

The clinical hallmark of HD is chorea, defined as uncontrolled movements flowing from one muscle group to another. Additional abnormal movements that are part of HD include dystonia, gait and postural instability, myoclonus, rigidity, and bradykinesia. These motor symptoms are often quite subtle as they become manifest, and no clear definitions exist for the severity or types of motor symptoms that must be present to make a firm diagnosis of clinical onset. In addition, it has become clear from studies of gene-positive individuals that the cognitive and behavioral symptoms of HD often precede the movement disorder by several years.[4–6]

The cognitive impairment seen in HD is thought to arise from dysfunction of frontal-subcortical pathways, thus giving rise to deficits in executive tasks (attention, concentration, planning, and multitasking) and other frontal features such as impulsivity. Recent clinical research studies (PREDICT and TRACK-HD) have followed premotor manifest HD subjects over time to capture which tasks or functions may be affected earliest. These studies have demonstrated impairment in the domains of executive function, memory, and visuospatial tasks. As the disease progresses, cognitive impairment worsens and most eventually meet criteria for dementia, with multiple domains being affected and contributing to functional decline.[7] However, even in late-stage HD, patients may maintain alertness and cognitive processing skills that allow them to understand what is happening around them but without the motor function to communicate. Health care providers must be aware of this and try to develop creative methods for communicating.

Behavioral symptoms of HD can present early and can be quite severe with significant impacts on interpersonal relationships and quality of life. The problems are diverse and vary among and within HD families. Depression is common in all stages of HD and has been estimated to occur in approximately 40% of patients.[8] Anxiety as well as obsessive-compulsive traits may be present and can be quite severe. Irritability and emotional dyscontrol leading sometimes to violent outbursts can occur and are also difficult to treat. Impulsivity may be present. These symptoms in combination with the other behavioral manifestations of the disease contributes to the higher rate of suicide attempts and ideation seen in the population with HD.[9] Patients with HD may also have various addiction problems including smoking, alcohol, and drugs. All behavioral manifestations are believed to result from disruption of frontal-subcortical circuits as well.

The phenotypic expression of HD varies widely among and within families of HD. Often a pattern evolves whereby in one family the behavioral manifestations are the earliest and most debilitating and in another the motor features present initially and are the greatest source of impairment. In addition, although these symptoms emerge gradually over time, they generally only come to attention when they begin to interfere with an individual's independent functioning. This functional impairment may be in the workplace or at home or in combination, and the threshold for "impairment" varies from person to person. Clinical studies have demonstrated that the first sign of diminished function in patients with HD is loss of employment.[10] This change in function is more closely tied to the cognitive and behavioral features of HD rather than the motor.

GENETICS AND DISEASE PATHOLOGY

In the centennial celebration of George Huntington's work, Dr Amerigo Negrette presented a paper describing a high prevalence of HD in people living in towns near Lake Maracaibo in Venezuela. Intrigued by this report, Dr Nancy Wexler of Columbia University organized the Venezuela Collaborative Huntington's Disease project with the goal of finding the cause of HD. In 1981, the first of 22 annual trips to the region occurred where large pedigrees were established and data collected including motor and neuropsychological testing as well as blood samples. This massive effort resulted in identification of the marker on chromosome 4 in 1983 and discovery of the causative gene mutation, an expanded CAG repeat in the IT-15 gene (now called the huntingtin gene), in 1993.[11] Since the identification of the HD gene mutation, there has been a wealth of research into the understanding of the role that this repeat expansion plays in the pathophysiology of the disease. The huntingtin gene is located on 4p16.3 and encodes the protein huntingtin. It belongs to a family of expanded CAG repeat disorders with spinal and bulbar muscular atrophy (Kennedy disease) being the first described.[12] Disease-causing mutations have a CAG repeat length of 40 and higher. There is an association with higher repeat lengths being associated with earlier age at onset but CAG repeat length only accounts for approximately 50% to 60% of predicted onset age.[13,14] Other genetic modifiers and environmental influences that contribute to HD onset are being sought in ongoing research efforts.

Huntingtin is a 348-kDa protein that is ubiquitously expressed, with the highest levels found in neurons. It is primarily cytoplasmic but also localizes to the nucleus and organelles.[15] The N-terminus contains a polyproline region in addition to the glutamine stretch resulting from the CAG expansion, which are both involved in the pathophysiology. The normal functions of huntingtin have not been completely elucidated, but it has thus far been found to play a role in a myriad of normal processes including axonal and vesicular transport, endocytosis, postsynaptic signaling, and cell survival pathways (reviewed in Ref.[16]).

Mutant huntingtin undergoes N-terminal cleavage, resulting in polyglutamine fragments, which can oligomerize and form aggregates, both cytoplasmic and nuclear. The N-terminal fragments, oligomers of these fragments, and the fully formed inclusions have been implicated in the toxicity of HD. It has been demonstrated that mutant huntingtin adversely affects a multitude of intracellular processes and causes widespread disruption including mitochondrial dysfunction, transcriptional dysregulation of various genes, altered axonal transport of critical factors, disrupted calcium signaling, abnormal protein interactions, alterations in proteosomal function, and autophagy. These diverse mechanisms are well reviewed by Zuccato and colleagues.[16]

The overall effects of mutant huntingtin expression are cell loss and gliosis in the brain, with the striatum being most affected by the disease. Jean-Paul Vonsattel developed the pathologic grading scheme for HD using striatal atrophy as the hallmark by which to characterize disease severity.[17] Grade 0 is defined by a normal gross appearance of the striatum but a 30% to 40% neuronal loss in the caudate nucleus, grade 1 exhibits atrophy of the tail of the caudate and 50% neuronal loss in the structure, grade 2 has mild-moderate gross atrophy of the caudate and even greater neuronal loss, grade 3 exhibits severe caudate atrophy with even greater neuronal loss, and grade 4 has severe atrophy with an obvious concave appearance of the caudate and greater than 95% neuronal loss (**Fig. 1**). In grades 3 and 4, there is notable cell loss of extrastriatal structures such as the cortex, globus pallidus, thalamus, subthalamic nucleus, substantia nigra, and cerebellum. Several elegant studies using magnetic resonance imaging have demonstrated progressive striatal atrophy first noted years before motor symptom onset in HD.[18] Cortical atrophy is also apparent before motor symptoms, with posterior frontal regions affected the earliest

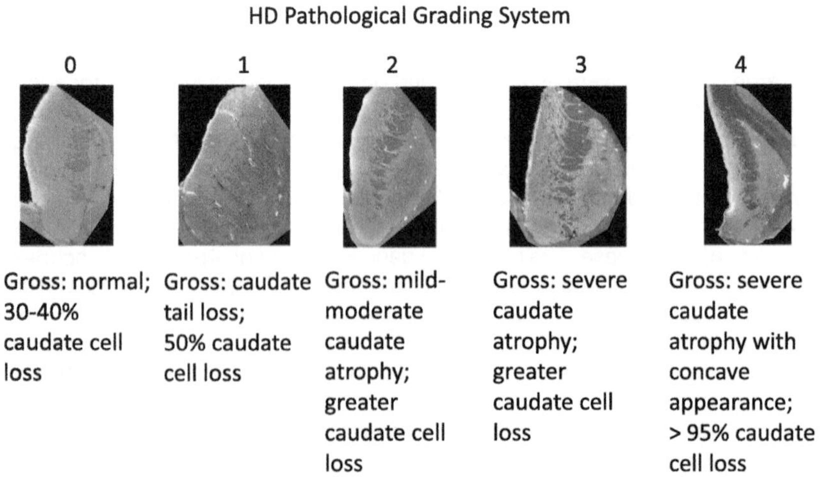

HD Pathological Grading System

0	1	2	3	4
Gross: normal; 30-40% caudate cell loss	Gross: caudate tail loss; 50% caudate cell loss	Gross: mild-moderate caudate atrophy; greater caudate cell loss	Gross: severe caudate atrophy; greater caudate cell loss	Gross: severe caudate atrophy with concave appearance; > 95% caudate cell loss

Fig. 1. Luxol fast blue with hematoxylin and eosin counterstained coronal sections of striatum from subjects with HD representative of each pathologic grade 0 to 4. (*Courtesy of* Jean-Paul Vonsattel, MD, Columbia University Medical Center.)

with progression to involve occipital, parietal, and other cortical regions eventually resulting in significant and widespread thinning.[19,20]

The medium-sized spiny gamma-aminobutyric acid (GABA) containing neurons of the striatum seem to be the most vulnerable to huntingtin toxicity. It has been proposed that the "indirect pathway" comprising GABAergic striatal projections to the external globus pallidus are affected earlier in the disease, thus resulting in loss of inhibition of this structure with resulting enhanced inhibition of GABAergic projections to the subthalamic nucleus. This in turn produces decreased excitation of the glutamatergic projections to the globus pallidus internus and overall diminished inhibitory GABAergic outflow to the thalamus. This disinhibition of the thalamus allows for enhanced excitatory outflow to the cortex resulting in hyperkinetic or uncontrolled movements, that is, chorea (**Fig. 2**). As the disease progresses into late stages the "direct pathway" also becomes profoundly affected, which results in loss of GABAergic inhibition of the internal globus pallidus and enhanced GABAergic inhibitory outflow to the thalamus. This thalamic inhibition of excitatory cortical connections produces a hypokinetic or akinetic state as seen in the last stages of HD (see **Fig. 2**).[21]

EVALUATION AND MANAGEMENT

The standard remains that symptomatic HD is diagnosed at the time of onset of the characteristic motor signs of the disease. However, since 1993, the genetic diagnosis of HD has been available, allowing for identification of individuals who carry the HD gene mutation but do not yet exhibit signs or symptoms of the disease. Titles for this population of gene-positive individuals have varied over time: presymptomatic, premanifest, premotor, and prodromal. All terms try to characterize a period of lack

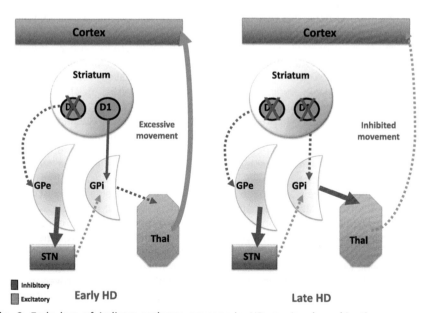

Fig. 2. Early loss of indirect pathway neurons in HD causing hyperkinetic movements (chorea) followed by later involvement of direct pathway neurons (akinesia). D1, D2, dopamine receptors; GPe, globus pallidus externus; GPi, globus pallidus internus; STN, subthalamic nucleus; Thal, thalamus.

of measurable deficits before actual disease onset. This technology thus becomes "heavily loaded" with information for at-risk individuals that affects (1) the future of their own health, career, and family planning; (2) other family members' risk status; and (3) their eligibility for obtaining life, long-term care, and possibly medical insurance in the future. (However, the federal Genetic Information Nondiscrimination Act passed in 2008 should prevent discrimination against persons with or at risk for genetic diseases by medical insurance providers and employers.)

These special circumstances have led to the development of HD genetic testing procedures in the at-risk population. It is advised that all at-risk persons speak with genetic counselors to discuss the full implications of obtaining the test before having the testing performed. Many clinical sites will also arrange meetings with neurologists or psychologists before testing and recommend that a family member or friend accompany the person to all appointments. The results are always given in person rather than by phone or mail to provide the best supportive environment possible in dealing with reactions to the genetic diagnosis. It must be emphasized that many patients who receive a negative result for the HD gene test also have problems managing their negative diagnosis given the guilt that accompanies it.

The gene test is reported as diagnostic for HD if the CAG repeat length in the huntingtin gene is 40 or greater and is normal if 26 or lower. Repeat lengths of 36 to 39 are "indeterminate," meaning they may have reduced penetrance, whereas intermediate repeat lengths of 27 to 35 may be normal or potentially disease-causing. Juvenile-onset HD typically occurs with repeat lengths of 50 and more. This condition occurs more commonly when the disease is inherited via the paternal line, as CAG repeat expansion may occur during spermatogenesis. There is a correlation between longer CAG repeat length and earlier onset of disease, but only approximately 50% to 60% of age of onset can be predicted by CAG repeat length.[14] Other as yet unidentified genetic or environmental modifiers may influence onset age as well.

Although the HD gene test has been available for some time, only a minority of at-risk people decide to obtain testing (estimated at 5% in the United States), as there are no known cures or treatments that delay the onset or progression of disease as yet.[22] Family planning issues are some of the major driving forces when persons at-risk for HD do decide to obtain genetic testing, and studies have revealed that women more often than men seek predictive testing.[23] Women who are at-risk for HD who are pregnant or are thinking about becoming pregnant can meet with genetic counselors to discuss testing options that are currently available. HD genetic testing can be obtained in utero through amniocentesis or chorionic villous sampling. Preimplantation genetic diagnosis (PGD) is performed utilizing in vitro fertilization technology.[24] Embryos are formed in vitro and tested for the HD gene at the 8-cell stage. Only those embryos not carrying the HD gene are implanted. This offers the advantage of not having to reveal the HD gene status to the at-risk parent. The downside is cost of the procedure and the failure rate of pregnancy with in vitro fertilization techniques.

Despite advances in testing options, there are few reports available documenting reproductive decision making in the population at risk for HD. Lesca and colleagues[25] showed that in a group of 868 at-risk couples, 5% requested presymptomatic testing while pregnant. Most of the couples (73%) decided to continue their pregnancy, and only 9% decided to do prenatal testing on their current pregnancy. Decruyenaere and colleagues[26] followed 89 subjects found to be carriers and 7 subjects with equivocal HD gene testing results for an average of 7 years after HD presymptomatic testing and reported on their reproductive decision making. They found that 48 subjects (46 gene positive and 2 equivocal) underwent gene testing for family planning reasons and 58% of them went on to have children with prenatal diagnosis or PGD. About 35% decided not have children after receiving their results and 7% remained undecided or did not have children for other reasons.

TREATMENT STRATEGIES

Despite the wealth of information learned during the past 2 decades on the function and dysfunction of mutant huntingtin, HD remains an incurable disease. However, symptomatic therapies are often used to provide some relief in the motor, behavioral, and cognitive symptoms.

Motor Symptoms

There are several medications that may alleviate chorea, but few controlled trials demonstrate their efficacy.[27,28] The American Academy of Neurology has published guidelines for chorea treatment in HD, but these are hampered by the paucity of randomized, placebo-controlled trials and comparisons among medications.[29] Tetrabenazine is a vesicular monoamine transport-2 inhibitor that causes presynaptic dopamine depletion and serves to ameliorate the chorea seen in HD. In fact, it is currently the only US Food and Drug Administration–approved medication for the treatment of HD. A placebo-controlled trial of tetrabenazine in HD demonstrated a significant reduction in chorea compared with placebo, with a 5-point decrease in chorea severity compared with 1.5-point improvement with placebo.[30] Amantadine has also been shown to provide improvement in chorea in HD presumably related to its antiglutamatergic action.[31,32] Both tetrabenazine and amantadine have level B evidence for chorea control per the American Academy of Neurology guidelines.[29] Dopamine receptor–blocking medications (neuroleptics) are also used to control chorea, although there are few studies to document whether any particular drug provides better symptom control than another. Both typical and atypical neuroleptics are used for chorea control, and selection depends on side-effect profile and availability. Benzodiazepines may also ameliorate chorea.

If dystonia predominates the motor manifestations of the disease, which may often happen in the later stages of disease, treatment with trihexiphenidyl, baclofen, benzodiazepines, or botulinum toxin injections for focal dystonia may be considered. Often, physical and occupational therapies are useful interventions to help the gait and balance difficulties, as well as the diminished motor control that accompanies HD progression. Speech and swallow therapies should be considered for dysarthria and dysphagia.

Behavioral Symptoms

The psychiatric manifestations of HD are wide ranging and include depression, anxiety, obsessive-compulsive symptoms, impulsivity, irritability, apathy, and psychosis. There is significant variability in the expression and severity of one or more of these symptoms in patients with HD, and evaluation and treatment of these symptoms must be individualized. There are few clinical trials that establish efficacy for any behavioral treatments in HD, but therapies are utilized alone or in combination in patients needing intervention. Selective serotonin reuptake inhibitors, serotonin-norepinephrine reuptake inhibitors, and other antidepressants are used in treatment of depression, anxiety, obsessive-compulsive symptoms, irritability, and impulsivity. A small study documented improvement in depression in subjects with HD with the use of venlafaxine XR.[33] Mood-stabilizing agents such as valproic acid as well as benzodiazepines may also be considered for anxiety and irritability. Neuroleptics are often used as agents that will help manage multiple HD symptoms. In addition to antichorea action, neuroleptics can also ameliorate irritability, psychosis, anxiety, and depression. Suicidal ideation is more common in the population with HD and must be addressed and risk factors (depression and impulsivity) treated aggressively. Concomitant psychotherapy including cognitive-behavioral therapy and counseling for patients and family members to handle these problems can provide significant improvement.

Cognitive Symptoms

Medications utilized in the treatment of Alzheimer disease have been explored for efficacy in HD-related cognitive impairment. The cholinesterase inhibitors including donepezil and rivastigmine may be used, but there is no evidence for established efficacy in HD.[27] Memantine may also be considered, but trials have not shown efficacy in cognitive symptomatology. Again, counseling patients and families may be of great benefit in managing these symptoms. Establishing routines, using novel communication strategies (centralized calendars), and close supervision are helpful.

FUTURE DIRECTIONS IN THERAPY

There is no therapy or intervention available that is proved to delay the onset or slow the progression of disease. This remains the primary focus of multiple studies in neurodegenerative diseases. HD stands out among these disorders as an ideal disease for potential neuroprotective or disease-modifying trials, as an identifiable presymptomatic subject population exists and is the target for such interventions. Studies are underway to assess the potential benefit of coenzyme Q10 and creatine as potential disease-modifying therapies given their role in addressing the energetic dysfunction present in HD.[27] Several other agents are being explored as well but have not yet moved into human clinical trials. The benefits of exercise are also being explored as an intervention that not only maintains mobility but may also serves to slow disease progression.

Many other strategies are being explored to modify the disease at the genetic level with HD again serving as an ideal disorder to study. Antisense oligonucleotides and RNA interference strategies that reduce expression of mutant huntingtin have been shown to ameliorate disease pathology and progression in HD transgenic mice.[34] These successes in animal models have spurred the design for human clinical trials using these interventions the start-ups of which are on the horizon.

Another exciting avenue of potential treatments incorporates the use of stem cell therapies. Previous studies utilized human fetal transplants in patients with HD, but clinical outcomes showed only mild, transient improvement, and follow-up at autopsy documented huntingtin inclusions in the transplanted tissue demonstrating spread of the pathologic condition.[35,36] However, many novel approaches are under development using a variety of stem cell sources including induced pluripotent stem cells, mesenchymal stem cells, neural stem cells, and embryonic stem cells. Such technologies are revealing further details of the pathophysiological mechanisms of disease in HD.[37] In addition, these techniques alone or in combination with gene therapy are being developed for human clinical trials in patients with HD.

SUMMARY

HD is an adult-onset, autosomal dominant, CAG repeat expansion disorder that results in progressive motor, behavioral, and cognitive decline related to striatal and cortical degeneration linked to pathologic inclusions of the huntingtin protein. HD serves as a model for genetic testing issues among dominantly inherited diseases.

In addition, it is ideal for investigating novel disease-modifying interventions including medications, gene silencing, gene therapy, and stem cell transplantation techniques.

REFERENCES

1. Huntington G. On chorea. The Medical and Surgical Reporter 1872;789:317–21.
2. Biglan KM, Shoulson I. Huntington's disease. In: Hallett M, Poewe W, editors. Therapeutics of Parkinson's disease and other movement disorders. Chicester (United Kingdom): John Wiley and Sons; 2008. p. 295–315.
3. Sackley C, Hoppitt TJ, Calvert M, et al. Huntington's disease: current epidemiology and pharmacological management in UK primary care. Neuroepidemiology 2011;37:216–21.
4. Stout JC, Paulsen JS, Queller S, et al. Neurocognitive signs in prodromal Huntington disease. Neuropsychology 2011;25:1–14.
5. Duff K, Paulsen JS, Beglinger LJ, et al. "Frontal" behaviors before the diagnosis of Huntington's disease and their relationship to markers of disease progression: evidence of early lack of awareness. J Neuropsychiatry Clin Neurosci 2010;22:196–207.
6. Tabrizi SJ, Scahill RJ, Durr A, et al. Biological and clinical changes in premanifest and early stage Huntington's disease in the TRACK-HD study: the 12-month longitudinal analysis. Lancet Neurol 2011;10:31–42.
7. Peavy GM, Jacobson MW, Goldstein JL, et al. Cognitive and functional decline in Huntington's disease: dementia criteria revisited. Mov Disord 2010;25:1163–9.
8. Paulsen JS, Nehl C, Hoth KF, et al. Depression and stages of Huntington's disease. J Neuropsychiatry Clin Neurosci 2005;17:496–502.
9. Paulsen JS, Hoth KF, Nehl C, et al. Critical periods of suicide risk in Huntington's disease. Am J Psychiatry 2005;162:725–31.
10. Paulsen JS, Wang C, Duff K, et al. Challenges assessing clinical end points in early Huntington disease. Mov Disord 2010;25:2595–603.
11. The Huntington's Disease Collaborative Research Group. A novel gene containing a trinucleotide repeat that is expanded and unstable on Huntington's disease chromosomes. Cell 1993;72:971–83.
12. La Spada AR, Wilson EM, Lubahn DB, et al. Androgen receptor gene mutations in X-linked spinal and bulbar muscular atrophy. Nature 1991;352:77–9.
13. Brinkman RR, Mezel MM, Theilmann J, et al. The likelihood of being affected with Huntington disease by a particular age, for a specific CAG size. Am J Hum Genet 1997;60:1202–10.
14. Wexler NS, Lorimer J, Porter J, et al. Venezuelan kindreds reveal that genetic and environmental factors modulate Huntington's disease age of onset. Proc Natl Acad Sci U S A 2004;101:3498–503.
15. DiFiglia M, Sapp E, Chase K, et al. Huntingtin is a cytoplasmic protein associated with vesicles in human and rat brain neurons. Neuron 1995;14:1075–81.
16. Zuccato C, Valenza M, Cattaneo E. Molecular mechanisms and potential therapeutical targets in Huntington's disease. Physiol Rev 2010;90:905–81.
17. Vonsattel JP, Myers RH, Stevens TJ, et al. Neuropathological classification of Huntington's disease. J Neuropathol Exp Neurol 1985;44:559–77.
18. Aylward EH, Liu D, Nopoulos PC, et al. Striatal volume contributes to the prediction of onset of Huntington disease in incident cases. Biol Psychiatry 2011;71(9):822–8.
19. Tabrizi SJ, Langbehn DR, Leavitt BR, et al. Biological and clinical manifestations of Huntington's disease in the longitudinal TRACK-HD study: cross-sectional analysis of baseline data. Lancet Neurol 2009;8:791–801.

20. Rosas HD, Salat DH, Lee SY, et al. Cerebral cortex and the clinical expression of Huntington's disease: complexity and heterogeneity. Brain 2008;131:1057–68.
21. Deng YP, Albin RL, Penney JB, et al. Differential loss of striatal projection systems in Huntington's disease: a quantitative immunohistochemical study. J Chem Neuroanat 2004;27:143–64.
22. Hayden MR. Predictive testing for Huntington's disease: a universal model? Lancet Neurol 2003;2:141–2.
23. Goizet C, Lesca G, Durr A. Presymptomatic testing in Huntington's disease and autosomal dominant cerebellar ataxias. Neurology 2002;59:1330–6.
24. Moutou C, Gardes N, Viville S. New tools for preimplantation genetic diagnosis of Huntington's disease and their clinical applications. Eur J Hum Genet 2004;12: 1007–14.
25. Lesca G, Goizet C, Durr A. Predictive testing in the context of pregnancy: experience in Huntington's disease and autosomal dominant cerebellar ataxia. J Med Genet 2002;39:522–5.
26. Decruyenaere M, Evers-Kiebooms G, Boogaerts A, et al. The complexity of reproductive decision-making in asymptomatic carriers of the Huntington mutation. Eur J Hum Genet 2007;15:453–62.
27. Venuto CS, McGarry A, Ma Q, et al. Pharmacologic approaches to the treatment of Huntington's disease. Mov Disord 2012;27:31–42.
28. Killoran A, Biglan KM. Therapeutics in Huntington's disease. Curr Treat Options Neurol 2012;14:137–49.
29. Armstrong MJ, Miyasaki JM. Evidence-based guideline: pharmacologic treatment of chorea in Huntington disease. Neurology 2012;79:597–603.
30. Huntington Study Group. Tetrabenazine as antichorea therapy in Huntington disease: a randomized control trial. Neurology 2006;66:366–72.
31. Verhagen Metman L, Morris MJ, Farmer C, et al. Huntington's disease: a randomized, controlled trial using the NMDA-antagonist amantadine. Neurology 2002;59: 694–9.
32. O'Suilleabhain P, Dewey RB Jr. A randomized trial of amantadine in Huntington disease. Arch Neurol 2003;60:996–8.
33. Holl AK, Wilkinson I, Painold A, et al. Combating depression in Huntington disease: effective antidepressive treatment with venlafaxine XR. Int Clin Psychopharmacol 2010;25:46–50.
34. Harper SQ. Progress and challenges in RNA interference therapy for Huntington disease. Arch Neurol 2009;66:933–8.
35. Bachoud-Levi AC, Gaura V, Brugieres P, et al. Effect of fetal neural transplants in patients with Huntington's disease 6 years after surgery: a long-term follow-up study. Lancet Neurol 2006;5:303–9.
36. Cicchetti F, Saporta S, Hauser RA, et al. Neural transplants in patients with Huntington's disease undergo disease-like neuronal degeneration. Proc Natl Acad Sci U S A 2009;106:12483–8.
37. Kaye JA, Finkbeiner S. Modeling Huntington's disease with induced pluripotent stem cells. Mol Cell Neurosci 2013;56C:50–64.

Clinical Neurogenetics
Friedreich Ataxia

Abigail Collins, MD

KEYWORDS

- Friedreich ataxia • Triplet repeat expansion • Autosomal recessive • Mitochondria
- Neurodegenerative disease

KEY POINTS

- Friedreich ataxia is the most common inherited ataxia in white people.
- Presentation is typically in adolescence, but can occur at any age.
- Signs and symptoms include posterior column and peripheral sensory neuropathy, areflexia, and ascending ataxia without cerebellar atrophy on brain magnetic resonance imaging, but less common phenotypes with preserved reflexes or progressive spastic paraplegia with less prominent ataxia also occur.
- Mortality is usually caused by cardiac morbidities, including arrhythmias or heart failure.
- Although there is no cure for Friedreich ataxia, management of comorbidities including scoliosis, dysphagia, sleep apnea, diabetes, cardiomyopathy, and arrhythmias can significantly improve quality of life and extend life expectancy.

INTRODUCTION

Definition

Friedreich ataxia is an autosomal recessive degenerative mitochondrial disorder affecting high-energy-use organs and tissues, including the heart and the central and peripheral nervous systems.[1] It is the most common cause of hereditary ataxia in the white population,[2] typically presenting in the first or second decade of life with slow progression.[3] In about 95% to 98% of affected individuals, the disease is caused by homozygous GAA TTC triplet repeat expansions in the first intron of the frataxin gene, *FXN*,[1] whereas point mutations or deletions in conjunction with an expanded triplet repeat account for the remainder of cases.[4,5] The expanded intronic alleles interfere with *FXN* transcription, decreasing the production of normally functioning frataxin protein to about 5% to 20% of normal.[6,7] Deficient frataxin levels result in excessive mitochondrial iron accumulation,[8,9] reduced iron-sulfur clusters vital for mitochondrial energy production,[10,11] and increased intracellular oxidative damage.[12–14] The consequence of these faulty cellular processes is inexorable cellular dysfunction, injury, and cell death producing the clinical phenotypes of this disease.[12,15] Treatments are supportive, and despite extensive ongoing research efforts there is currently no disease-modifying therapies or cure for Friedreich ataxia.

Funding Source: None.
Conflicts of Interest: The author has nothing to disclose.
Pediatrics and Neurology, Children's Hospital Colorado, University of Colorado, Denver, School of Medicine, 13123 East 16th Avenue, B155, Aurora, CO 80045, USA
E-mail address: abigail.collins@ucdenver.edu

Neurol Clin 31 (2013) 1095–1120
http://dx.doi.org/10.1016/j.ncl.2013.05.002
0733-8619/13/$ – see front matter © 2013 Elsevier Inc. All rights reserved.

SYMPTOMS AND CLINICAL COURSE

- Neurologic symptoms
  - Progressive gait instability and ataxia in 99% to 100% of patients, most often presenting in adolescence, resulting in loss of ambulation and unsupported sitting typically 10 to 15 years after onset of symptoms, although slower and faster progression are possible, and are related to repeat number and age of onset.[3,16–20]
  - Lower limb then upper limb incoordination and ataxia in 99% to 100% of patients.[3,16,18]
  - Weakness in feet and legs in 67% to 88% of patients,[3,16,19] followed in late disease by weakness in hands and arms.
  - Dysarthria typically early in the course, with slow, jerky speech, present in 91% to 97% of patients.[3,16,18,20]
  - Impaired sensation in feet in 73% to 92% of patients, followed by cool temperature and purple discoloration late in the course.[3,16,18–20]
  - Dysphagia in 27% to 64% of patients[16,19,20] worsening with advanced disease, particularly for thin liquids.
  - Impaired visual fixation and tracking.[20]
  - Decreased visual acuity in 13% to 27% of patients.[16,19]
  - Decreased hearing in 8% to 22% of patients.[3,16,19]
  - Urinary urgency then incontinence in late disease in 23% to 53% of patients.[16,18,19]
  - Preserved cognition, with mild executive dysfunction.[20]
  - Daytime fatigue caused by central sleep apnea.
- Cardiac symptoms
  - Palpitations caused by arrhythmias.[20]
  - Shortness of breath and exercise intolerance caused by hypertrophic cardiomyopathy, typically present but often asymptomatic until late in the course.[20] Cardiomyopathy is the cause of death in about 65% of people with Friedreich ataxia.[20]
- Skeletal symptoms
  - Kyphoscoliosis may be an early presenting feature with higher prevalence of double thoracic and lumbar curves in 60% to 79% of patients.[3,16,18–20]
  - Foot deformities in 52% to 74% of patients.[3,16,18–20]
- Endocrinologic symptoms
  - Excessive thirst and urination caused by glucose intolerance or frank diabetes mellitus in 8% to 32% of patients.[3,16,18]

EPIDEMIOLOGY

- Most common inherited ataxia, accounting for up to half of all genetic ataxias and as much as three-quarters of inherited ataxia in individuals younger than 25 years of age.[2,21]
- Prevalence rate is 1 in 30,000 to 50,000 people of white descent.[2]
- Approximately 1 in 100 people carry a mutant copy of FXN.[21]
- Most prevalent in the Americas, Europe, Australia, Asia, the Middle East, North Africa, and India because of a founder mutation in the white population with spread to these regions. It is least prevalent in China, Japan and Central Africa.[22]
- Onset typically in early teens, although may range from 2 years of age to the early 70s.[16]
- Disease duration: 75% survive longer than 34 years from onset of symptoms.[17]

- Median latency from symptom onset to confinement in a wheelchair is 11 years.[17]
- Mean age of death is 37 years.[3,20]

CLINICAL FINDINGS
Physical Examination

- General physical examination
  - Scoliosis in children (60%–79%).[3,16,18,19]
  - Bilateral pes cavus (52%–75%)[3,16,18,19] with equinovarus deformities (about 50%).[20]
  - Cool feet with purple discoloration and markedly prolonged capillary refill time.[20]
  - Soft heart sounds, peripheral edema, weak distal pulses, and increased jugular venous pulsations if significant cardiomyopathy (20%).[20]
- Neurologic examination
  - Normal mental status and apparent normal cognitive function but, on formal neuropsychological testing, impaired verbal fluency, attention, and working memory; reduced speed of information processing; and impaired visuoconstructive, visuoperceptive, and visuospatial reasoning may be present.[20]
  - Square wave jerks with fixation, slow extraocular movements, saccadic smooth pursuit in 12% to 30% of patients,[3,16] and horizontal nystagmus in 20% to 40% of patients.[3,16,20] Optic atrophy in 30% of patients and decreased visual acuity or loss in 13% to 27%, sometimes with a sudden onset.[3,16,18]
  - Ataxic speech (91%–97%) and slow lateral tongue movements.[3,16,18,20]
  - Hearing impairments (8%–22%).[3,16,19]
  - Limb weakness in an upper motor neuron pattern in 67% to 88% of patients with decreased distal bulk in lower limbs in 39% to 54% and upper limbs in 25% to 49%.[3,16,19]
  - Posterior column sensory neuropathy with impaired vibration sense initially present in feet and progressing rostrally in 73% to 92% of patients.[3,16,19]
  - Lower limb areflexia in 74% to 99% of patients with extensor plantar responses in 79% to 90%, and retained reflexes in 10%.[3,16,18–20]
  - Gait ataxia in 100% of patients[3,16,18–20] progressing to truncal ataxia with titubation requiring support.
  - Limb dysdiadochokinesis with rapid alternating movements in 99% to 100% of patients.[3,16] Dysmetria and intention tremor with reaching.

Imaging

Brain magnetic resonance Imaging (MRI) findings in Friedreich ataxia include atrophy of the spinal cord and medulla (**Fig. 1**),[23] and occasionally atrophy of the cerebellum, although this is an uncommon finding early in the course of disease.[24] Most often the cerebellum appears to be normal on conventional imaging without prominent atrophy early in the course of disease.[25–27] Brain MRI is typically obtained early in the course of an evaluation for individuals presenting with ataxia, and the absence of cerebellar atrophy supports Friedreich ataxia as a possible cause.

Research imaging techniques have been able to identify and quantify more subtle regions of gray and white matter atrophy, and determine correlations between disease severity and imaging findings. A volumetric-based MRI study confirmed atrophy of the dorsal medulla, and was able to show atrophy of the rostral cerebellar vermis, inferomedial cerebellar hemispheres, and of the peridentate white matter, but not of the dentate nucleus. The degree of atrophy in the involved brain regions correlated with

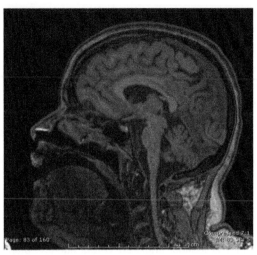

Fig. 1. Brain MRI in Friedreich ataxia. An 18-year-old woman with Friedreich ataxia showing characteristic findings of Friedreich ataxia with cervical cord atrophy and minimal cerebellar atrophy.

disease severity and duration.[28] Another study examined the superior cerebellar peduncle (SCP) cross-sectional area in patients with Friedreich ataxia and found them to be significantly smaller compared with controls, and that the SCP volumes were negatively correlated with disease severity and duration, and positively correlated with the age of disease onset.[29] MRI multigradient echo sequences showed significantly increased R2* values in the dentate nucleus of patients with Friedreich ataxia relative to controls, correlating with increased iron accumulation in this brain region.[30] MRI diffusion-tensor imaging, used to investigate white matter atrophy, found that, compared with control subjects, patients with Friedreich ataxia had white matter atrophy in the central portion of the medulla oblongata, the dorsal pons, central midbrain, bilateral peridentate region, superior cerebellar peduncles, medial right cerebral peduncle, and optic chiasm. The disease severity correlated significantly with atrophy of the bilateral peridentate white matter and the SCP decussation in the central midbrain.[31] Another study used diffusion-weighted imaging to assess neurodegeneration by measuring the mean diffusivity (MD) of water in the brain, because reduced integrity of brain tissue allows increased movement of water through the brain. This study found significantly higher MD values in patients with Friedreich ataxia compared with controls in the medulla, inferior cerebellar peduncle, middle cerebellar peduncle, SCP, optic radiations, brainstem, cerebellar hemispheres, and most prominently in the cerebellar vermis. The MD values were strongly correlated with disease duration and disease severity in patients as measured by an ataxia severity rating score.[32] Taken together, these studies using research imaging techniques show more widespread neurodegeneration of the white matter, especially of the brainstem and cerebellum, and cerebellar gray matter structures in patients with Friedreich ataxia than is apparent on conventional MRI imaging.

DISEASE PATHOLOGY

Within the central and peripheral nervous systems there is a selective vulnerability of specific types of motor and sensory neurons in Friedreich ataxia.[33] Early in the course of disease, the primary large myelinated sensory neurons of the dorsal root ganglia conveying proprioceptive, pressure, and vibration sense degenerate, resulting in an axonal peripheral neuropathy. The efferent components of these neurons enter the spinal cord where they either synapse in the Clark nucleus, which conveys unconscious sensory inputs to the cerebellum, or they ascend via the dorsal columns to synapse in the gracile or cuneate nuclei in the caudal medulla, which relay sensory information to both the ipsilateral cerebellum and the contralateral sensory cortex. The degeneration of the efferent components of the dorsal root ganglia sensory neurons produces atrophy of the dorsal columns, the spinocerebellar tract nuclei, and their outputs to the cerebellum and cortex. This degeneration results in profound impairment of proprioception and vibration, and accounts for the sensory ataxia of Friedreich ataxia. Other sensory neurons, including those of the auditory and visual systems, may also be affected and degenerate.[3]

Motor neurons are another vulnerable population of cells in Friedreich ataxia, particularly those originating from the primary motor cortex descending as the lateral corticospinal tracts of the spinal cord. Degeneration of these neurons results in atrophy of the corticospinal tracts and, symptomatically, upper motor neuron weakness.[33] The combined atrophy of the dorsal columns and corticospinal tracts of the spinal cord in Friedreich ataxia is highly characteristic, easily recognized, and commonly tested (**Fig. 2**). Within the cerebellum there is atrophy of the dentate nucleus, which results in the loss of cerebellar outputs and, thus, produces the cerebellar component of ataxia.[33] Heart disorders occur in most affected individuals, with early hypertrophy

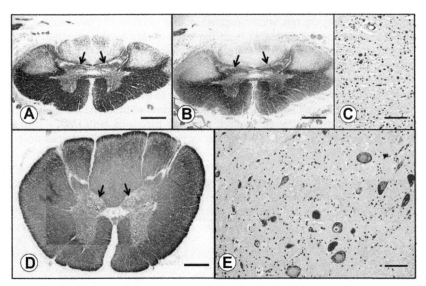

Fig. 2. Upper lumbar spinal cord in Friedreich ataxia. (*A–C*) Friedreich ataxia; (*D–E*) normal control. (*A, D*) Immunostain of myelin basic protein; (*B*) immunostain of phosphorylated neurofilament protein in axons; (*C, E*) cresyl violet. The overall area of the spinal cord in Friedreich ataxia (*A, B*) is greatly reduced in comparison with a normal control (*D*). In Friedreich ataxia, the nucleus dorsalis of Clarke (*C*) is devoid of large round chromatin-rich neurons. (*E*) The normal nucleus. Atrophy of the dorsal nuclei in Friedreich ataxia is also apparent on low-power magnification of the spinal cord (*arrows in A, B*). In the normal spinal cord, dorsal nuclei show a distinct bulge (*arrows in D*). Bars: (*A, B, D*), 1 mm; (*C, D*) 100 μm. (*From* Koeppen AH. Friedreich's ataxia: pathology, pathogenesis, and molecular genetics. J Neurol Sci 2011;303:1–12; with permission.)

of cardiac myocytes, particularly in the left ventricular wall and septum, followed by loss of myocytes and progressive replacement by connective tissue (**Fig. 3**).[34] End-stage cardiac disease results in dilatation of the heart with heart failure and iron deposits in surviving myocardial cells.[35]

GENETICS
Genetic Basis of Disease

Friedreich ataxia is an autosomal recessive disorder caused by homozygous triplet repeat expansions in the first intron of the frataxin gene, *FXN*, in 95% to 98% of affected individuals.[1] The remaining 2% to 5% are compound heterozygotes with one expanded allele and a second allele containing a point mutation or deletion.[1] *FXN* is located on chromosome 9q13 in humans, and encodes the highly conserved protein, frataxin (OMIM 606829; http://omim.org/entry/606829).[1,36] The frataxin gene contains 5 exons that encode a 210 amino acid mitochondrial matrix protein.[8] It is therefore an autosomal recessive mitochondrial disorder caused by mutations in a nuclear DNA gene that encodes for a mitochondrial protein.

The GAA TTC repeat tract within the first *FXN* intron is polymorphic in the human population with normal alleles containing 8 to approximately 38 repeats.[1] The critical pathologic triplet repeat threshold in Friedreich ataxia is approximately 90 repeats, with expansions reported in affected individuals ranging from about 90 to more than 1000 repeats; however, between 600 and 900 repeats most frequently are observed.[1] Because of a founder mutation in the white population, about 1 in 100 white people carry an expanded allele; however, heterozygous carriers of 1 expanded allele, point mutation, or deletion do not show features of the disease.[21] Transmission of the expanded triplet repeat is unstable from parent to child.[1] When inherited from the mother, contractions or expansions are equally common, whereas inheritance from the father more often results in contractions.[37] The expanded triplet repeat is also unstable within somatic cells, including postmitotic cells, and is theorized to account for the selective vulnerability of specific cell types, such as the dorsal root ganglia sensory neurons and motor cortex neurons.[38] The mechanisms of the dynamic triplet repeat instability have not been fully elucidated, although problems with DNA replication, recombination events, and aberrant DNA repair have all been postulated as potential explanations.[39]

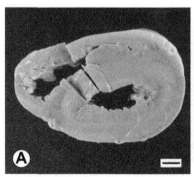 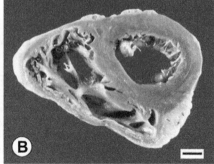

Fig. 3. Gross appearance of the heart in Friedreich ataxia. (*A*) Concentric cardiac hypertrophy and discoloration of the myocardium. In this case, the ventricles are narrowed. (*B*) Cardiac hypertrophy affecting only the left ventricular wall and interventricular septum. The right ventricle is dilated. Bars: 1 cm. (*From* Koeppen AH. Friedreich's ataxia: pathology, pathogenesis, and molecular genetics. J Neurol Sci 2011;303:1–12; with permission.)

The intronic triplet repeat expansion in Friedreich ataxia produces partial gene silencing, and results in a significantly reduced quantity of structurally and functionally normal frataxin to about 5% to 20% of normal levels.[6,7] In contrast, missense or null alleles are thought to result in nonfunctional or only partially functional frataxin and have never been observed to occur in a homozygous state.[1,4,21,40] The degree of partial *FXN* gene silencing is inversely correlated with the number of expanded triplet repeats, such that the higher the number of repeats, the lower the amount of frataxin produced.[7] In an individual with expanded alleles of 2 different sizes, the smaller allele determines the amount of residual frataxin production, and is clearly associated with the age of onset (but not severity) of disease.[7,41] Higher GAA repeat numbers in the smaller allele show earlier onset, more rapid disease progression, cardiomyopathy, and presence of associated nonuniversal disease manifestations such as diabetes, optic atrophy, and hearing loss.[42] However, copy number only accounts for 46% of the age of diagnosis, and other genetic and environmental factors play an important role in disease severity and progression.[43]

Patients with point mutations in combination with an expanded allele typically have a standard Friedreich ataxia phenotype caused by the triplet repeat expansion number, although a few specific missense mutations (D122Y, R165P, and G130V) cause an atypical and milder phenotype with early-onset spastic gait, slow disease progression, retained or brisk reflexes, normal speech, and minimal or absent ataxia.[4] This is thought to be caused by residual frataxin function of these missense mutations.

Molecular Pathogenesis: Frataxin Production and Function

There are several mechanisms by which triplet repeat expansions in an intron result in partial gene silencing and reduced frataxin production. These seem to occur at the level of transcription and/or pre-mRNA stability and processing rather than bring caused by posttranscriptional events, resulting in a deficiency of *FXN* mRNA levels to 4% to 29% of normal.[6,44] Blockage of transcription elongation by unusual DNA structures and epigenetic changes of the DNA interfering with transcription initiation seem to play a role. Evidence for altered splicing of mRNA transcripts suggests that this mechanism is not involved in diminished frataxin production.[45]

In vitro studies in Friedreich ataxia model systems provide evidence for the existence of preformed unusual secondary DNA structures. Triplexes occur when a single strand of the GAA TTC triplet repeat DNA binds to a double helix of the same GAA TTC triplet repeat, hairpin turns form from a single strand of expanded triplet repeat DNA that folds back and anneals to itself, and sticky DNA forms when the expanded triplet repeat region forms a triplex by binding 2 separate triplet repeat DNA segments and linking them.[46–51] These preexisting secondary structures seem to inhibit transcription by sequestering transcription factors and RNA polymerase, and by inhibiting the transcription complex from unwinding the DNA template.[52,53] There is in vitro evidence to suggest that R-loops form in which DNA triplet repeat triplexes are generated during transcription, allowing the unpaired strand of pyrimidine-rich triplet repeat DNA to anneal with the nascent RNA, resulting in an RNA:DNA hybrid that blocks transcription and traps RNA polymerase on the DNA template.[46,47,54]

Epigenetic changes as shown in **Fig. 4** are another mechanism of gene silencing in Friedreich ataxia, whereby the increased GAA TTC triplet repeats induce local heterochromatin that is transcriptionally repressed.[45,55] Heterochromatin formation is secondary to increased DNA methylation of DNA sequences adjacent to the expanded triplet repeat region, and decreased histone acetylation in the same region. The compact chromatin configuration prevents binding of transcription factors, thereby inhibiting transcription initiation and elongation.[56–60] The exact mechanisms of

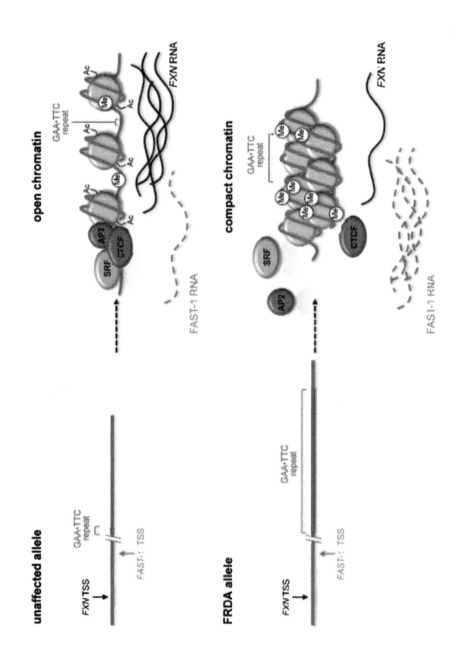

heterochromatin formation are not clearly elucidated, but the net impact is a significant reduction in the amount of *FXN* RNA.[45]

Although the exact function of frataxin is unknown, data support a role in iron metabolism as outlined in **Fig. 5**.[61,62] Frataxin is vital for cellular function, as shown by constitutional knockout experiments in which a complete lack of frataxin results in embryonic lethality in all investigated multicellular organisms.[63–66] Frataxin has an important role in the biogenesis of iron-sulfur clusters, which are necessary for mitochondrial respiratory chain complexes I, II, III, and the Krebs cycle enzyme aconitase function.[11] Iron-sulfur cluster biogenesis occurs in the mitochondria, and, in addition to reduced energy production, a deficiency of frataxin results in mitochondrial iron accumulation because of an excess of unincorporated iron in the iron-sulfur clusters.[8,9,11,67–69] Iron homeostasis is also disturbed because of the lack of feedback inhibition of iron-sulfur clusters on the iron regulatory protein that inhibits cellular iron uptake.[70,71] The result is constitutive iron uptake, which contributes to ongoing intracellular injury because of oxidative stress. Iron enters the mitochondria as reduced iron, which, if not rapidly incorporated into metabolic pathways, may react with hydrogen peroxide to form insoluble intramitochondrial iron precipitates, and generate hydroxyl radicals in the process.[33,72,73] Because of the deficiency of iron-sulfur clusters, mitochondrial respiratory chain complexes I, II, and III cannot function adequately and leak electrons across the inner mitochondrial membrane.[11,73] These react with molecular oxygen to ultimately form hydrogen peroxide, which oxidizes reduced iron to generate more hydroxyl radicals.[73] Free radicals damage a host of intracellular proteins, lipids, and DNA, and stimulate cell signaling pathways including stress responses, resulting in cellular injury and ultimately cell death through apoptosis.[73] The deficiency of this small, ubiquitous protein causes intracellular cataclysm and metabolic apocalypse.

Genomics

Although triplet repeat size has a significant influence on the phenotype of Friedreich ataxia, it accounts for only about 46% of the variability in the age of onset, indicating that there are other genetic or environmental factors involved.[43] Mitochondrial DNA

Fig. 4. An epigenetic model for Friedreich ataxia. Not shown to scale. Unaffected alleles are aberrantly methylated in the region flanking the repeat. Nonetheless, the 5′ end of the gene is associated with histones that are enriched for marks of active chromatin. In particular, acetylation of histone H3 and H4 is high. The net result is that the chromatin is open and permissive for transcription. Transcription factors including serum response factor (SRF), activator protein 2 (AP2)[33] and CCCTC-binding factor (CTCF)[25] associate with the 5′ end of the gene. An early growth response protein 3 (EGR3)-like factor binds to the 5′ end of intron 1[33] and an E-box binding protein[48] bind to the region immediately upstream of the repeat. Under these conditions transcription initiation and elongation takes place normally. In contrast, Friedreich ataxia alleles become associated with histones that are hypoacetylated and show more extensive DNA methylation in the region flanking the repeat. The net effect of these and other histone changes is the formation of a compact chromatin configuration, which reduces binding of transcription factors and both frataxin (*FXN*) transcription initiation and elongation are reduced. Loss of CTCF binding is correlated with an increase in the amount of FXN antisense transcript-1 (FAST-1) RNA that is transcribed antisense to *FXN*, but how this relates to silencing is unclear. TSS, transcription start site. (*Reproduced from* Kumari D, Usdin K. Is Friedreich ataxia an epigenetic disorder? Clin Epigenetics 2012;4(1):2. Available at: http://www.clinicalepigeneticsjournal.com/content/4/1/2; with permission.)

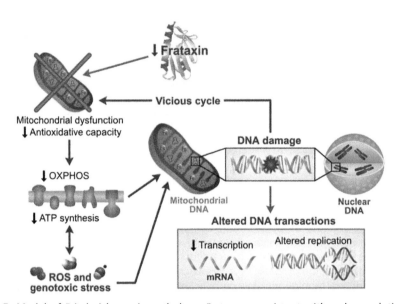

Fig. 5. Model of Friedreich ataxia pathology. Data are consistent with a dysregulation of mitochondrial function, decreased oxidative phosphorylation, increased reactive oxygen species (ROS) production, and subsequent mitochondrial and nuclear DNA damage. These factors contribute to decreased signaling and altered DNA transactions, which are likely to result in subsequent loss of protein synthesis and decreased protein degradation, as suggested in the transcription profiling. These alterations may cause tissue damage, altered immune response, and the clinical pathology associated with Friedreich ataxia. OXPHOS, oxidative phosphorylation. (*Reproduced from* Haugen AC, Di Prospero NA, Parker JS, et al. Altered gene expression and DNA damage in peripheral blood cells from Friedreich's ataxia patients: cellular model of pathology. PLoS Genet 2010;6(1):e1000812. http://dx.doi.org/10.1371/journal.pgen.1000812; with permission.)

has been investigated in this regard because it is polymorphic within the population, and specific haplotypes can be identified from maternal inheritance patterns.[74] The groups of particular haplotypes are called mtDNA haplogroups, and are known to influence polymorphic biological features of healthy individuals, such as sperm motility[75] and longevity,[76] as well as disease expression in disorders such as Leber hereditary optic neuropathy[77] and late-onset Alzheimer disease.[78] A study by Giacchietti investigated the influence of mitochondrial haplogroups on the Friedreich ataxia phenotype and found that haplogroup U, commonly found in European populations, had a delay in the age of disease onset and a lower rate of cardiomyopathy.[79] Other genomic factors influencing frataxin transcription and disease phenotype have not yet been identified.

Relevant Disease Models

Numerous models have been developed to study Friedreich ataxia and the consequences of frataxin deficiency including yeast,[8,9] *Caenorhabditis elegans*,[80–82] zebrafish,[83] mice,[84–89] and, more recently, human induced pluripotent stem cells (iPSCs) from affected individuals.[90] The *FXN*-knockout mouse model shows embryonic lethality,[63] whereas the KIKI (double knock-in) and KIKO (simple knock-in crossed with a knockout) mouse models with 230 GAA repeats have no overt disease phenotype but are useful for studying involved biologic pathways.[88] The YG8R mouse model containing the full human *FXN* locus with a triplet repeat expansion and deleted for the endogenous murine frataxin gene partially recapitulates disease phenotype with ataxia and DRG (dorsal root ganglia) pathology, but lacks cardiomyopathy.[89] Conditional mouse models of *FXN* deletion have been useful for studying postembryonic effects of absent frataxin in specific organs and tissues depending on the promoter used, but so far no model accurately recapitulates the partial frataxin deficiency and human disease phenotype. This is an active area of ongoing research. Of the numerous cellular models, the iPSC-derived cells are an exciting new research tool that shows decreased *FXN* expression, markers of heterochromatin at the GAA TTC expansion, as well as expansion instability of the GAA TTC repeat with mitosis.[90] Research efforts to generate specific neuronal cells and cardiomyocytes from iPSCs are underway. This disease-in-a-dish model will allow ongoing study of the underlying genetic and intracellular underpinnings of Friedreich ataxia, as well as providing a screening tool to assess the effect of medications and drugs.[83]

EVALUATION AND MANAGEMENT
Strategies for Diagnosis

Any patient with apparent sporadic or autosomal recessive progressive ataxia should be tested for Friedreich ataxia, and this diagnosis should be considered in patients with apparent sporadic or autosomal recessive hereditary spastic paraplegia with negative testing for causative genes. The commonly associated clinical features of Friedreich ataxia are variable, including impaired vibration and joint position sense, absent deep tendon reflexes, and adolescent age of onset, and the lack of these typical features does not exclude Friedreich ataxia as a possible diagnosis given the broadening phenotypic spectrum of this disorder. Testing should be sent for the triplet repeat expansions in the first intron of the *FXN* gene first. If this is nondiagnostic because of the presence of only 1 expanded allele, there are 2 options for additional testing. Frataxin protein levels can be easily and inexpensively measured clinically, and, if in the affected range, would support further gene studies.[91] As an alternative, gene studies could be sent without measuring frataxin, including sequencing of the *FXN* gene for point mutations, and, if negative, deletion analysis performed in patients with atypical phenotypes. Brain MRI is recommended to evaluate atrophy of the cerebellum, medulla, and spinal cord in all patients presenting with ataxia. Presence of significant cerebellar atrophy early in the course, which is an atypical finding, does not exclude the diagnosis. Nerve conduction velocity studies may show a large fiber sensory axonal neuropathy and provide further support for the diagnosis, but absence of neuropathy does not exclude the diagnosis, and is not routinely recommended given the availability of genetic testing.

There are several other genetic ataxias that may present with similar clinical features to Friedreich ataxia with decreased or absent reflexes, young age of onset, and lack of brain MRI cerebellar atrophy, as reviewed by Fogel and Perlman.[92] Ataxia with vitamin E deficiency typically manifests before 20 years of age, most commonly in individuals of North African origin. Cardiomyopathy is less common than in Friedreich ataxia, and retinitis pigmentosa or deficits in visual acuity may be early presenting features. Head titubation is prominent, and there is less neuropathy and a slower disease progression than is seen in Friedreich ataxia. Serum vitamin E levels are reduced because of a mutation in the alpha-tocopherol transfer protein. Treatment with vitamin E halts disease progression and can improve ataxia symptoms. Abetalipoproteinemia also presents typically before the age of 20 years, but, in addition to the phenotypic overlap with Friedreich ataxia, abetalipoproteinemia is typically associated with lipid malabsorption, diarrhea, acanthocytosis, hypocholesterolemia, and retinitis pigmentosa caused by deficiencies of fat-soluble vitamins, particularly vitamin E. The underlying genetic defect is caused by a mutation in the gene that encodes the large subunit of the microsomal triglyceride transfer protein. This protein functions in the assembly of apolipoprotein-B, which transports very-low-density lipoproteins and chylomicrons. Dietary modifications and fat-soluble vitamin supplementation may prevent neurologic complications if started early in the course of disease. In addition, Refsum disease has a complex phenotype with cerebellar ataxia without atrophy on imaging studies, peripheral neuropathy, sensorineural deafness, retinitis pigmentosa, anosmia, skeletal anomalies, ichthyosis, progressive renal insufficiency, cardiomyopathy, and/or arrhythmias. It is a progressive storage disorder caused by abnormalities of peroxisomal metabolism with insufficient branched-chain fatty acid oxidation of unusual fats found in dairy, meat, and fish. It is diagnosed by abnormalities in very-long-chain fatty acids, pristanic acid, and/or phytanic acid. The accumulation of unmetabolized fat in the peroxisomes of myelinated neurons disrupts their function through an unknown mechanism. Dietary restrictions of very-long-chain fatty acids, phytanic acid, and pristanic acid may be helpful to slow disease progression.

Current Management Strategies and Therapeutic Options

Once a diagnosis is made, the most important aspect of care for an individual with Friedreich ataxia is to screen for treatable comorbidities that can affect both morbidity and mortality. The following are recommended[93]:

- Swallow study to assess for dysphagia and aspiration at baseline and as needed for concerns of swallowing impairment thereafter with referral to speech and swallow therapist.
- Scoliosis series radiographs to screen for scoliosis annually in any child presenting at less than the age of 18 years, as an initial baseline in anyone presenting at more than 18 years of age, and referral to orthopedics for any abnormality for ongoing monitoring and management.
- Echocardiogram is the routine imaging technique of choice to evaluate for left ventricular and septal hypertrophy, and annual monitoring for the development of cardiomyopathy, because the severity of ataxia does not correlate with severity of cardiomyopathy. Cardiac MRI (cMRI) has been shown to be more sensitive and accurate in determining the severity of cardiac remodeling in patients with Friedreich ataxia, but may not be available in all locations.[94] Abnormalities detected on echocardiogram or cMRI should result in a cardiology referral for ongoing evaluation and management.
- Electrocardiogram annually to evaluate for repolarization abnormalities that could give rise to arrhythmias, and cardiology referral for any abnormalities.
- Holter monitor and referral to cardiology for patients experiencing palpitations.
- Screening for diabetes mellitus by glycosylated hemoglobin annually, and, if abnormally increased, a glucose tolerance test and referral to endocrinology.
- Neuropsychological testing at baseline, and as needed depending on concerns about executive function, judgment, and for abnormal score on Montreal Cognitive Assessment.
- Referral to genetic counselor or geneticist to discuss inheritance patterns and familial implications.
- Ophthalmology referral to evaluate for optic atrophy at baseline and as needed for visual impairments.
- Audiology referral to evaluate for hearing loss at baseline and as needed for hearing impairments.
- Sleep study to evaluate for sleep apnea (central or peripheral) and referral to pulmonologist or otolaryngologist to treat as indicated if abnormal.

- Urodynamic studies if urinary urgency or incontinence, and a referral to urology if symptoms are significant.
- Physical medicine and rehabilitation evaluation for equipment needs, a home safety evaluation, and referral to physical and occupational therapy.
- Screening for depression and social and economic stressors, and referral to mental health services and involvement of social work as needed.
- Referral to community-based ataxia support groups, such as the National Ataxia Foundation (www.ataxia.org) or the Friedreich Ataxia Research Alliance (www. curefa.org)

There are currently no medications approved to treat Friedreich ataxia, prolong the life of an individual with Friedreich ataxia, or cure the condition. Nonetheless, there are a host of medications that may be used off-label to treat comorbid symptoms, and thereby improve quality of life significantly. Many patients with ataxia can be more sensitive to the side effects of medications, just as older people may be more sensitive and need lower doses of medications. Symptoms that can be managed include depression, excessive daytime sleepiness, erectile dysfunction, fatigue, imbalance and incoordination, muscle cramps or spasms, weakness, neuropathy, nystagmus, overactive bladder, restless leg syndrome, stiffness, spasticity, rigidity, dystonia, and tremor (**Table 1**).[95]

Exercise and physical therapy should be prescribed to all patients with Friedreich ataxia based on available data. Moderate exercise was studied in a rat model of ataxia with reduced lifespan, and it increased lifespan compared with nonexercising control mutant rats by about 13%, improved motor function, and improved cerebellar Purkinje cell survival by 62%.[96] Human studies investigating the benefits of intensive physiotherapy in patients with degenerative cerebellar diseases showed a short-term benefit in balance and gait, and, more importantly, sustained improvements in more than half of the participants at 24 weeks from completion of the exercise regimen.[97] Children with ataxia showed improved motor performance despite progressive cerebellar degeneration by using directed training of whole-body-controlled video games; a highly motivational, economical, and accessible strategy to train dynamic balance and interactions with dynamic environments.[98] As opposed to medications, exercise and physiotherapy are the only known treatments for ataxia that can improve symptoms regardless of cause and may be able to slow disease progression. I recommend a minimum of 20 minutes of aerobic exercise per day for every patient with ataxia and/ or mitochondrial disorders, especially walking or a stationary bike to increase the heart rate; strengthening exercises of core muscle groups and legs; and stretching exercises of shoulders, hips, and hamstrings. In addition, balance exercises focused on proper flexed posture of the knees and arms in which the center of gravity is purposefully and in a controlled fashion taken away from midline and back again. See **Table 2** for specific physical therapy recommendations designed by Dr Broetz[99] for patients with ataxia, although these were not designed specifically for patients with Friedreich ataxia and have not been validated in clinical trials.

Future Directions in Therapy and Diagnosis

Although there are currently no treatments for Friedreich ataxia approved by the US Food and Drug Administration, there are several drugs being studied in both preclinical and clinical trials to address the underlying pathologic mechanisms, including decreased frataxin expression, mitochondrial iron accumulation, and oxidative stress, as shown in **Table 3**. As discussed earlier, the expanded intronic triplet repeats in Friedreich ataxia cause partial gene silencing, but the frataxin that is produced is

Table 1
Medications for symptoms associated with ataxia. There are no treatments approved by the US Food and Drug Administration for the symptom of ataxia. However, there are many other symptoms that commonly accompany ataxic disorders, and, in combination with adequate therapy and referral to appropriate medical specialists, medications may be useful to treat these accompanying symptoms. Many of these medications are being used off-label, and have been reported in the medical literature and by ataxia clinicians as being useful. Patients with ataxia are particularly sensitive to medications that act on the central nervous system, and doses should be adjusted accordingly. These medications should only be used under a doctor's supervision

Symptom	Medication Options
Depression	Class: SSRIs Class: SNRIs
Dizziness/vertigo	Acetazolamide 4-Aminopyridine Baclofen Clonazepam Flunarizine Gabapentin Meclizine Memantine Ondansetron Scopolamine
Excessive daytime sleepiness	Modafinil Armodafinil
Erectile dysfunction	Tadalafil Vardenafil Sildenafil
Fatigue	Amantadine Atomoxetine Buproprion Carnitine Creatine Modafanil Armodafinil Pyridostigmine Selegiline Venlafaxine Desvenlafaxine Class: SSRIs Class: SNRIs
Imbalance/incoordination	Amantadine Buspirone Riluzole Varenicline
Memory or cognitive impairment	Class: cholinesterase inhibitors Memantine
Muscle cramps or spasms	Baclofen Tizanidine
Weakness	Creatine
Neuropathy	Duloxetine Gabapentin Pregabalin Class: antiseizure medications Class: tricyclic antidepressants

(continued on next page)

Table 1 (continued)	
Symptom	**Medication Options**
Nystagmus	Acetazolamide 4-Aminopyridine Baclofen Carbamazepine Clonazepam Gabapentin Isoniazid Memantine
Overactive bladder	Class: anticholinergic medications Botulinum toxin injections
Speech and swallowing impairments	Fluoxetine
Stiffness/dystonia/spasticity	Amantadine Baclofen Botulinum toxin injections Dantrolene sodium Diazepam Carbidopa-levodopa Pramipexole Ropinirole Tizanidine Trihexyphenidyl
Action or rest tremor	Amantadine Botulinum toxin Injections Carbamazepine Clonazepam Flunarizine Gabapentin Isoniazid Levetiracetam Carbidopa-levodopa Ondansetron Pramipexole Primidone Propranolol Ropinirole Topiramate Valproic acid Deep brain stimulation Surgery

Abbreviations: SNRI, serotonin-norepinephrine reuptake inhibitor; SSRI, selective serotonin reuptake inhibitor.

Reproduced from the National Ataxia Foundation; with permission.

structurally and functionally normal for most affected individuals with 2 homozygous expanded alleles. A feasible therapeutic approach is to increase *FXN* transcription to correct the frataxin deficiency. Because histone hypoacetylation is associated with heterochromatin formation and transcriptional silencing in expanded *FXN* alleles, histone deactylase (HDAC) inhibitors are being actively investigated as a mechanism to induce an active chromatin conformation, and thereby increase frataxin expression.[100] HDAC inhibitors have been shown to increase frataxin levels in blood lymphocytes of patients with Friedreich ataxia in vitro,[58] and in an in vivo mouse model of Friedreich ataxia without acute toxicity.[101] Preclinical toxicity and phase I clinical

Table 2
Exercises for ataxia. The goal of physical therapy exercises is to improve static and dynamic balance, improve coordination, and reduce stiffness and fear of falling. Exercises that cannot be performed without risk of falling should be performed with a therapist. Those exercises that can be safely performed without supervision should be done every day. Most importantly, exercises should be performed without holding on to anything and as fluidly as possible. Difficulty can be increased as goals are met, with the ultimate goal of reacting more flexibly when balance is lost

Exercise/Goal	Duration or Repetitions	Instructions
Walking • Dynamic balance • Conditioning	30 min per day minimum	Starting and stopping: bend your knees, face forward, relax your arms and stay flexible Changing direction: lift feet while changing direction, take several steps, always in a forward direction, bend your knees Walking on different surfaces: walk on uneven ground, walk with a partner, but do not hold on to anything, walk uphill and downhill on cement or tarmac
Back extension lying prone • Flexibility	5–10 repetitions	Lie prone on stomach with elbows bent and hands flat on ground below shoulders Straighten your arms to lift torso off the floor. The legs and pelvis should remain on the floor Relax your back and gluteal muscles, and extend long through the legs, pointing your toes Lower yourself back into the prone position
Back rotation lying on back • Flexibility	10 repetitions to each side	Lie on your back with your legs bent, feet on the floor, arms to the side of your head with your elbows bent at the ears and hands above head Tilt your knees to one side while simultaneously turning your head in the opposite direction Bring your knees and head back to the midline, and repeat to the other side
Shoulder range of motion lying on back • Flexibility	10 repetitions	Lie on your back with your arms by your side, palms down Lift your arms and rest them on the floor on either side of your head with your elbows slightly bent, palms up Extend your arms, straightening the elbows With your hands on the floor, bring your arms down toward your sides, palms down
Leg and arm extension from all fours • Flexibility • Coordination	5 repetitions on each side	Kneel down, and place your palms on the floor, shoulder with apart directly under your shoulders in a table position Touch your left elbow to your right knee underneath your belly, rounding your back as you do so Without touching the floor, extend your left arm and right leg, holding them at least parallel with the ground, while balancing on your supporting leg and arm

(continued on next page)

Table 2
(continued)

Exercise/Goal	Duration or Repetitions	Instructions
Forward bend from sitting • Flexibility • Coordination	5 repetitions	Sit on a comfortable chair with your feet touching the floor Bend forward as far as you can, relaxing your arms, then straighten up into a seated position Variations with increased difficulty: Bend forward and touch your toes, sit back up Bend forward and touch the floor, lift buttocks off chair and stand up
Weight shifting from sitting • Flexibility • Coordination	5 repetitions to each side	Sit on a comfortable chair with your feet touching the floor Hold your arms extended to your sides, shoulder height Shift your upper body to the right side, keeping your buttocks in place, then come back to sitting position. Repeat 5 times Shift your upper body to the left side, keeping your buttocks in place, then come back to sitting position. Repeat 5 times
Standing and sitting • Flexibility • Coordination	10 repetitions	Sit on a comfortable chair with your feet touching the floor Bend your back forward slightly, and shift your weight onto your feet Stand up, keeping your back and knees slightly bent Sit back down slowly without collapsing into the chair
Standing from bear crawl • Flexibility • Coordination	5 repetitions	Stand in a comfortable position, bend your knees and spine forward until you are touching the floor with your hands and feet (quadruped position) Straighten your legs while keeping your hands on the ground Lift your hands off the ground and stand again, keeping your weight forward and your knees and back slightly bent
Kneeling leg forward extension • Flexibility • Coordination	5 repetitions to each side	Kneel on a comfortable surface Move 1 leg forward and place your foot in front of you with the knee bent, in a marriage-proposal position. Try not to touch the floor with your toes as you move your foot forward Move back into a kneeling position
Kneeling leg sideways extension • Flexibility • Coordination	5 repetitions to each side	Kneel on a comfortable surface Straighten 1 leg to the side and tap the ground with your toes Move back into a kneeling position
Stand from kneeling • Flexibility • Coordination	5 repetitions to each side	Kneel on a comfortable surface Move 1 leg forward and place your foot in front of you with the knee bent, in a marriage-proposal position Stand up shifting your weight forward Bring your hind leg next to the forward leg

(continued on next page)

	Table 2 (continued)		

Table 2 (continued)

Exercise/Goal	Duration or Repetitions	Instructions
Knee bends • Static balance • Coordination • Leg strengthening	5 repetitions	Stand upright, feet hip width apart, with knees slightly bent and upper body upright Lift your heels off the ground Squat as far as possible while continuing to keep your torso erect Stand
Knee bounce and arm swing • Static balance • Coordination • Leg strengthening	30 s	Stand upright, feet hip width apart Gently bob up and down at the knees Swing your arms back and forth while bobbing
Side steps • Dynamic balance training	20 repetitions with each leg	Stand upright, feet hip width apart Take a big step to the side Bring your leg back to the original position
Forward steps • Dynamic balance training	20 repetitions with each leg	Stand upright, feet hip width apart Take a big step forward Bring your leg back to the original position
Backward steps • Dynamic balance training	20 repetitions with each leg	Stand upright, feet hip width apart Take a big step backward Bring your leg back to the original position
Cross-step front • Dynamic balance training	20 repetitions with each leg	Stand upright, feet hip width apart Take a step crossing one leg in front of the other Bring your leg back to the original position
Cross-step back • Dynamic balance training	20 repetitions with each leg	Stand upright, feet hip width apart Take a step crossing one leg in back of the other Bring your leg back to the original position

Adapted from Doris Broetz, Physiotherapy. Available at: www.broetz-physiotherapie.de; with permission.

trials of the most promising HDAC inhibitors are currently being developed.[102] Other medications that are being studied to increase *FXN* transcription include recombinant human erythropoietin in vitro[103] and in human trials,[41,104,105] PPARg (Peroxisome Proliferator-Activated Receptors gamma) agonists including pioglitazone in a proof-of-concept human trial in France, resveratrol in vitro,[106] and interferon gamma both in vitro and in a mouse model.[107] Another approach to increase intracellular frataxin is to supply the deficient frataxin protein via a TAT-frataxin fusion protein. This protein has been shown to enter mitochondria in cells cultured from patients and in a mouse model of Friedreich ataxia, resulting in improved growth, lifespan, and cardiac function.[108]

A second approach is to decrease the downstream effects of frataxin deficiency, such as mitochondrial iron accumulation and cytosolic iron deficits. Deferiprone has been the most studied medication in this regard, and is a lipid-soluble iron chelator that can be taken orally. It is currently used to treat iron overload in transfusion-dependent patients. Although there were initial suggestions that deferiprone reduced dentate nucleus iron in small open-label human trials,[30,109] a subsequent trial did not confirm this and suggested that the iron had shifted into ferritin in non-neuronal cells.[110] An open-label trial of 20 affected individuals showed stabilization in ataxia

Table 3
Investigational therapies for the treatment of Friedreich ataxia

Investigational Therapy	Category	Mechanism of Action
HDAC inhibitors	Transcriptional activator	Inhibit histone deacetylase enzymes to increase histone acetylation in the region of the *FXN* gene, which reduces heterochromatin, increases transcription, and increases frataxin protein levels within the cell
Recombinant human erythropoietin	Transcriptional activator	Increases intracellular frataxin levels without increasing *FXN* mRNA, suggesting a posttranscriptional effect
PPAR-gamma agonists	Transcriptional activator	PPARs are nuclear hormone receptors that stimulate transcription. PGC-1α functions as a transcriptional coactivator of PPAR-gamma and regulates genes involved in energy metabolism, including mitochondrial biogenesis and function. PGC-1α expression is downregulated in cells of patients with Friedreich ataxia. Bypassing this defect with a PPAR-gamma agonist, such as pioglitazone, increases mitochondrial biogenesis and proteins involved in their function, including frataxin
Interferon gamma	Transcriptional activator	Regulates iron distribution by directly modulating the expression of proteins involved in iron metabolism, including increasing *FXN* expression
TAT-frataxin fusion protein	Protein Replacement	A fusion protein synthesized by joining frataxin to the protein transduction domain of the TAT protein, which successfully delivers it to the mitochondria where it restores deficient frataxin levels
Deferiprone	Iron chelator	Deferiprone is an iron chelator that can cross cell membranes. It reduces intracellular iron and decreases intracellular iron accumulation
Resveratrol	Antioxidant	Interferes with Bax expression, an activator of the intrinsic apoptosis pathway to prevent cell death from oxidative stress
Idebenone	Antioxidant	Idebenone is an antioxidant that carries electrons and is a CoQ10 analogue. It facilitates mitochondrial respiratory chain function to improve mitochondrial ATP production and reduce oxidative stress from free radicals. It also interferes with apoptosis
EPI-743	Antioxidant	CoQ10 and idebenone analogue that is approximately 1000-fold to 10,000-fold more potent than CoQ10 or idebenone in protecting cells subjected to oxidative stress in patient fibroblasts

Abbreviations: CoQ10, coenzyme Q10; HDAC, histone deacetlyase; PGC-1α, PPAR-gamma coactivator-1 protein; PPAR, peroxisome proliferator-activated receptors.

scales over 11 months, and a decrease in cardiac wall thickness.[111] A larger double-blind, randomized, placebo-controlled phase II trial in 80 individuals with Friedreich ataxia was recently completed, and did not show an improvement in ataxia scale scores during the study, although a decrease in mass of the left ventricle was found.[102] Nonetheless, the risk of agranulocytosis makes this drug risky to use in the long term and necessitates weekly blood counts.

Reducing oxidative stress is another approach to treatment. Idebenone has been studied extensively for treatment of Friedreich ataxia in phase III clinical trials and open-label extension studies, and showed a trend toward improvement in ataxia scale scores and cardiac hypertrophy, but no end point was statistically significant.[112–114] Other antioxidants are being developed, including EPI-743, a highly fat-soluble antioxidant that has shown surprising clinical benefit in patients with mitochondrial disorders in phase I toxicity and phase IIa clinical trials.[115,116] A phase IIb clinical trial with EPI-743 is currently underway for individuals with Friedreich ataxia.

A combination of therapies will likely be adopted in the future to address each significant area of cellular disorder with the goal of maximizing benefits and reducing toxicity of any one agent. If successful treatment can be achieved to improve clinical symptoms and, more importantly, modify disease progression, there would be a rationale for presymptomatic diagnosis and management to prevent the development of symptoms of Friedreich ataxia in at-risk individuals. With the breadth of therapeutic approaches and rapid pace of development, this seems to be an achievable goal.

SUMMARY

Friedreich ataxia is the most common hereditary ataxia, especially in people of white descent. The unique genetics of this condition result in transcriptional inhibition of an otherwise structurally and functionally normal frataxin protein, whose role in mitochondrial energy production and intracellular metabolic processes is vital for cell survival. Important advances have been made in understanding the underlying molecular processes since the discovery of the gene in 1996, but the only treatments currently available that may improve the clinical manifestations or slow disease progression of this neurodegenerative disorder are exercise and physiotherapy. Management of non-neurologic symptoms improves quality and duration of life, and every neurologist managing patients with Friedreich ataxia should be familiar with appropriate interventions and treatment options. In addition, all individuals affected by Friedreich ataxia, including patients, their families, and their loved ones, should be offered hope for the future of Friedreich ataxia, because potential therapies are now being developed.

REFERENCES

1. Campuzano V, Montermini L, Molto M, et al. Friedreich's ataxia: autosomal recessive disease caused by an intronic GAA triplet repeat expansion. Science 1996;271:1423–7.
2. Cossée M, Schmitt M, Campuzano V, et al. Evolution of the Friedreich's ataxia trinucleotide repeat expansion: founder effect and permutations. Proc Natl Acad Sci U S A 1997;94:7452–7.
3. Harding AE. Friedreich's ataxia: a clinical and genetic study of 90 families with analysis of early diagnostic criteria and intrafamilial clustering of clinical features. Brain 1981;104:589–620.
4. Cossée M, Dürr A, Schmitt M, et al. Frataxin point mutations and clinical presentation of compound heterozygous Friedreich ataxia patients. Ann Neurol 1999;43:200–6.

5. Bichichandani S, Ashizawa T, Patel P. Atypical Friedreich ataxia caused by compound heterozygosity for a novel missense mutation and GAA triplet-repeat expansion. Am J Hum Genet 1997;60:1251–6.

6. Campuzano V, Montermini L, Lutz Y, et al. Frataxin is reduced in Friedreich ataxia patients and is associated with mitochondrial membranes. Hum Mol Genet 1997;6:1771–80.

7. Deutsch E, Santani A, Perlman S, et al. A rapid, noninvasive immunoassay for frataxin: utility in assessment of Friedreich ataxia. Mol Genet Metab 2010;101: 238–45.

8. Babcock M, de Silva D, Oaks R, et al. Regulation of mitochondrial iron accumulation by Yfh1, a putative homolog of frataxin. Science 1997;276:1709–12.

9. Foury F, Cazzalini O. Deletion of the yeast homologue of the human gene associated with Friedreich's ataxia elicits iron accumulation in mitochondria. FEBS Lett 1997;411:373–7.

10. Stehling O, Elsasser H, Bruckel B, et al. Iron-sulfur protein maturation in human cells: evidence for a function of frataxin. Hum Mol Genet 2004;13:3007–15.

11. Rötig A, de Lonlay P, Chretien D, et al. Frataxin gene expansion causes aconitase and mitochondrial iron-sulfur cluster protein deficiency in Friedreich ataxia. Nat Genet 1997;17:215–7.

12. Gakh O, Park S, Liu G, et al. Mitochondrial iron detoxification is a primary function of frataxin that limits oxidative damage and preserves cell longevity. Hum Mol Genet 2006;15:467–79.

13. Chantrel-Groussard K, Geromel V, Puccio H, et al. Disabled early recruitment of antioxidant defenses in Friedreich's ataxia. Hum Mol Genet 2001;10:2061–7.

14. Schulz J, Dehmer T, Schöls L, et al. Oxidative stress in patients with Friedreich ataxia. Neurology 2000;55:1719–21.

15. Santos M, Oshima K, Pandolfo M. Frataxin deficiency enhances apoptosis in cells differentiating into neuroectoderm. Hum Mol Genet 2001;10:1935–44.

16. Dürr A, Cossée M, Agid Y, et al. Clinical and genetic abnormalities in patients with Friedreich ataxia. N Engl J Med 1996;335:1169–75.

17. Klockgether T, Lüdtke R, Kramer B, et al. The natural history of degenerative ataxia: a retrospective study in 466 patients. Brain 1998;121:589–600.

18. Delatycki M, Paris D, McKinlay Gardner R. Clinical and genetic study of Friedreich ataxia in an Australian population. Am J Med Genet 1999;87: 168–74.

19. Ribaï P, Pousset F, Tanguy ML, et al. Neurological, cardiological and oculomotor progression in 104 patients with Friedreich ataxia during long-term follow-up. Arch Neurol 2007;64:558–64.

20. Delatycki M, Corben L. Clinical features of Friedreich ataxia. J Child Neurol 2012;27(9):1133–7.

21. Pandolfo M. Friedreich ataxia. Arch Neurol 2008;65:1296–303.

22. Labuda M, Labuda D, Miranda B, et al. Unique origin and specific ethnic distribution of the Friedreich ataxia GAA expansion. Neurology 2000;54:2322–4.

23. Wullner U, Klockgether T, Petersen D, et al. Magnetic resonance imaging in hereditary and idiopathic ataxia. Neurology 1993;43:318–25.

24. Junck L, Gilman S, Gebarski SS, et al. Structural and functional brain imaging in Friedreich's ataxia. Arch Neurol 1994;51:349–55.

25. Langelier R, Bouchard J, Bouchard R. Computer tomography of posterior fossa in hereditary ataxias. Can J Neurol Sci 1979;6:195–8.

26. Gyldensted C, Pedersen L. Computer tomography in hereditary ataxias. Neuroradiology 1978;16:327–8.

27. Wessel K, Schroth G, Diener H, et al. Significance of MRI-confirmed atrophy of the cranial spinal cord in Friedreich ataxia. Eur Arch Psychiatry Neurol Sci 1989; 238:225–30.

28. Della Nave R, Ginestroni A, Giannelli M, et al. Brain structural damage in Friedreich ataxia. J Neurol Neurosurg Psychiatry 2008;79(1):82–5.

29. Akhlaghi H, Corben L, Georgiou-Karistianis N. Superior cerebellar peduncle atrophy in Friedreich's ataxia correlate with disease symptoms. Cerebellum 2011;10:81–7.

30. Waldvogel D, van Gelderen P, Hallett M. Increased iron in the dentate nucleus of patients with Friedreich's ataxia. Ann Neurol 1999;46:123–5.

31. Pagani E, Ginestroni A, Della Nave R. Assessment of brain white matter fiber bundle atrophy in patients with Friedreich's ataxia. Radiology 2010;255:882–9.

32. Rizzo G, Tonon C, Valentino M, et al. Brain diffusion-weighted imaging in Friedreich's ataxia. Mov Disord 2011;26:705–12.

33. Koeppen A. Friedreich's ataxia: pathology, pathogenesis, and molecular genetics. J Neurol Sci 2011;303:1–12.

34. Casazza F, Morpurgo M. The varying evaluation of Friedreich's ataxia cardiomyopathy. Am J Cardiol 1996;77:895–8.

35. Lamarche JB, Cote M, Lamiuex B. The cardiomyopathy of Friedreich's ataxia morphological observations in 3 cases. Can J Neurol Sci 1980;7:389–96.

36. Chamberlain S, Shaw J, Rowland A, et al. Mapping of mutation causing Friedreich's ataxia to human chromosome 9. Nature 1988;334:248–50.

37. Pianese L, Cavalcanti F, De Michele G, et al. The effect of parental gender on the GAA dynamic mutation in the FRDA gene. Am J Hum Genet 1997;60:460–3.

38. De Biase I, Rasmussen A, Endres D, et al. Progressive GAA expansions in dorsal root ganglia of Friedreich's ataxia patients. Ann Neurol 2007;61:55–60.

39. Pearson CE, Nichol Edamura K, Cleary JD. Repeat instability: mechanisms of dynamic mutations. Nat Rev Genet 2005;6:729–42.

40. Correia A, Adinolfi S, Pastore A, et al. Conformational stability of human frataxin and effect of Friedreich's ataxia-related mutations on protein folding. Biochem J 2006;398:605–11.

41. Sacca F, Puorro G, Antenora A, et al. A combined nucleic acid and protein analysis in Friedreich ataxia: implications for diagnosis, pathogenesis and clinical trial design. PLoS One 2011;6:e17627, 1-9.

42. Montermini L, Richter A, Morgan K, et al. Phenotypic variability in Friedreich ataxia: role of the associated GAA triplet repeat expansion. Ann Neurol 1997; 41:675–82.

43. La Pean A, Jeffries N, Grow C, et al. Predictors of progression in patients with Friedreich ataxia. Mov Disord 2008;23:2026–32.

44. Punga T, Buhler M. Long intronic GAA repeats causing Friedreich ataxia impede transcription elongation. EMBO Mol Med 2010;2:120–9.

45. Kumari D, Usdin K. Is Friedreich ataxia an epigenetic disorder? Clin Epigenetics 2012;4(1):2. Available at: http://www.clinicalepigeneticsjournal.com/content/4/1/2.

46. Grabczyk E, Usdin K. The GAA*TTC triplet repeat expanded in Friedreich's ataxia impedes transcription elongation by T7 RNA polymerase in a length and supercoil dependent manner. Nucleic Acids Res 2000;28:2815–22.

47. Grabczyk E, Usdin K. Alleviating transcript insufficiency caused by Friedreich's ataxia triplet repeats. Nucleic Acids Res 2000;28:4930–7.

48. Jain A, Rajaswari M, Ahmed F. Formation and thermodynamic stability of intermolecular (R*R*Y) DNA triplex in GAA/TTC repeats associated with Friedreich's ataxia. J Biomol Struct Dyn 2002;19:691–9.

49. Mariappan S, Catasti P, Silks L, et al. The high-resolution structure of the triplex formed by the GAA/TTC triplet-repeat associated with Friedreich's ataxia. J Mol Biol 1999;285:2035–52.

50. Potaman V, Oussatcheva E, Lyubchenko Y, et al. Length-dependent structure formation in Friedreich ataxia (GAA)n*(TTC)n repeats at neutral pH. Nucleic Acids Res 2004;32:1224–31.

51. Sakamoto N, Chastain P, Parniewski P, et al. Sticky DNA: self-association properties of long GAA.TTC repeats in R.R.Y triplex structures from Friedreich's ataxia. Mol Cell 1999;3:465–75.

52. Kohwi Y, Kohwi-Shigematsu T. Altered gene expression correlates with DNA structure. Genes Dev 1991;5:2547–54.

53. Sakamoto N, Ohshima K, Montermini L, et al. Sticky DNA, a self-associated complex formed at long GAA*TTC repeats in intron 1 of the frataxin gene, inhibits transcription. J Biol Chem 2001;276:27171–7.

54. Grabczyk E, Mancuso M, Sammarco M. A persistent RNA.DNA hybrid formed by transcription of the Friedreich ataxia triplet repeat in live bacteria, and by T7 RNAP in vitro. Nucleic Acids Res 2007;35:5351–9.

55. Festenstein R. Breaking the silence in Friedreich's ataxia. Nat Chem Biol 2006;2:512–3.

56. Castaldo I, Pinelli M, Monticelli A, et al. DNA methylation in intron 1 of the frataxin gene is related to GAA repeat length and age of onset in Friedreich ataxia patients. J Med Genet 2008;45:808–12.

57. Greene E, Mahishi L, Entezam A, et al. Repeat-induced epigenetic changes in intron 1 of the frataxin gene and its consequences in Friedreich ataxia. Nucleic Acids Res 2007;35:3383–90.

58. Herman D, Jenssen K, Burnett R, et al. Histone deacetylase inhibitors reverse gene silencing in Friedreich's ataxia. Nat Chem Biol 2006;2:551–8.

59. Kim E, Napierala M, Dent S. Hyperexpansion of GAA repeats affects post-initiation steps of FXN transcription in Friedreich's ataxia. Nucleic Acids Res 2011;39:8366–77.

60. Kumari D, Biacsi R, Usdin K. Repeat expansion affects both transcription initiation and elongation in Friedreich ataxia cells. J Biol Chem 2011;286:4209–15.

61. Pandolfo M, Pastore A. The pathogenesis of Friedreich ataxia and the structure and function of frataxin. J Neurol 2009;256(Suppl 1):9–17.

62. Haugen A, Di Prospero N, Parker J, et al. Altered gene expression and DNA damage in peripheral blood cells from Friedreich's ataxia patients: cellular model of pathology. PLoS Genet 2010;6:e1000812. http://dx.doi.org/10.1371/journal.pgen.1000812.

63. Cossée M, Puccio H, Gansmuller A, et al. Inactivation of Friedreich ataxia mouse gene leads to early embryonic lethality without iron accumulation. Hum Mol Genet 2000;9:1219–26.

64. Ventura N, Rea S, Henderson S, et al. Reduced expression of frataxin extends the lifespan of Caenorhabditis elegans. Aging Cell 2005;4:109–12.

65. Anderson P, Kirby K, Hilliker A, et al. RNAi-mediated suppression of the mitochondrial iron chaperone, frataxin, in Drosophila. Hum Mol Genet 2005;14:3397–405.

66. Vazzola V, Losa A, Soave C, et al. Knockout of frataxin gene causes embryo lethality in Arabidopsis. FEBS Lett 2007;581:667–72.

67. Wilson R, Roof D. Respiratory deficiency due to loss of mitochondrial DNA in yeast lacking the frataxin homologue. Nat Genet 1997;16:352–7.

68. Lodi R, Cooper J, Bradley J, et al. Deficit of in vivo mitochondrial ATP production in patients with Friedreich ataxia. Proc Natl Acad Sci U S A 1999;96:11492–5.
69. Delatycki M, Camakaris J, Brooks H, et al. Direct evidence that mitochondrial accumulation occurs in Friedreich ataxia. Ann Neurol 1999;45:673–5.
70. Li L, Kaplan J. A mitochondrial-vacuolar signaling pathway in yeast that affects iron and copper metabolism. J Biol Chem 2004;279:33653–61.
71. Rouault T. The role of iron regulatory proteins in mammalian iron homeostasis and disease. Nat Chem Biol 2006;2:406–14.
72. Horton A, Fairhurst S. Lipid peroxidation and mechanisms of toxicity. CRC Crit Rev Toxicol 1987;18:27–79.
73. Pandolfo M. Friedreich ataxia: new pathways. J Child Neurol 2012;27:1204–11.
74. Torroni A, Huoponen K, Francalacci P, et al. Classification of European mtDNAs from an analysis of three European populations. Genetics 1996;144:1835–50.
75. Ruiz-Pesini E, Lapena A, Diez-Sanchez C, et al. Human mtDNA haplogroups associated with high or reduced spermatozoa motility. Am J Hum Genet 2000;67:682–96.
76. De Benedictis G, Rose G, Carrieri G, et al. Mitochondrial DNA inherited variants are associated with successful aging and longevity in humans. FASEB J 1999;13:1532–6.
77. Howell N, Oostra R, Bolhuis P, et al. Sequence analysis of the mitochondrial genomes from Dutch pedigrees with Leber hereditary optic neuropathy. Am J Hum Genet 2003;72:1460–9.
78. Shoffner J, Brown M, Torroni A, et al. Mitochondrial DNA variants observed in Alzheimer disease and Parkinson disease patients. Genomics 1993;17:171–84.
79. Giacchetti M, Monticelli A, De Biase I, et al. Mitochondrial DNA haplogroups influence the Friedreich's ataxia phenotype. J Med Genet 2004;41:293–5.
80. Vasquez-Manrique R, Gonzalez-Cabo P, Ros S, et al. Reduction of Caenorhabditis elegans frataxin increases sensitivity to oxidative stress, reduces lifespan, and causes lethality in a mitochondrial complex II mutant. FASEB J 2006;20:172–4.
81. Ventura N, Rea S, Testi R. Long-lived C. elegans mitochondrial mutants as a model for human mitochondrial-associated diseases. Exp Gerontol 2006;41:974–91.
82. Zarse K, Schulz T, Birringer M, et al. Impaired respiration is positively correlated with decreased life span in Caenorhabditis elegans models of Friedreich ataxia. FASEB J 2007;21:1271–5.
83. Yanicoustas C, as presented at the 4th International Friedreich's Ataxia Conference, as reviewed in (91) Martelli A, Napierala M, Puccio H. Understanding the genetic and molecular pathogenesis of Friedreich's ataxia through animal and cellular models. Dis Model Mech 2012;5:165–76.
84. Puccio H, Simon D, Cossée M, et al. Mouse models for Friedreich ataxia exhibit cardiomyopathy, sensory nerve deficit and Fe-S enzyme deficiency followed by intramitochondrial iron deposits. Nat Genet 2001;27:181–6.
85. Simon D, Seznec H, Gansmuller A, et al. Friedreich ataxia mouse models with progressive cerebellar and sensory ataxia reveal autophagic neurodegeneration in dorsal root ganglia. J Neurosci 2004;24:1987–95.
86. Ristow M, Mulder H, Pomplun D, et al. Frataxin deficiency in pancreatic islets causes diabetes due to loss of beta cell mass. J Clin Invest 2003;112:527–34.
87. Thierbach R, Schulz T, Isken F, et al. Targeted disruption of hepatic frataxin expression causes impaired mitochondrial function, decreased life span and tumor growth in mice. Hum Mol Genet 2005;14:3857–64.

88. Miranda C, Santos M, Ohshima K, et al. Frataxin knockin mouse. FEBS Lett 2002;512:291–7.
89. Al-Mahdawi S, Pinto R, Varshney D, et al. GAA repeat expansion mutation mouse models of Friedreich ataxia exhibit oxidative stress leading to progressive neuronal and cardiac pathology. Genomics 2006;88:580–90.
90. Ku S, Soragni E, Campau E, et al. Friedreich's ataxia induced pluripotent stem cells model intergenerational GAATTC triplet repeat instability. Cell Stem Cell 2010;7:631–7.
91. Brigatti K, Deutsch E, Lynch D, et al. Novel diagnostic paradigms for Friedreich ataxia. J Child Neurol 2012;27:1146–51.
92. Fogel B, Perlman S. Clinical features and molecular genetics of autosomal recessive cerebellar ataxias. Lancet Neurol 2007;6:245–57.
93. Bidichandani S, Delatycki M. Friedreich ataxia. In: Pagon R, Bird T, Dolan C, et al, editors. Gene reviews [Internet]. Seattle (WA): University of Washington, Seattle; 2012.
94. Meyer C, Schmid G, Gorlitz S, et al. Cardiomyopathy in Friedreich's ataxia: assessment by cardiac MRI. Mov Disord 2007;22:1615–22.
95. Medications for ataxia symptoms. Available at: http://www.ataxia.org/pdf/Medications_for_ataxia_symptoms.pdf.
96. Uhlendorf T, Van Kummer B, Yaspelkis B, et al. Neuroprotective effects of moderate aerobic exercise on the spastic Han-Wistar rat, a model of ataxia. Brain Res 2011;1369:216–22.
97. Miyai I, Ito M, Hattori N, et al, Cerebellar Ataxia Rehabilitation Trialists Collaboration. Cerebellar ataxia rehabilitation trial in degenerative cerebellar diseases. Neurorehabil Neural Repair 2012;26:515–22.
98. Ilg W, Schatton C, Schicks J, et al. Video game-based coordinative training improves ataxia in children with degenerative ataxia. Neurology 2012;79:2056–60.
99. Doris Broetz. Physiotherapy. Available at: www.broetz-physiotherapie.de.
100. Gottesfeld J. Small molecules affecting transcription in Friedreich ataxia. Pharmacol Ther 2007;116:236–48.
101. Rai M, Soragni E, Jenssen K, et al. HDAC inhibitors correct frataxin deficiency in a Friedreich ataxia mouse model. PLoS One 2008;3:e1958.
102. Arpa and colleagues, Fourth International Friedreich's Ataxia Conference Abstracts, www.curefa.org, as reviewed in (100) Wilson R. Therapeutic developments in Friedreich ataxia. J Child Neurol 2012;27(9):1212–6.
103. Sturm B, Stupphann D, Kaun C, et al. Recombinant human erythropoietin: effects on frataxin production in vitro. Eur J Clin Invest 2005;35:711–7.
104. Boesch S, Sturm B, Hering S, et al. Friedreich's ataxia: clinical pilot trial with recombinant human erythropoietin. Ann Neurol 2007;62:521–4.
105. Boesch S, Sturm B, Hering S, et al. Neurological effects of recombinant human erythropoietin in Friedreich's ataxia: a clinical pilot trial. Mov Disord 2008;23:1940–4.
106. Sarsero J, Li L, Warden H, et al. Upregulation of expression from the FRDA genomic locus for the therapy of Friedreich ataxia. J Gene Med 2003;5:72–81.
107. Tomassini B, Arcuri G, Fortuni S, et al. Interferon gamma upregulates frataxin and corrects the functional deficits in a Friedreich ataxia model. Hum Mol Genet 2012;21:2855–61.
108. Vyas P, Tomamichel W, Pride P, et al. A TAT-frataxin fusion protein increases lifespan and cardiac function in a conditional Friedreich's ataxia mouse model. Hum Mol Genet 2012;21:1230–47.

109. Boddaert N, Le Quan Sang K, Rötig A, et al. Selective iron chelation in Friedreich ataxia. Biological and clinical implications. Blood 2007;110:401–8.
110. Koeppen A, Micheal S, Knutson M, et al. The dentate nucleus in Friedreich's ataxia: the role of iron-responsive proteins. Acta Neuropathol 2007;114:163–73.
111. Velasco-Sanchez D, Aracil A, Montero R, et al. Combined therapy with idebenone and deferiprone in patients with Friedreich's ataxia. Cerebellum 2011;10:1–8.
112. Lynch D, Perlman S, Meier T. A phase 3, double-blind, placebo-controlled trial of idebenone in Friedreich ataxia. Arch Neurol 2010;67:941–7.
113. Meier T, Perlman S, Rummey C, et al. Assessment of neurological efficacy of idebenone in pediatric patients with Friedreich's ataxia: data from a 6-month controlled study followed by a 12-month open-label extension study. J Neurol 2012;259:284–91.
114. Lagedrost S, Sutton M, Cohen M, et al. Idebenone in Friedreich ataxia cardiomyopathy-results from a 6-month phase III study (IONIA). Am Heart J 2011;161:639–45.
115. Enns G, Kinsman S, Perlman S, et al. Initial experience in the treatment of inherited mitochondrial disease with EPI-743. Mol Genet Metab 2012;105:91–102.
116. Martinelli D, Catteruccia M, Piemonte F, et al. EPI-743 reverses the progression of the pediatric mitochondrial disease–genetically defined Leigh syndrome. Mol Genet Metab 2012;107:383–8.

Clinical Neurogenetics
Behavioral Management of Inherited Neurodegenerative Disease

Eric Wexler, MD, PhD

KEYWORDS

- Major depression • Psychosis • Impulse-control disorder • Bipolar • Aggression

KEY POINTS

- Pharmacologic treatments often require 3 months to be effective.
- Using validated rating scales guides treatment by quantitatively tracking progress.
- Psychiatric symptoms cluster differently in adult neurogenetic disorders.
- Psychiatric symptoms in these patients are more resistant to treatment.
- Psychotropic side effects are unavoidable, sometimes intolerable, and may even be life-threatening.

INTRODUCTION

Clinical case

"In neurogenetics, all is not in the genes." Patients A.Z. and B.Z. are Hispanic, full brothers in their late 30s who paternally inherited a 2700 pentanucleotide intronic expansion in the Ataxin-10 gene. Superficially, they are clinically similar, each experiencing ataxia and seizures, and both have been hospitalized for acute psychosis. However, a more careful review of their history reveals the following critical differences: Patient A.Z. developed seizures in his early 20s, but was free of balance problems for over a decade. A.Z. was seizure free on a regimen of zonisamide and carbamazepine when he abruptly developed paranoid delusions, auditory hallucination, visual illusions, and aggressive behavior. EEG and laboratory testing revealed no evidence of seizures, encephalopathy, or metabolic derangement. Risperidone therapy was initiated and lamotrigene was substituted for zonisamide to rule out the latter as a cause of his psychosis. Over the next 6 months, the patient's psychotic symptoms gradually resolved. In contrast, Patient B.Z. developed balance problems in his late 20s and then developed seizures a full 5 years later. His seizures were initially controlled with levetiracetam monotherapy, but 3 years later he developed breakthrough seizures, despite the addition of carbamazepine to his regimen. His refractory seizure necessitated acute hospitalization, where he was started on lacosamide and eventually became seizure free. On the day following his last witnessed

Department of Psychiatry, Center for Neurobehavioral Genetics, Semel Institute, University of California Los Angeles School of Medicine, 695 Charles Young Drive South, Gonda Room 2309, Los Angeles, CA 90024-1759, USA
E-mail address: ewexler@ucla.edu

Neurol Clin 31 (2013) 1121–1144
http://dx.doi.org/10.1016/j.ncl.2013.04.016
0733-8619/13/$ – see front matter © 2013 Elsevier Inc. All rights reserved.

large seizure, he became acutely psychotic and violent. This prompted the addition of the anti-psychotic Quetiapine to his regimen and his psychiatric symptoms resolved within 48 hours. Although he was seizure and psychosis free on discharge, he was exhibiting significant cognitive blunting and substantial difficulty ambulating. After being psychosis free on low-dose quetiapine for over 3 months, it was decided to taper off the antipsychotic, because it was likely contributing to both his cognitive impairment and his walking difficulties.

Behavioral changes are well-established features of degenerative diseases like Parkinson disease (PD), frontotemporal dementia (FTD), and Alzheimer disease. However, psychiatric symptoms are important features of many adult-onset neurogenetic disorders, including Huntington disease (HD), non-HD basal ganglia diseases (eg, Fahr), a subset of spinocerebellar ataxias,[1,2] rapid-onset dystonia-parkinsons,[3] late-onset Tay-Sachs,[4] mitochondrial disorders,[1] inherited prion diseases,[5] etc. An expanded summary of the most frequently observed psychiatric manifestations of "common" neurogenetic disease is found in **Table 1**. The behavioral changes associated with these disorders are often equally or more disabling than the classic cognitive and motor symptoms. When left untreated, these symptoms increase the rates of both medical and psychiatric hospital admissions, substantially elevate suicidality, exacerbate caregiver stress, and, overall, greatly worsen the financial and societal burden of these diseases.

Individuals with inherited neurodegenerative disorders represent some of the more challenging psychiatric patients, from the perspective of both diagnosis and treatment. Some of the difficulties in treating these patients are illustrated by the case titled: "*In neurogenetics, all is not in the genes*" in the boxed inset above. Despite the fact that they were afflicted with epilepsy, a progressive ataxia, and refractory psychosis requiring acute hospitalization, theirs is a relatively straightforward case of psychiatric management. Many neurogenetics patients exhibit multiple concurrent psychiatric symptoms, each requiring a separate, targeted management approach. This article discusses the diagnostic challenges faced and provides practical, sequenced treatment plans for mitigating these psychiatric symptoms.

CLINICAL FINDINGS

The neuropsychiatric symptoms of neurogenetics patients are similar to those seen in the general population. What distinguishes the adult neurodegenerative disease population is that they experience psychiatric symptoms more frequently, in different combinations, and are more treatment resistant than otherwise normal age-matched individuals. This section provides simple operational definitions for the primary symptoms, as well as clarifying some of the more frequently confused symptom classes.

Major Depression

The cardinal symptoms of major depressive disorder are affective in nature and include persistent sad mood or anhedonia, in the context of other neurovegetative signs or cognitive distortions (eg, inappropriate guilt, worthlessness, hopelessness, changes in sleep or appetite, etc). The diagnosis of major depression can be aided by the use of a semi-structured clinical interview like the Inventory of Depressive Symptomatology, Clinician Rating (IDS-C) and Self-Report (IDS-SR).[6] In turn, the severity of depressive symptoms can be effectively quantified during the course of treatment using a host of patient self-rated scales, including: (1) IDS-SR, (2) Geriatric Depression Scale-30 Questions: self-report scale validated in the elderly, Alzheimer

Table 1
Psychiatric symptoms among common adult neurogenetic disorders

Neurogenetic Disorder	Psychiatric Symptoms
Inborn errors of metabolism[61,62]	
Adrenoleukodystophy[63,64]	Dep, I/D
Metachromatic leukodystrophy[62]	Psy
Ceroid lipofuscinosis[62]	Dep
Neiman-Pick type C[65–67]	Dep, Man, Psy
Late-onset Tay-Sachs[4,68–70]	Dep, Man, Psy
Fabry disease[62]	Dep, I/D
Acute porphyria[62]	Dep, Psy
Wilson disease[62,71–73]	Dep, Man, I/D, OCD, Psy
Cerebellar degenerations (pooled)[74–76]	Dep, Psy
SCA1[77–80]	Dep
SCA3[76–80]	Dep
SCA10[2]	Psy
SCA12[81]	Dep, Anx
Cortical degeneration	
FTD (eg, inherited mutations in MAPT, GRN, TDP-43, VCP, CHMP2b)[82–87]	Dep, I/D
Prion disease (eg, GSS)[88,89]	Dep, Psy
Striatum	
Parkinson disease[90–92]	Dep, Ap, I/D, Psy
Myoclonus dystonia[81,93]	Anx, OCD
Early-onset primary dystonia (DYT1)[94]	Dep
Basal ganglia[74,95]	
Fahr disease[95]	Dep, OCD
Huntington chorea (HD)[96–98]	Dep, Ap, I/D, OCD, Psy
HD-like disorders[99–102] (eg, DRPLA, HDL-1, -2, -3, NBIA, PKAN, SCA-17)	Dep, I/D, OCD, Psy
Mitochondrial disorders (eg, MELAS)[1]	Dep, Psy

Abbreviations: Anx, anxiety; Ap, apathy; CHMP2b, charged multivesicular body protein 2b; Dep, depression; DRPLA, dentatorubral-pallidoluysian atrophy; GRN, progranulin; GSS, Gerstmann–Sträussler–Scheinker syndrome; HDL-1, -2, -3, Huntington's disease-like syndromes-1, -2, -3; I/D, impulsivity/disinhibition; Man, mania; MAPT, microtubule-associated protein Tau; NBIA, neurodegeneration with brain iron accumulation; NBIA2, neuroferritinopathy; OCD, obsessions or compulsions/perseveration; PKAN, pantothenate-kinase-associated neurodegeneration; Psy, psychosis; SCA-17, spinocerebellar ataxia-17; TDP-43, TAR DNA-binding protein 43; VCP, valosin containing protein.

disease, and PD[7]; (3) Hospital Anxiety and Depression Scale as self-report scale validated in HD[8]; (4) Burns Depression checklist-25,[9] a free, self-report scale that is more easily understood by patients than the more common Beck Depression Inventory. (The Beck Depression Inventory and the Hamilton Depression Scale are among the most commonly encountered rating scales in the general depression literature, but neither performs well for evaluating patients whose depression is dominated by anhedonia or somatic complaints, as in the case of degenerative disorders like HD.[8,10])

Apathy

Patients with isolated apathy or anhedonia are often misdiagnosed with the syndrome of major depression, even by seasoned clinicians. In contrast to major depression, apathy is the specific lack of motivation relative to the patient's previous level of functioning concomitant with each of the following: (1) blunting of affect or emotion, (2) lack of novelty seeking or interest in personal problems, and (3) decreased goal-directed behavior, not resulting from physical fatigue. It is important to distinguish between apathetic major depression and isolated apathy found in HD and PD,[11] because the latter generally does not respond to classic antidepressant therapy. The severity of isolated apathy may be gauged using the Apathy Evaluation Scale, for which self-rated and clinician rating scales are available.[12–15]

Mania and Bipolar Affective Disorder

The diagnosis of bipolar affective disorder is given to all patients with a history of a spontaneous manic or hypomanic episode, irrespective of whether they have suffered a major depressive episode, provided it is not substance induced. Mania is defined as a distinct period of elevated or irritable mood that is almost indistinguishable from acute amphetamine intoxication. During this period, patients may also experience inflated self-esteem or grandiose delusions, racing thoughts, pressured speech, poor attention span, a decreased need for sleep, increased goals-directed activity including hypersexuality, increased risky behavior (eg, compulsive spending, gambling, promiscuity, drug use, poor business decisions, reckless driving, etc), and frank psychosis (eg, paranoia). It is worth noting that irritable mania can coexist with symptoms of major depression (ie, mixed episode). Two neurogenetic populations that show a greater incidence of manic symptoms are (1) adult patients with hexosaminidase-A deficiency (late-onset Tay-Sachs), whereby upwards of 50% will be diagnosed as bipolar during their lifetime, and (2) PD patients who develop manic-like symptoms in response to treatment with dopaminergic agonists. The severity of manic symptoms can be assessed using the Young Mania Rating Scale.[16]

Attention Deficit-hyperactivity Disorder Versus Bipolar Affective Disorder

Attention deficit-hyperactivity disorder (ADHD) patients exhibit symptoms of inattention, hyperactivity, and impulsivity leading to poor or reckless decision-making and can seem superficially similar to bipolar affective disorder patients. ADHD is a long-standing cognitive and behavioral disorder that is the patient's baseline (ie, relatively stable over time). This long-term persistence of symptoms distinguishes it from bipolar affective disorder, which is an abrupt change in mood and behavior. It is important to make this distinction because the primary treatments for ADHD (psychostimulants and noradrenergic antidepressants) can precipitate mania in bipolar patients.

Obsessions and Compulsions Versus Impulsions

Patients with true obsessive-compulsive disorder (OCD) perform rituals in an effort to reduce anxiety—they "need" to perform the ritual. These thoughts and actions are considered egodystonic, meaning that they are not consistent with the individual's idealized self-perception. For example, a patient with obsessive fears of contamination must wash their hands after touching a light switch. To do otherwise would cause unbearable anxiety out of fear they may contract a horrible disease. Patients with impulse control problems also have trouble controlling execution of some learned task; however, each type of impulsion can be distinguished from compulsions. Among egodystonic impulsions, any anxiety present is created by the patient's inability not control their actions (ie, like a tic, they do not need to do it, they just cannot stop themselves). Alternatively, the impulsive act might be gratifying, and like addiction, self-reinforcing (ie, they may not try resisting because they like it). For example, the kleptomaniac enjoys the feeling when they do not resist pocketing a bobble at the local store, making this act egosyntonic. These differences are not without distinction. For example, compulsions and egodystonic impulsions generally respond well to serotonergic agents, while egosyntonic impulsions often do not. The Yale-Brown Obsessive Compulsive Scale Checklist can be used initially to screen rapidly for the presence of a broader range of compulsions and impulsions[17,18] than other commonly used screening tools (eg, Questionnaire for Impulsive-Compulsive Disorders in Parkinson's disease rating scale[19]). In higher functioning patients the Barratt Impulsivity Scale may be used to assess the patient's overall level of impulsivity, at the time of their initial visit.[20]

Obsessions Versus Perseveration

Obsessions and compulsions differ significantly from perseverative behaviors, even though both are "sticky" thoughts. Although obsessions and compulsions are driven by a need to reduce anxiety, perseveration is an involuntary continuation of ideas or experiences due to a breakdown in automatic regulatory mechanisms of executive functioning. The OCD patient does not want to be angst-ridden over their fears, whereas the perseverative patient cannot think about anything else and does not want to. For example, a Huntington patient who does nothing but talk about eating at a popular fast-food restaurant and then jumps out of the car when she sees one is suffering from an impulse control disorder with perseveration, as well as impaired executive planning function, but not OCD, which is an important distinction because much of what gets labeled as OCD in many neurogenetics patients (eg, HD) is not really true obsessions and compulsions, but rather perseveration and stereotypy or punding.[21]

Irritability and Aggression

Operationally, the term irritable means impatience, intolerance, and reduced control over temper, which can progress to angry and aggressive verbal or behavioral outbursts.[22] In contrast, aggression refers to behaviors that intentionally harm persons or property. Patients who are irritable, a mood state, may act aggressively or violently toward others in certain social situations. Similarly, patients with persecutory delusions or command hallucinations may become aggressive secondary to their psychosis. Conversely, those with intermittent explosive disorder may seem calm until the moment when they fail to control their impulse to do harm to others. The important distinction here is between aggression that arises secondary to another psychiatric symptom versus a violent impulse control disorder, both being common in patients suffering from degenerative disorders like PD, HD, or FTD. Aggression may be tracked using the Overt Aggression Scale-Modified for outpatient use.[23,24]

Anxiety Versus Akathisia

Anxiety is the unpleasant mood characterized by fear, uneasiness, concern, or dread that often induces restlessness. General anxiety symptoms can occur in isolation, but often accompany other psychiatric conditions (eg, major depression). These symptoms may be tracked during the course of treatment using the Burns,[9] Sheehan,[25] or Zung[26] anxiety rating scales. In contrast, akathisia is the sense of inner restlessness induced by dopamine receptor antagonists (antipsychotics and some antiemetics), and to a lesser degree, many antidepressants.

Suicidality

Increased suicidal ideation is a common feature of many neurodegenerative diseases, particularly in the context of other psychiatric symptoms (eg, impulsivity). Contrary to common belief, a sad mood alone is not a strong predictor of completed suicide. The 4 most common features of patients that attempt suicide are hopelessness, impulsivity, agitation/anxiety, and aggression. The presence of any one of these should be considered a warning sign that warrants further investigation. There are many well-known risk factors for suicide, but because of their number, it is easy to forget to inquire about all of them during the standard clinical interview. One alternative is to use a standardized rating scale like the Columbia Suicide Severity Rating Scale.[27]

EVALUATION AND MANAGEMENT

This treatment primer is guided by the principle of evidence-based practice; however, it is not a strictly evidence-based tutorial—it cannot be. The literature is largely silent on how to treat psychiatric disorders in specific neurodegenerative diseases, with the possible exception of PD. Even for this relatively common neurodegenerative disorder, most trials are uninterpretable because they were either too short in duration or too underpowered to detect responses.[28] In lieu of focused primary trials data to guide treatment, the clinical approaches presented in this article were synthesized from the results of large-scale trials conducted among the general psychiatric population and shaped by the clinical experience of treating neurogenetics patients. For example, the depression treatment algorithms presented in **Figs. 2–5** are largely based on 3 sources: Sequenced Treatment Alternatives to Relieve Depression,[29,30] Combining Medications to Enhance Depression Outcomes trials, and the Texas Medication Algorithm Project.[31–33] Medication titration schedules for each treatment plan can be found in **Box 1**.

Effective Treatment Planning Will Include the Following Components

First, distinguish what needs to be treated first from their list of complaints. This triage should include an assessment of symptom severity using a combination of clinician-rated and patient self-reporting standardized rating scales. These tools provide the means to track patient progress during the course of treatment. In addition, they can help the clinician refine their diagnosis. For example, these symptom inventories will help to distinguish major depression from its mimics like isolated apathy, which is common among patients with frontal lobe dysfunction. The best-validated rating scales for general clinical screening include the following: (1) Neuropsychiatric Inventory,[34] and (2) the Brief Psychiatric Rating Scale,[35,36] both being a clinician-rated scale, (3) SCL-90 symptom checklist,[37] and (4) the Brief Symptom Inventory,[38] both patient self-rating scales, as well as (5) the Mini-International Neuropsychiatric Interview; a validated 15-minute structured psychiatric interview.[39,40]

Second, decide what can be treated most easily and address that first.

Third, determine what psychosocial factors might be either worsening their symptoms or could impede treatment (eg, they are anxious because they cannot afford the medication).

Fourth, establish whether the patient will tolerate the proposed treatment and if not figure out if there is a way to mitigate the harm caused by treatment.

Fifth, adhere to the principle of "don't miss the obvious." When a patient has an established genetic diagnosis that can explain their new symptoms, it is easy to become complacent and miss the better (correct) diagnosis. For example, a young adult who recently gene-tested positive for HD and is now exhibiting erratic behavior

---

Box 1
Dosing regimens for the most commonly used psychopharmacologic agents

Drug: Titration schedule

Aripiprazole: 5 mg QAM × 1 wk then increase by 5 mg/d/wk using the best tolerated BID dosing strategy to target of 20–30 mg/d

Buproprion SR: (150 mg QAM × 3–7 d → 150 mg QAM/Qnoon × 4–6 wk → 200 mg BID)

Buspirone: 20–30 mg BID to TID

Citalopram: 10 mg and increase by 10 mg/d/wk until a maximum of 40 mg QAM

Cloazapine: 25 mg QHS → increase by 25 mg/d/wk to 50 mg/d. Continue titrating by 25 mg/d/mo until target symptoms improve or side effects are intolerable, Max = 400–450 mg/d in divided dosing.

> Notes. Neurodegenerative disease patients often require much lower doses of clozapine than young and otherwise healthy schizophrenics. For example, approximately 50 mg/d was all that was needed, on average, to treat PD patients with medication induced psychosis.[103]

> White blood cell counts (total and absolute neutrophil count) are required weekly for first 6 mo, biweekly for the next 6 mo, and then monthly thereafter. This presumes no interruption of Clozapine dosing because of low cell counts (ie, WBC <3000 or ANC <1500) or the need for continued weekly monitoring because of borderline low white counts (WBC <3500 or ANC <2000). Monitoring is more thoroughly reviewed in Ref.[104] and online at www.clozaril.com.

Clomipramine: Initiate clomipramine 25 mg QD × 3 days then increase by 25 mg/day every 3–7 days until achieving 100 mg/day then check blood level and EKG. Next, add Fluvoxamine (1A2 + 2D6 antagonist) 25 mg QD then titrate by 25 mg/d/wk according to Clomipramine (CMI): desmethylclomipramine (DMC) blood levels, to achieve a target CMI:DMC ratio >1 and combined levels below the toxic range (CMI + DMC <500 ng/mL)[105–108]

> Unmetabolized clomipramine is essentially a selective serotonin reuptake inhibitor. However, CMI is metabolized by p450 1A2 and 2D6 into DMC, which is a relatively pure selective norepinephrine reuptake inhibitor. Therefore, the goal is to maximize the amount of unmetabolized CMI by inhibiting its metabolism, using a supplemental inhibitor of 1A2 or 2D6 (eg, Fluvoxamine inhibits 1A2 and 2D6, Paroxetine and Fluoxetine inhibit 2D6).

Cytomel: 25 mcg QD × 1–2 wk → 50 μg QAM

Duloxetine: 30 mg QAM × 7 d → 30 mg QAM/Qnoon × 2–3 wk → 60 mg QAM + 30 mg Q1200 × 4 wk → 60 mg QAM/Q1200

Fluoxetine: 10 mg and increase by 10 mg/d/wk intil target of 40–60 mg, QAM, as tolerated; max = 60–80 mg/d.

Gabapentin: 100 mg TID × 3 d → 300 mg TID × 2 wk → 400 mg TID × 2 wk → 600 mg TID × 2 wk → 800 mg TID[109–111]

Insoitol: 1 g (1 level tablespoon) QD then increase to 1 g TID-QID as rapidly as tolerated[39,112]

Lamotrigene: 5 mg/d to start then increase by 5 mg/d every weekday (stay at same dose on weekend) for 2 wk then increase by 25 mg/d/wk targeting 200 mg/d (max = 600 mg/d or blood level <14 μg/mL)[39,112]

> Concomitant valproic acid (VPA) use can effectively double Lamotrigene (LTG) blood levels. When combining VPA + LTG, make initial increases 5 mg every other day × 2 wk, then increase by 12.5 mg (half of a 25 mg) every wk with target of 50–200 mg, or a blood level not to exceed 14 μg/mL

> Slow titration reduces, but does not eliminate, the risk of either annoying rashes or a dermatologic emergency (eg, Stevens-Johnson reaction). The former (junk rashes) can be further minimized by adhering to a regimen of "antigen precautions" that include refraining from changing their personal hygiene products, laundry detergents, etc. This protocol is reviewed elsewhere by Ketter and colleagues[113]

Lithium: 300 mg QHS × 1 wk → increase by 150–300 mg/d/wk to achieve a target blood level of 0.8–1 mEq/L

Milnacipran: 12.5 mg × 3 d → 12.5 mg BID × 4 d → increase by 25 mg/d every 2 wk. Target = 150 mg/d total. Max = 200 mg/d[114,115]

Mirtazapine: 15 mg QHS × 1–2 wk → 30 mg QHS × 2–3 wk → 45 mg QHS × 4 wk → 60 mg QHS Good choice for patients with insomnia.

Nortriptyline: 25 mg QAM 3–7 d → 50 mg × 3–7 d → 75 mg × 2–3 wk → 100 mg × 4 wk → 150 mg. During titration, check nortriptyline blood levels and document EKG.

Olanzapine: 5 mg → increase by 2.5 mg/d/wk → target = 15–30 mg/d

> The long-acting depot formulation is not recommended because it seems to exhibit highly variable pharmacokinetics and can induce a postinjection delirium/sedation syndrome (<2%), necessitating observation of each patient for 3 h after each injection[116]

Oxcarbazine: 150 mg QD × 3 d → 150 mg BID × 1 wk → Increases by 150–300 mg/d/wk; Target = 600–1200 mg BID

Phenytoin: 100 mg TID → Increase by 30 mg/d/wk × 3 wk (390 mg/d)

> Maintain serum trough <20 μg/mL

Pramipexole: 0.125 mg TID → increase by 0.125 mg TID every 4–7 d to maximum of 1 mg TID; Target = 0.75 g TID

Propranolol: Akathisia: 10 mg TID. Aggression: 10 mg TID → increase by 10 mg TID every 3 d, max = 40 mg TID

Quetiapine: 25 mg QHS × 1 wk → increase by 25 mg/d/wk to 200–300 mg

Selegeline TD: 6 mg patch QD × 1–2 wk → 9 mg QD × 8 wk → 12 mg QD

> L-Methamphetamine metabolite has low biologic activity, but is mistaken for D-amphetamine on drug tests.

Tiagabine: Insomnia: 2 mg QHS → Increase every other day by 2 mg/d; target = 8–12 mg/d

Topiramate: 50 mg BID → Increase by 50 mg/d/wk → Target = 100–150 mg BID

Tranylcypromine: 10 mg QAM × 2 wk → increase by 10 mg/d every 1–2 wk until the patient reaches 60 mg QD or is unable to tolerate side effects

Valproic acid: 250 mg QHS → increase by 250 mg/d/wk to target a blood level of 90–100 μg/mL

> VPA frequently causes an asymptomatic increase in serum ammonia levels, in the context of normal liver function and VPA blood levels that are within the normal range. In rare cases, VPA-induced hyperammonemia causes an emergent encephalopathy (VHE). The early signs of VHE are lethargy, confusion, reduced motor activity, and possible seizures. Unfortunately, signs of VHE can be misattributed to worsening mania, depression, or baseline psychosis in the psychiatric population. Reviewed by Lewis and colleagues[117–130]

Venlafaxine XR: Start at 37.5 mg QAM × 3 d → 75 mg QAM × 4 d → 150 mg/d × 1 wk → 225 mg QAM × 2 wk → if tolerated → 300 mg QAM × 2 wk → if tolerated → 375 mg QAM + monitor blood pressure/heart rate.

and problems in school may be displaying the early onset of personality-related HD symptoms, but recreational drug use is still more likely.

Once the primary symptoms have been identified, the clinician can begin to implement the treatment plans presented in **Figs. 1–6**. These figures provide detailed, sequential pharmacologic treatment algorithms for addressing the most commonly encountered symptom clusters: unipolar major depression (see **Fig. 1**), bipolar depression (see **Fig. 2**), aggression without psychosis (see **Fig. 3**), impulse control

Unipolar Major Depression

Trial 1. Start SSRI (Fluoxetine or Citalopram)
  • All SSRIs are equally effective, on a population basis
  • Fluoxetine *non-compliant patients who tolerate higher doses, may be considered for once or twice weekly administration.*
  • Citalopram *Inexpensive and has few P450 interactions*

Treatment comliance is greatly enhanced by warning about common SSRI side effects, especially increased anxiety. (See Figure 6)

Assess symptoms at regular intervals over 12 weeks
  • Use MADRS & GDS-30 assess symtpoms.
  • 30-50% of eventual responders show little significant benefit before 8 weeks!!! [29,30]

**Recurrently suicidal patients should be referred for electroconvusive therapy (ECT). Impulsive depressed or manic patients with recurrent suicidal ideation are at high risk of imminent self-harm. ECT is the fastest biological depression treatment, with symptom resolution in 2-4 weeks, on average.*

Trial 2. Medication Switch vs Augmentation [120]
  A. Partial response + Tolerable side effects ⇨ Augment
  • Aripiprazole
  • Buproprion SR
  • Buspirone
  • Cytomel
  • Mirtazapine
  • Lithium
  • Pramipexole *Best evidence in PD [118,119]*
  B. Heavy side-effect burden ⇨ Switch to non-serotonergic agent (see Table 1)
  • Mirtazapine *Good choice for patients with insomnia.*
  • Nortriptyline *high-quality support for efficacy in PD [28]*
  • Buproprion SR *Best tolerated*
  C. Poor SSRI response, Tolerable side effects ⇨ Switch to dual acting agents
  • Venlafaxine XR *Generic available*
  • Duloxetine
  • Milnacipran *Fewest drug-drug interactions*
  • Mirtazapine, Nortriptyline, Desipramine or Buproprion may also be considered

---

Regularly assess symptom severity over 12

Trial 3. Medication Switch vs Augmentation.
  A. Reconsider Diagnosis of bipolar depression
  B. Non-responders ⇨ Switch
  • Mirtazapine + Venlafaxine XR, Duloxetine or Milnacipran
  • Tranylcypromine
  • Consider ECT for severely depressed or debilitated patients
  C. Partial responders: Repeat 2B or 2C or use bipolar depression protocol (Figure 3.)

Fig. 1. Multistage sequential approach to managing new-onset and refractory unipolar major depression.

disorders (see **Fig. 4**), medication-induced acute anxiety (see **Fig. 5**), and psychosis (see **Fig. 6**).

ADVERSE EFFECTS

This section presents some of the psychopharmacologic pitfalls the practicing neurologist may encounter, but are inadequately addressed by other similar reviews. For a summary of the more pertinent psychotropic side effects, the reader should consult **Box 1** and **Tables 1–3** or one of the many excellent reviews.[41–43]

Bipolar-spectrum Depression

Step 1. Start Lithium or Valproic Acid as mood stabilizer

• The primary treatments for bipolar depression are mood stabilizers, not antidepressants [121].
  • Lithium
  • Valproic Acid
  • Carbamazepine and Oxcarbazine *No weight gain, but are less effective primary mood stabilizers.*

Step 2. Wait 12 weeks and reassess

Step 3. Partial response for depression: Augment

• Lamotrigene *emergent-rash risk mandates slow titration [39].*
  • Aripiprazole *Risk of dyskinesias*
  • Quetiapine *Significant sedation*
  • Olanzapine *Good choice in HD, but avoid in PD, inherited dystonia and Late-onset Tay Sachs due to relatively high D2 receptor blockade*
   • Clozapine *Most effective atypical antipsychotic, but it has a panoply of poorly tolerated side-effects (See Table 1)*
   • Pramipexole [113]
   • Insoitol *few side effects other than mild bloating.* **Superior to risperidone, but inferior to lamotrigene in a head-to-head blinded trial [122].**

Fig. 2. Managing bipolar-associated major depression.

Serotonin Syndrome

Serotonin syndrome (SS) is a predictable, but often missed, potentially life-threatening adverse reaction to many common psychotropic agents. SS, which is characterized by hyperthermia, rigidity, and changes in mental status, can be confused with neuroleptic malignant syndrome, which is an uncommon idiopathic reaction to dopamine receptor blockade. In contrast to neuroleptic malignant syndrome, SS is neither rare nor idiopathic, yet most cases are missed because they are fortunately mild and easily explained away by both the clinician and the patient; this is especially true for patients with degenerative movement disorders like HD or PD because they may already be experiencing rigidity, impaired communication, or mental status changes.

SS has been documented after ingesting a single serotonergic agent, yet most reported cases have occurred in the context of polypharmacy, most commonly when one of the agents was an irreversible monoamine oxidase inhibitor, like the antidepressant phenelzine.[44] The list of modern serotonergic agents is extensive and includes virtually all antidepressants, recreational drugs like amphetamine or "ecstasy" (MDMA), opiates like meperidine or other inhibitors of monamine oxidase like selegiline procarbazine, the antibiotics linezolid, furazolidone, and to a lesser extent isoniazid, or the herbal supplement Syrian Rue. (More complete lists can be found in Refs.[45,46]). (Adding a drug that broadly inhibits p450 metabolism [eg, the antiviral ritinovir] has the potential to raise the level of many psychotropics and can thus precipitate SS.) The risk of missing the diagnosis is that small increases in serotonergic medication doses can precipitate a clinical emergency. For example, in these severe cases it is not uncommon for the patient's core temperatures to exceed 41°C (>106°C). Clinicians can reasonably diagnose even mild cases of SS in a patient that recently used a serotonin-altering drug if they exhibits one of the following signs: (1) tremor and hyperreflexia; (2) spontaneous clonus; (3) muscle rigidity + temperature >38°C + either ocular clonus or inducible clonus; (4) ocular clonus + agitation or diaphoresis; or (5) inducible clonus + agitation or diaphoresis.[45]

Agression ± psychosis

Step 1. Start Atypical Antipsychotic
• The initial goal is to tranquilize the erratic and potentially violent patient (See Table 3: Antipsychotic side effects)
  • Olanzapine *more calming*
  • Quetiapine *most sedating*
  • If aggression is the result of irritability then symptoms may fully resolve with antipsychotic therapy alone, within 2 weeks
  • For Impulsive agression (Intermittant Explosive Disorder) See Figure 4. Managment of Impulse Control Disorders

Step 2. Start SSRI.
  • Fluoxetine is best supported by the literature [123]
  • Monitor aggression severity using (OAS-M) during 12 week stabilization period.
  • Increased anxiety due to SSRI can be controlled with either increasing dose of atypical antipsychotic or adding clonazepam 0.5-1 mg TID

Step 3. Augment SSRI with mood stabilizer [23,124]
  • Phenytoin
  • Oxcarbazine *Monitor for hyponatremia
  • Carbamazepine
  • Lithium
  Avoid use of pro-aggressive agents like Levetiracetam

Step 4. Swap first-line agents

Step 5. Switch to second-line agents
  • Propranolol
  • Topiramate
  • Valproic Acid
  • Lamotrigene

Fig. 3. Sequenced management of comorbid psychosis and aggression.

Antidepressant Withdrawal Syndrome

Antidepressant withdrawal syndrome (AWS) may occur is upwards of 1 in 5 patients who abruptly discontinue an antidepressant, primarily those with serotonergic activity.[47,48] This syndrome is characterized by the following: dizziness, nausea, sleep disturbances, flulike symptoms, parasthesias, anxiety, agitation, irritability, dysphoria, or crying spells. Although not life threatening to the patient, it is quite unpleasant. When patients are not warned about the possibility of AWS, the sudden and unpleasant onset of symptoms can quickly erode the patient's trust in their treating physician. A given drug's propensity to induce AWS is primarily linked to its half-life and whether that drug has any active metabolites. For example, paroxetine has a short half-life (as low as 3 hours among fast metabolizers) and no active metabolites and is thought by many to have the highest incidence of AWS. In contrast, fluoxetine has a half-life on the order of 5 days, a potent active metabolite, and is rarely associated with AWS. Unfortunately, there is no specific treatment for AWS except supportive measures or restarting another serotonergic drug.

Antidepressant-induced Sexual Dysfunction

Antidepressants are among the most common causes of medication-induced sexual dysfunction, a constellation of symptoms that may include a decreased libido, erectile

Impulse control disorders (ICDs)

Step 1. Start with SSRI + Cognitive Behavioral Therapy   • Warn patient about side effects, especially increased anxiety   • Maximize dose *Effective treatment of OCD and ICDs are usually higher than what is considered maximum for treating mood disorders (e.g. 80m/day Fluoxetine, 300 mg/day Sertraline   • Montior common ICD symptoms using QUIP [19]   *ICD treatment reviewed in [125]

Step 2. Optimize treatment of comorbid anxiety   • Comorbid anxiety worsens impulse control and compulsions   • Clonazepam   • Gabapentin   • Buspirone   • Valproate   • Atypical Antipsychotic

Step 3.   Swap SSRI or Switch to Clomipramine

Step 4.   Start Clomipramine + SSRI   • Titrate fluvoxamine to achieve a target CMI:DMC ratio > 1 and combined levels below the toxic range (CMI+DMC < 500 ng/ml)   • Document EKG

Step 5. Treatment resistant augmentation strategies   • Mirtazapine   • Quetiapine   • Buspirone   • Morphine (30mg Q3days-Qweek)   • Naltrexone   • Inositol

Fig. 4. Managing nonaggressive impulsivity.

dysfunction or reduced vaginal lubrication, or difficulty in achieving orgasm. Iatrogenic sexual dysfunction can easily worsen patients' already fragile mood state and encourage medication noncompliance. Worse yet, antidepressant-induced sexual dysfunction usually does not remit with time, unlike many antidepressant-induced side effects. This highly troubling situation is often missed because clinicians do not ask about it, out of their embarrassment, fear of embarrassing the patient, or simply because of the time constraints of a busy clinic. For example, in one study among

Medication Induced Acute Anxiety

• Clonazepam 0.5-1mg TID   • Gabapentin 300-800 mg TID   • Trazadone 25mg prn   • Quetiapine 25mg prn   • Propranolol 10 mg TID starting dose, MDD=320mg   • Hydroxyzine 50-100mg QID   • Diphenhydramine 25-50mg prn   • Olanzapine 2.5-5 mg   • Haldol 0.5-2 mg

Fig. 5. Common treatments for iatrogenic anxiety.

Psychosis

Psychosis (uncomplicated) [19]
- Ziprasidone *No weight gain*
- Aripiprazole *No weight gain*
- Olanzapine *generic available*
- Clozapine *Most effective for negative & positive symptoms
- Residual negative-symptoms:Duloxetine or Milacipran [127]
- Residual cognitive impairment: Augment with acetylcholinesterase inhibitors and/or memantine [128]

Metformin 1000mg QD (500 BID) can help reverse antipsychotic-induced weight gain, improve insulin resistance iand restore menstruation in (female) patients with schizophrenia [129,130]

Dopamine induced Psychosis
- Quetiapine
- Clozapine *most effective [28]*

* See Table 3: for a comparison of antipsychotic side-effects

Psychosis with Dystonia or Dyskinesia
- Quetiapine
- Clozapine *most effective

Psychosis with Chorea
- Olanzapine *generic available
- Risperidone *generic avaliable
- Clozapine

* Symptoms may be tracked using the Positive and Negative Symptom Scale (PANSS) [19]

Psychosis with residual negative symptoms
- switch to clozapine [63]
- augment with lamotrigene
- augment with duloxetine [64]
- augment with cholinesterase inhibitor [??]
- augment with methylphenidate

Fig. 6. Treatments for psychosis, an overview.

depressed patients treated with selective serotonin reuptake inhibitors, greater than 50% endorsed sexual dysfunction, but less than 15% spontaneously reported symptoms without prompting. As a corollary, it is equally important to discern whether the onset of sexual dysfunction occurs after the start of antidepressant therapy, and not vice versa (ie, sexual dysfunction is common in many psychiatric disorders, even before the initiation of treatment).

There are numerous approaches to treating antidepressant-induced sexual dysfunction[49] documented in the literature; however, they all fall into 5 basic categories:

1. Switch: The most effective treatment for sexual dysfunction is to switch to a nonserotonergic antidepressant, either Buproprion SR or Mirtazepine.
2. Reduce and augment: Another approach is to reduce substantially the dose of serotonergic antidepressant and to supplement with another agent that is known to augment antidepressant efficacy. Some antidepressant augmenters are Buproprion SR, Buspirone, Mirtazapine, Cytomel, either individually or in combination.

Table 2
Antidepressant side effects

	Drug	Weight Gain	Sedation	Insomnia Akathisia	Postural Hypotension	GI	Anticholinergic	Sexual Dysfunction	Transmitters Affected
SSRI	Citalopram (Celexa)	++	+	++	++	++	+	++++	5HT
	Escitalopram (Lexapro)	++	+	++	++	++	+	++++	5HT
	Fluoxetine (Prozac)	++	+	+++	++	++	+	++++	5HT
	Fluvoxamine (Luvox)	++	++	++	++	++	+	++++	5HT
	Paroxetine (Paxil)	+++	++	++	+++	++	++	+++++	5HT
	Sertraline (Zoloft)	++	+	+++	++	+++	+	++++	5HT
SNRI	Venlafaxine (Effexor XR)	+	+	+++	+	++	+	++++	5HT > NE
	Desvenlafaxine (Pristiq)	+	+	+++	+	++	+	++++	5HT > NE
	Duloxetine (Cymbalta)	+	+	+++	+	+++	+	++++	5HT = NE
	Milnacipran (Savella)	+	++	+	+	+++	++	++	5HT = NE
NRI	Atomoxetine (Strattera)	+	+	+	+	+	+	+	NE >> 5HT
TCA	Nortriptyline (Pamelor)	++	+++	+	++	+	+++	++	NE = 5HT
	Desipramine (Norpramin)	++	+	+	+	++	+	++	NE >> 5HT
	Clomipramine (Anafranil)	+++++	+++++	++	+++	++	+++++	+++++	5HT = NE
MAOI	Phenelzine (Nardil)	+++	+++	++	++++	++	++	+++++	5HT, DA, NE
	Selegiline Transdermal (Emsam)	+	+	++	++	+	++	+	DA > 5HT + NE
	Tranylcypromine (Parnate)	++	++	+++	+++	++	++	+++++	5HT + DA > NE
Miscellaneous	Bupropion (Wellbutrin SR)	+	+	+++	+	++	+	+	???
Receptor antagonists	Trazodone (Desyrel)	++	+++++	+	++	++	+	++	5HTR
	Vilazodone (Vybrid)	+	+	+++	+	+++	+	+++	5HT, 5HTR
	Mirtazapine (Remeron)	+++++	+++++	+	+	+	++	++	NER

Abbreviations: 5HT, serotonin; 5HTR, serotonin receptor partial agonist; Anticholinergic, inhibition of binding or transduction through muscarinic acetylcholine receptors; DA, dopamine; GI, gastrointestinal; MAOI, monoamine oxidase inhibitor; NE, norepinephrine; NER, norepinephrine receptor; NRI, selective norepinephrine reuptake inhibitor; SNRI, serotonin and norepinephrine reuptake inhibitor; SSRI, selective serotonin reuptake inhibitor; TCA, tricyclic antidepressant.

Table 3
Side effects of most commonly used antipsychotics

Drug	Weight Gain	Sedation	Metabolic Syndrome	TD or EPS	Postural Hypotension	Anticholinergic	↑Prolactin
Aripiprazole (Abilify)	+	++	+	++	+	+	+
Asenapine (Saphris)	+/++	+++	+/++	+/++	++	+	+
Clozapine (Cozaril)	++++	++++	+++	+	++++	++++	+
Haloperidol (Haldol)	+	+++	+	++++	+	+	++++
Iloperidone (Fanapt)	++	++	++	++	++++	++	+
Olanzapine (Zyprexa)	++++	+++	+++	++	+++	+++	+
Paliperidone (Invega)	+++	++	++	++	+	+	+
Quetiapine (Seroquel)	+++	+++	++	+/++	++	++	+
Risperidone (Risperdal)	+++	++	++	+++	+	+	++++
Ziprasidone (Geodon)	+	++	+	+++	++	+	++
Lurasidone (Latuda)	+/++	++/+++	+	++	+	++	++

Abbreviations: Anticholinergic, inhibition of binding or transduction through muscarinic acetylcholine receptors; EPS, extrapyramidal symptoms; TD, tardive dyskinesia.

3. Drug holiday: If a serotonergic antidepressant is required (eg, treatment of OCD), then judiciously planned "drug holidays" can be tested. This approach is most effective when the patient is using a relatively short half-life selective serotonin re-uptake inhibitor like venlafaxine or paroxetine. One common implementation has the patient skip their Friday morning dose of medication, with the intention of engaging in intercourse Saturday night, which is enough time for their blood levels to drop by more than half, potentially allowing their central serotonin levels to drop below the threshold that is inducing sexual dysfunction.
4. *Serotonin blockade*: When drug holidays are partially effective, it is reasonable to prescribe the short-acting anti-serotonergic antihistamine Cyproheptadine (Periac-tin; 4–16 mg) 1 to 2 hours before coitus, to further reduce the effective serotonin levels.
5. Antidotes: When all else fails, it is reasonable to proceed through a sequence of "antidote" trials, the most commonly used is as follows: (1) dopaminergic agents like Dexadrine IR (2.5–5 mg BID), Methylphenidate (10–30 mg), or Amantadine (100–200 mg BID); (2) Yohimbine (5.4 mg TID); (3) Sildenafil (50–200 mg 1-2 h before coitus); (4) Nefazadone (50–150 mg QD); as well as the previously mentioned agents (5) Cyproheptadine; (6) Buspirone; (7) Buproprion; and (8) Mirtazapine.

Lithium Toxicity

Lithium's effectiveness in treating manic-depression was first published in the medical literature in the mid-19th century,[50] yet its use has fallen out of favor among clinicians because of its narrow therapeutic window. It remains a highly effective agent for treat-ing a wide range of psychiatric conditions, including impulsive aggression and refrac-tory depression, and probably has greater efficacy as an antimanic agent than more modern treatments, like valproic acid.[51] Moreover, there is preliminary evidence that long-term lithium treatment is protective against developing Alzheimer dementia.[52–54] It is worth noting that lithium is a good example of a drug whereby patient concerns differ sharply from those of the prescribing physician. Clinicians will often neglect patient concerns about short-term quality-of-life issues. As a result, patients will often quickly discontinue lithium if they experience weight gain, skin blemishes, upset stom-achs, unsightly tremors, or memory problems.

To take advantage of this multifunctional drug, the outpatient clinician needs to be aware of both acute and chronic toxicity issues, which can become life-threatening. Nearly every patient will experience mild to moderate acute toxicity, most often the result of inadvertent dehydration (eg, during strenuous activity). Patients often report the rapid emergence of the symptoms of acute toxicity, which include the loss of fine hand-eye coordination, tremor, "fuzzy" thinking, or nausea and vomiting. If left un-treated, toxicity can progress to the development of emergent cardiac symptoms (arrhythmias and bradycardia), seizures, and encephalopathy, some of which may take months to resolve fully. Other more permanent side effects include thyroid dysfunction, nephrogenic diabetes insipidus, and tubular renal failure, although the latter seems to be relatively uncommon. As a general precaution, it is recommended that thyroid and renal function be tested 4 times the first year and then yearly there-after. A more complete discussion of lithium's adverse effects is reviewed in Refs.[55–57]

Dopamine Dysregulation Syndrome

Dopamine dysregulation syndrome occurs in patients receiving dopamine agonists for the treatment of PD or dystonia (inherited or sporadic). DDS symptoms may include excessive shopping, gambling, or hypersexuality, expansive, euphoric, or irritable moods, medication abuse, and complex compulsions (ie, punding). Although the medical literature often refers to excessive shopping, gambling, or hypersexuality as "compulsions," they are not. Among the general population, these symptoms are best described as behavioral addictions, whereby they may respond to the drugs naloxone, Acamprosate, or other "anticraving" treatments. The use of dopaminergic agents may activate a predilection toward these addictive behaviors. However, these goal-directed behaviors are also the most common symptoms of mania, exhibited by bipolar patients and amphetamine abusers. This distinction is important because common treatments for compulsions (ie, serotonergic antidepressants) or addictions are usually ineffective and may even worsen symptoms. In contrast, there is some evidence for the efficacy of the antimanic agents valproic acid, quetiapine, and clozapine.[58–60]

SUMMARY

Psychiatric symptoms often manifest years before overt neurologic signs in patients with inherited neurodegenerative disease. The most frequently cited example of this phenomenon is the early onset of personality changes in "presymptomatic" Huntington patients. In some cases the changes in mood and cognition are even more debilitating than their neurologic symptoms. These patients represent some of the more challenging patients that a clinician will face from the perspective of both psychiatric diagnosis and treatment; yet it is their neurologist, not a psychiatrist, who is responsible for their care. This article serves as a primer to the diagnosis, sequenced treatment, and longitudinal assessment of the most common psychopathology encountered among these patients, while still being concise enough to be applied in a busy neurology clinic or private practice.

REFERENCES

1. Anglin RE, Tarnopolsky MA, Mazurek MF, et al. The psychiatric presentation of mitochondrial disorders in adults. J Neuropsychiatry Clin Neurosci 2012;24(4): 394–409.
2. Wexler E, Fogel BL. New-onset psychosis in a patient with spinocerebellar ataxia type 10. Am J Psychiatry 2011;168(12):1339–40.
3. Brashear A, Cook JF, Hill DF, et al. Psychiatric disorders in rapid-onset dystonia-parkinsonism. Neurology 2012;79(11):1168–73.
4. Shapiro BE, Hatters-Friedman S, Fernandes-Filho JA, et al. Late-onset Tay-Sachs disease: adverse effects of medications and implications for treatment. Neurology 2006;67(5):875–7.
5. De Michele G, Pocchiari M, Petraroli R, et al. Variable phenotype in a P102L Gerstmann-Straussler-Scheinker Italian family. Can J Neurol Sci 2003;30(3): 233–6.
6. Trivedi MH, Rush AJ, Ibrahim HM, et al. The Inventory of Depressive Symptomatology, Clinician Rating (IDS-C) and Self-Report (IDS-SR), and the Quick Inventory of Depressive Symptomatology, Clinician Rating (QIDS-C) and Self-Report (QIDS-SR) in public sector patients with mood disorders: a psychometric evaluation. Psychol Med 2004;34(1):73–82.
7. Williams JR, Hirsch ES, Anderson K, et al. A comparison of nine scales to detect depression in Parkinson disease: which scale to use? Neurology 2012;78(13): 998–1006.
8. De Souza J, Jones LA, Rickards H. Validation of self-report depression rating scales in Huntington's disease. Mov Disord 2010;25(1):91–6.
9. Burns DD. The feeling good handbook. New York: Plume; 1999.

10. Rickards H, De Souza J, Crooks J, et al. Discriminant analysis of Beck depression inventory and Hamilton rating scale for depression in Huntington's disease. J Neuropsychiatry Clin Neurosci 2011;23(4):399–402.

11. Krishnamoorthy A, Craufurd D. Treatment of apathy in Huntington's disease and other movement disorders. Curr Treat Options Neurol 2011;13(5): 508–19.

12. Marin RS, Firinciogullari S, Biedrzycki RC. Group differences in the relationship between apathy and depression. J Nerv Ment Dis 1994;182(4):235–9.

13. Marin RS, Firinciogullari S, Biedrzycki RC. The sources of convergence between measures of apathy and depression. J Affect Disord 1993;28(2):117–24.

14. Marin RS, Biedrzycki RC, Firinciogullari S. Reliability and validity of the Apathy evaluation scale. Psychiatry Res 1991;38(2):143–62.

15. Clarke DE, Ko JY, Kuhl EA, et al. Are the available apathy measures reliable and valid? A review of the psychometric evidence. J Psychosom Res 2011;70(1): 73–97.

16. Young RC, Biggs JT, Ziegler VE, et al. A rating scale for mania: reliability, validity and sensitivity. Br J Psychiatry 1978;133:429–35.

17. Mollard E, Cottraux J, Bouvard M. French version of the Yale-Brown Obsessive Compulsive Scale. Encephale 1989;15(3):335–41.

18. Goodman WK, Price LH, Rasmussen SA, et al. The Yale-Brown obsessive compulsive scale. I. Development, use, and reliability. Arch Gen Psychiatry 1989;46(11):1006–11.

19. Stroup TS, Lieberman JA, McEvoy JP, et al. Results of phase 3 of the CATIE schizophrenia trial. Schizophr Res 2009;107(1):1–12.

20. Patton JH, Stanford MS, Barratt ES. Factor structure of the Barratt impulsiveness scale. J Clin Psychol 1995;51(6):768–74.

21. Lim SY, Evans AH, Miyasaki JM. Impulse control and related disorders in Parkinson's disease: review. Ann N Y Acad Sci 2008;1142:85–107.

22. Snaith RP, Taylor CM. Irritability: definition, assessment and associated factors. Br J Psychiatry 1985;147:127–36.

23. Olvera RL. Intermittent explosive disorder: epidemiology, diagnosis and management. CNS Drugs 2002;16(8):517–26.

24. Weintraub D, Mamikonyan E, Papay K, et al. Questionnaire for impulsive-compulsive disorders in Parkinson's disease-rating scale. Mov Disord 2012; 27(2):242–7.

25. Kick SD, Bell JA, Norris JM, et al. Validation of two anxiety scales in a university primary care clinic. Psychosom Med 1994;56(6):570–6.

26. Zung WW. A rating instrument for anxiety disorders. Psychosomatics 1971; 12(6):371–9.

27. Posner K, Brown GK, Stanley B, et al. The Columbia-suicide severity rating scale: initial validity and internal consistency findings from three multisite studies with adolescents and adults. Am J Psychiatry 2011;168(12):1266–77.

28. Seppi K, Weintraub D, Coelho M, et al. The Movement Disorder Society evidence-based medicine review update: treatments for the non-motor symptoms of Parkinson's disease. Mov Disord 2011;26(Suppl 3):S42–80.

29. Gaynes BN, Warden D, Trivedi MH, et al. What did STAR*D teach us? Results from a large-scale, practical, clinical trial for patients with depression. Psychiatr Serv 2009;60(11):1439–45.

30. Gaynes BN, Rush AJ, Trivedi MH, et al. The STAR*D study: treating depression in the real world. Cleve Clin J Med 2008;75(1):57–66.

31. Morris DW, Budhwar N, Husain M, et al. Depression treatment in patients with general medical conditions: results from the CO-MED trial. Ann Fam Med 2012;10(1):23–33.
32. Bobo WV, Chen H, Trivedi MH, et al. Randomized comparison of selective serotonin reuptake inhibitor (escitalopram) monotherapy and antidepressant combination pharmacotherapy for major depressive disorder with melancholic features: a CO-MED report. J Affect Disord 2011;133(3):467–76.
33. Rush AJ, Trivedi MH, Stewart JW, et al. Combining medications to enhance depression outcomes (CO-MED): acute and long-term outcomes of a single-blind randomized study. Am J Psychiatry 2011;168(7):689–701.
34. Cummings JL, Mega M, Gray K, et al. The neuropsychiatric inventory: comprehensive assessment of psychopathology in dementia. Neurology 1994;44(12):2308–14.
35. Velligan D, Prihoda T, Dennehy E, et al. Brief psychiatric rating scale expanded version: how do new items affect factor structure? Psychiatry Res 2005;135(3):217–28.
36. Flemenbaum A, Zimmermann RL. Inter- and intra-rater reliability of the brief psychiatric rating scale. Psychol Rep 1973;32(3):783–92.
37. Derogatis LR, Lipman RS, Covi L. SCL-90: an outpatient psychiatric rating scale–preliminary report. Psychopharmacol Bull 1973;9(1):13–28.
38. Morlan KK, Tan SY. Comparison of the brief psychiatric rating scale and the brief symptom inventory. J Clin Psychol 1998;54(7):885–94.
39. Nierenberg AA, Ostacher MJ, Calabrese JR, et al. Treatment-resistant bipolar depression: a STEP-BD equipoise randomized effectiveness trial of antidepressant augmentation with lamotrigine, inositol, or risperidone. Am J Psychiatry 2006;163(2):210–6.
40. Sheehan DV, Lecrubier Y, Sheehan KH, et al. The Mini-International Neuropsychiatric Interview (M.I.N.I.): the development and validation of a structured diagnostic psychiatric interview for DSM-IV and ICD-10. J Clin Psychiatry 1998;59(Suppl 20):22–33 [quiz: 34–57].
41. Preskorn SH, Flockhart D. 2010 Guide to Psychiatric Drug Interactions. Prim Psychiatr 2009;16(12):45–74.
42. Sirven JI, Noe K, Hoerth M, et al. Antiepileptic drugs 2012: recent advances and trends. Mayo Clin Proc 2012;87(9):879–89.
43. Perucca P, Gilliam FG. Adverse effects of antiepileptic drugs. Lancet Neurol 2012;11(9):792–802.
44. Culpepper L. The use of monoamine oxidase inhibitors in primary care. J Clin Psychiatry 2012;73(Suppl 1):37–41.
45. Boyer EW, Shannon M. The serotonin syndrome. N Engl J Med 2005;352(11):1112–20.
46. Bienvenu OJ, Neufeld KJ, Needham DM. Treatment of four psychiatric emergencies in the intensive care unit. Crit Care Med 2012;40(9):2662–70.
47. Schatzberg AF, Blier P, Delgado PL, et al. Antidepressant discontinuation syndrome: consensus panel recommendations for clinical management and additional research. J Clin Psychiatry 2006;67(Suppl 4):27–30.
48. Warner CH, Bobo W, Warner C, et al. Antidepressant discontinuation syndrome. Am Fam Physician 2006;74(3):449–56.
49. Koran LM. Obsessive-compulsive and related disorders in adults: a comprehensive clinical guide. Cambridge (United Kingdom), New York: Cambridge University Press; 1999.

50. Healy D. Some continuities and discontinuities in the pharmacotherapy of nervous conditions before and after chlorpromazine and imipramine. Hist Psychiatr 2000;11(44):393–412.

51. BALANCE investigators and collaborators, Geddes JR, Goodwin GM, Rendell J, et al. Lithium plus valproate combination therapy versus monotherapy for relapse prevention in bipolar I disorder (BALANCE): a randomised open-label trial. Lancet 2010;375(9712):385–95.

52. Forlenza OV, de Paula VJ, Machado-Vieira R, et al. Does lithium prevent Alzheimer's disease? Drugs Aging 2012;29(5):335–42.

53. Forlenza OV, Diniz BS, Radanovic M, et al. Disease-modifying properties of long-term lithium treatment for amnestic mild cognitive impairment: randomised controlled trial. Br J Psychiatry 2011;198(5):351–6.

54. Nunes PV, Forlenza OV, Gattaz WF. Lithium and risk for Alzheimer's disease in elderly patients with bipolar disorder. Br J Psychiatry 2007;190: 359–60.

55. McKnight RF, Adida M, Budge K, et al. Lithium toxicity profile: a systematic review and meta-analysis. Lancet 2012;379(9817):721–8.

56. Grunfeld JP, Rossier BC. Lithium nephrotoxicity revisited. Nat Rev Nephrol 2009; 5(5):270–6.

57. Freeman MP, Freeman SA. Lithium: clinical considerations in internal medicine. Am J Med 2006;119(6):478–81.

58. Sriram A, Ward HE, Hassan A, et al. Valproate as a treatment for dopamine dysregulation syndrome (DDS) in Parkinson's disease. J Neurol 2013;260(2): 521–7.

59. Fasano A, Ricciardi L, Pettorruso M, et al. Management of punding in Parkinson's disease: an open-label prospective study. J Neurol 2011;258(4):656–60.

60. Fasano A, Petrovic I. Insights into pathophysiology of punding reveal possible treatment strategies. Mol Psychiatry 2010;15(6):560–73.

61. Pan L, Vockley J. Neuropsychiatric symptoms in inborn errors of metabolism: incorporation of genomic and metabolomic analysis into therapeutics and prevention. Curr Genet Med Rep 2013;1(1):65–70.

62. Sedel F, Baumann N, Turpin JC, et al. Psychiatric manifestations revealing inborn errors of metabolism in adolescents and adults. J Inherit Metab Dis 2007;30(5):631–41.

63. Garside S, Rosebush PI, Levinson AJ, et al. Late-onset adrenoleukodystrophy associated with long-standing psychiatric symptoms. J Clin Psychiatry 1999; 60(7):460–8.

64. Rosebush PI, Garside S, Levinson AJ, et al. The neuropsychiatry of adult-onset adrenoleukodystrophy. J Neuropsychiatry Clin Neurosci 1999;11(3):315–27.

65. Sevin M, Lesca G, Baumann N, et al. The adult form of Niemann-Pick disease type C. Brain 2007;130(Pt 1):120–33.

66. Patterson MC, Hendriksz CJ, Walterfang M, et al. Recommendations for the diagnosis and management of Niemann-Pick disease type C: an update. Mol Genet Metab 2012;106(3):330–44.

67. Walterfang M, Fietz M, Fahey M, et al. The neuropsychiatry of Niemann-Pick type C disease in adulthood. J Neuropsychiatry Clin Neurosci 2006;18(2): 158–70.

68. Zaroff CM, Neudorfer O, Morrison C, et al. Neuropsychological assessment of patients with late onset GM2 gangliosidosis. Neurology 2004;62(12):2283–6.

69. Navon R, Argov Z, Frisch A. Hexosaminidase A deficiency in adults. Am J Med Genet 1986;24(1):179–96.

70. Neudorfer O, Pastores GM, Zeng BJ, et al. Late-onset Tay-Sachs disease: phenotypic characterization and genotypic correlations in 21 affected patients. Genet Med 2005;7(2):119–23.

71. Carta MG, Sorbello O, Moro MF, et al. Bipolar disorders and Wilson's disease. BMC Psychiatry 2012;12:52.

72. Shanmugiah A, Sinha S, Taly AB, et al. Psychiatric manifestations in Wilson's disease: a cross-sectional analysis. J Neuropsychiatry Clin Neurosci 2008;20(1): 81–5.

73. Taly AB, Meenakshi-Sundaram S, Sinha S, et al. Wilson disease: description of 282 patients evaluated over 3 decades. Medicine (Baltimore) 2007;86(2): 112–21.

74. Liszewski CM, O'Hearn E, Leroi I, et al. Cognitive impairment and psychiatric symptoms in 133 patients with diseases associated with cerebellar degeneration. J Neuropsychiatry Clin Neurosci 2004;16(1):109–12.

75. Leroi I, O'Hearn E, Marsh L, et al. Psychopathology in patients with degenerative cerebellar diseases: a comparison to Huntington's disease. Am J Psychiatry 2002;159(8):1306–14.

76. McMurtray AM, Clark DG, Flood MK, et al. Depressive and memory symptoms as presenting features of spinocerebellar ataxia. J Neuropsychiatry Clin Neurosci 2006;18(3):420–2.

77. Braga-Neto P, Pedroso JL, Alessi H, et al. Cerebellar cognitive affective syndrome in Machado Joseph disease: core clinical features. Cerebellum 2012; 11(2):549–56.

78. Schmitz-Hubsch T, Coudert M, Tezenas du Montcel S, et al. Depression comorbidity in spinocerebellar ataxia. Mov Disord 2011;26(5):870–6.

79. Klinke I, Minnerop M, Schmitz-Hubsch T, et al. Neuropsychological features of patients with spinocerebellar ataxia (SCA) types 1, 2, 3, and 6. Cerebellum 2010;9(3):433–42.

80. Schmitz-Hubsch T, Coudert M, Bauer P, et al. Spinocerebellar ataxia types 1, 2, 3, and 6: disease severity and nonataxia symptoms. Neurology 2008;71(13): 982–9.

81. O'Hearn E, Holmes SE, Calvert PC, et al. SCA-12: tremor with cerebellar and cortical atrophy is associated with a CAG repeat expansion. Neurology 2001; 56(3):299–303.

82. Duker AP, Espay AJ, Wszolek ZK, et al. Atypical motor and behavioral presentations of Alzheimer disease: a case-based approach. Neurologist 2012;18(5): 266–72.

83. Raaphorst J, Beeldman E, De Visser M, et al. A systematic review of behavioural changes in motor neuron disease. Amyotroph Lateral Scler 2012;13(6):493–501.

84. Rohrer JD. Behavioural variant frontotemporal dementia–defining genetic and pathological subtypes. J Mol Neurosci 2011;45(3):583–8.

85. Arvanitakis Z. Update on frontotemporal dementia. Neurologist 2010;16(1): 16–22.

86. Caycedo AM, Miller B, Kramer J, et al. Early features in frontotemporal dementia. Curr Alzheimer Res 2009;6(4):337–40.

87. Zamboni G, Huey ED, Krueger F, et al. Apathy and disinhibition in frontotemporal dementia: insights into their neural correlates. Neurology 2008;71(10): 736–42.

88. Laplanche JL, Hachimi KH, Durieux I, et al. Prominent psychiatric features and early onset in an inherited prion disease with a new insertional mutation in the prion protein gene. Brain 1999;122(Pt 12):2375–86.

89. Martorell L, Valero J, Mulet B, et al. M129V variation in the prion protein gene and psychotic disorders: relationship to neuropsychological and psychopathological measures. J Psychiatr Res 2007;41(10):885–92.

90. Starkstein SE, Brockman S, Hayhow BD. Psychiatric syndromes in Parkinson's disease. Curr Opin Psychiatry 2012;25(6):468–72.

91. Muller T, Gerlach M, Youdim MB, et al. Psychiatric, nonmotor aspects of Parkinson's disease. Handb Clin Neurol 2012;106:477–90.

92. Hattori N. Autosomal dominant parkinsonism: its etiologies and differential diagnoses. Parkinsonism Relat Disord 2012;18(Suppl 1):S1–3.

93. Weissbach A, Kasten M, Grunewald A, et al. Prominent psychiatric comorbidity in the dominantly inherited movement disorder myoclonus-dystonia. Parkinsonism Relat Disord 2013;19(4):422–5.

94. Heiman GA, Ottman R, Saunders-Pullman RJ, et al. Increased risk for recurrent major depression in DYT1 dystonia mutation carriers. Neurology 2004;63(4):631–7.

95. Vlastelica M. Psychiatric aspects of basal ganglia diseases. Psychiatr Danub 2011;23(2):152–6.

96. Thompson JC, Harris J, Sollom AC, et al. Longitudinal evaluation of neuropsychiatric symptoms in Huntington's disease. J Neuropsychiatry Clin Neurosci 2012;24(1):53–60.

97. Paulsen JS, Ready RE, Hamilton JM, et al. Neuropsychiatric aspects of Huntington's disease. J Neurol Neurosurg Psychiatry 2001;71(3):310–4.

98. Rosenblatt A, Leroi I. Neuropsychiatry of Huntington's disease and other basal ganglia disorders. Psychosomatics 2000;41(1):24–30.

99. Schneider SA, Bhatia KP. Huntington's disease look-alikes. Handb Clin Neurol 2011;100:101–12.

100. Wild EJ, Tabrizi SJ. Huntington's disease phenocopy syndromes. Curr Opin Neurol 2007;20(6):681–7.

101. Schneider SA, Walker RH, Bhatia KP. The Huntington's disease-like syndromes: what to consider in patients with a negative Huntington's disease gene test. Nat Clin Pract Neurol 2007;3(9):517–25.

102. Fischer CA, Licht EA, Mendez MF. The neuropsychiatric manifestations of Huntington's disease-like 2. J Neuropsychiatry Clin Neurosci 2012;24(4):489–92.

103. Anon. Low-dose clozapine for the treatment of drug-induced psychosis in Parkinson's disease. The Parkinson Study Group. N Engl J Med 1999;340(10):757–63.

104. Schulte P. Risk of clozapine-associated agranulocytosis and mandatory white blood cell monitoring. Ann Pharmacother 2006;40(4):683–8.

105. Szegedi A, Wetzel H, Leal M, et al. Combination treatment with clomipramine and fluvoxamine: drug monitoring, safety, and tolerability data. J Clin Psychiatry 1996;57(6):257–64.

106. Conus P, Bondolfi G, Eap CB, et al. Pharmacokinetic fluvoxamine-clomipramine interaction with favorable therapeutic consequences in therapy-resistant depressive patient. Pharmacopsychiatry 1996;29(3):108–10.

107. Figueroa Y, Rosenberg DR, Birmaher B, et al. Combination treatment with clomipramine and selective serotonin reuptake inhibitors for obsessive-compulsive disorder in children and adolescents. J Child Adolesc Psychopharmacol 1998;8(1):61–7.

108. Mavissakalian M, Jones B, Olson S, et al. The relationship of plasma clomipramine and N-desmethylclomipramine to response in obsessive-compulsive disorder. Psychopharmacol Bull 1990;26(1):119–22.

109. Pollack MH, Matthews J, Scott EL. Gabapentin as a potential treatment for anxiety disorders. Am J Psychiatry 1998;155(7):992–3.
110. Lavigne JE, Heckler C, Mathews JL, et al. A randomized, controlled, double-blinded clinical trial of gabapentin 300 versus 900 mg versus placebo for anxiety symptoms in breast cancer survivors. Breast Cancer Res Treat 2012; 136(2):479–86.
111. Blanco C, Antia SX, Liebowitz MR. Pharmacotherapy of social anxiety disorder. Biol Psychiatry 2002;51(1):109–20.
112. Sienaert P, Lambrichts L, Dols A, et al. Evidence-based treatment strategies for treatment-resistant bipolar depression: a systematic review. Bipolar Disord 2013;15(1):61–9.
113. Ketter TA, Wang PW, Chandler RA, et al. Dermatology precautions and slower titration yield low incidence of lamotrigine treatment-emergent rash. J Clin Psychiatry 2005;66(5):642–5.
114. Olie JP, Gourion D, Montagne A, et al. Milnacipran and venlafaxine at flexible doses (up to 200 mg/d) in the outpatient treatment of adults with moderate-to-severe major depressive disorder: a 24-week randomised, double blind exploratory study. Encephale 2009;35(6):595–604.
115. Boku S, Inoue T, Honma H, et al. Olanzapine augmentation of milnacipran for stage 2 treatment-resistant major depression: an open study. Hum Psychopharmacol 2011;26(3):237–41.
116. Detke HC, Zhao F, Witte MM. Efficacy of olanzapine long-acting injection in patients with acutely exacerbated schizophrenia: an insight from effect size comparison with historical oral data. BMC Psychiatry 2012;12:51.
117. Lewis C, Deshpande A, Tesar GE, et al. Valproate-induced hyperammonemic encephalopathy: a brief review. Curr Med Res Opin 2012;28(6):1039–42.
118. Barone P. Treatment of depressive symptoms in Parkinson's disease. Eur J Neurol 2011;18(Suppl 1):11–5.
119. Barone P, Poewe W, Albrecht S, et al. Pramipexole for the treatment of depressive symptoms in patients with Parkinson's disease: a randomised, double-blind, placebo-controlled trial. Lancet Neurol 2010;9(6):573–80.
120. Gaynes BN, Dusetzina SB, Ellis AR, et al. Treating depression after initial treatment failure: directly comparing switch and augmenting strategies in STAR*D. J Clin Psychopharmacol 2012;32(1):114–9.
121. Goldberg JF, Perlis RH, Ghaemi SN, et al. Adjunctive antidepressant use and symptomatic recovery among bipolar depressed patients with concomitant manic symptoms: findings from the STEP-BD. Am J Psychiatry 2007;164(9): 1348–55.
122. Swartz HA, Thase ME. Pharmacotherapy for the treatment of acute bipolar II depression: current evidence. J Clin Psychiatry 2011;72(3):356–66.
123. Coccaro EF. Intermittent explosive disorder as a disorder of impulsive aggression for DSM-5. Am J Psychiatry 2012;169(6):577–88.
124. Jones RM, Arlidge J, Gillham R, et al. Efficacy of mood stabilisers in the treatment of impulsive or repetitive aggression: systematic review and meta-analysis. Br J Psychiatry 2011;198(2):93–8.
125. Aboujaoude E, Koran LM. Impulse control disorders. New York: Cambridge University Press; 2010.
126. Hicks CW, Pandya MM, Itin I, et al. Valproate for the treatment of medication-induced impulse-control disorders in three patients with Parkinson's disease. Parkinsonism Relat Disord 2011;17(5):379–81.

127. Mico U, Bruno A, Pandolfo G, et al. Duloxetine as adjunctive treatment to clozapine in patients with schizophrenia: a randomized, placebo-controlled trial. Int Clin Psychopharmacol 2011;26(6):303–10.

128. Singh J, Kour K, Jayaram MB. Acetylcholinesterase inhibitors for schizophrenia. Cochrane Database Syst Rev 2012;(1):CD007967.

129. Smith RC. Metformin as a treatment for antipsychotic drug side effects: special focus on women with schizophrenia. Am J Psychiatry 2012;169(8):774–6.

130. Praharaj SK, Jana AK, Goyal N, et al. Metformin for olanzapine-induced weight gain: a systematic review and meta-analysis. Br J Clin Pharmacol 2011;71(3): 377–82.

Index

Note: Page numbers of article titles are in **boldface** type.

A

Acidemia(s)
    organic, 1035–1039
ADHD. *See* Attention deficit-hyperactivity disorder (ADHD)
Aggression
    inherited neurodegenerative diseases and, 1125
Akathsia
    anxiety *vs.,* 1125
ALS. *See* Amyotrophic lateral sclerosis (ALS)
Amino acid metabolism
    defects of, 1032–1041
        aminoacidopathies, 1039–1041
        clinical aspects of, 1032–1035
        organic acidemias, 1035–1039
        urea cycle defects, 1041
Aminoacidopathies, 1039–1041
Amyotrophic lateral sclerosis (ALS), **929–950**
    clinical course of, 929–931
    clinical findings in, 931–932
    defined, 929
    diagnosis of, 932, 939–940
    evaluation of, 939–940
    genetic basis of, 932–939
        ANG, 938
        C90RF72, 933
        FUS, 936–937
        OPTN, 938
        PFN1, 937–938
        SETX, 938
        SOD1, 933, 936
        TARDBP, 936
        UBQLN2, 937
        VAPB, 939
        VCP, 938
    genomics/risk variants for, 939
    incidence of, 931
    management of, 940
    nature of, 931
    physical examination in, 931
    symptoms of, 929–931
Antidepressant-induced sexual dysfunction
    inherited neurodegenerative disease management and, 1131–1136

http://dx.doi.org/10.1016/S0733-8619(13)00105-9
0733-8619/13/$ – see front matter © 2013 Elsevier Inc. All rights reserved.

Antidepressant withdrawal syndrome (AWS)
    inherited neurodegenerative disease management and, 1131
Anxiety
    akathsia *vs.,* 1125
Apathy
    inherited neurodegenerative diseases and, 1124
ASDs. *See* Autism spectrum disorders (ASDs)
Ataxia(s)
    defined, 988
    Friedreich, **1095–1120**. *See also* Friedreich ataxia
Attention deficit-hyperactivity disorder (ADHD)
    bipolar affective disorder *vs.,* 1124
    inherited neurodegenerative diseases and, 1124
Autism spectrum disorders (ASDs), **951–968**
    clinical course of, 952–953
    clinical findings in, 954
    defined, 951–952
    described, 951–952
    diagnosis of, 957
    evaluation of, 957
    genetic testing in, 957–962
    genetics of, 954–955
    incidence of, 951
    introduction, 951–952
    management of, 957
    nature of, 953
    pathology of, 955–957
    psychiatric comorbidities, 953
    symptoms of, 952–953
Autophagic vacuolar myopathies, 1022
Autosomal dominant spinocerebellar ataxias (SCAs), **987–1007**
    clinical course of, 988
    clinical findings in, 988
    defined, 987
    genetics of, 988–993
    genomics of, 996
    models of, 996–1002
    molecular pathogenesis of, 988, 994–995
        ion-channel mutations/dysfunction, 994–995
        noncoding repeats/RNA toxicity, 995
        polyglutamine ataxias, 994
        signal transduction, 995
    physical examination in, 988
    symptoms of, 988
AWS. *See* Antidepressant withdrawal syndrome (AWS)

B

Becker muscular dystrophy (BMD), 1010–1011
Benign familial neonatal epilepsy, 893
Benign infantile epilepsy, 893

Bipolar affective disorder
    ADHD *vs.,* 1124
    inherited neurodegenerative diseases and, 1124
BMD. *See* Becker muscular dystrophy (BMD)

C

Cerebrovascular disorders
    genetic architecture of, 920–923
        ischemic stroke, 920–921
Channelopathy(ies)
    muscle, 1022
Compulsion(s)
    impulsions *vs.,* 1124–1125
    inherited neurodegenerative diseases and, 1124–1125
Congenital muscular dystrophies, 1017
Congenital myasthenic syndromes, 1017
Congenital myopathies, 1017

D

Depression
    inherited neurodegenerative diseases and, 1122–1123
Distal myopathies, 1015, 1016
DMD. *See* Duchenne muscular dystrophy (DMD)
Dopamine dysregulation syndrome
    inherited neurodegenerative disease management and, 1136–1137
Dravet syndrome, 893, 897
Duchenne muscular dystrophy (DMD), 1010–1011
Dystonia, **969–986**
    clinical course of, 970–974
    clinical findings in, 975–978
    defined, 969
    diagnostic modalities in, 976–978
    genetics of, 979–980
    imaging in, 976
    introduction, 969–975
    management of
        medical, 980
        surgical, 980–982
    nature of, 975
    pathology of, 978–979
    physical examination in, 975
    symptoms of, 970–974

E

Early infantile epileptic encephalopathy (EIEE), 893
EDMD. *See* Emery-Dreifuss muscular dystrophy (EDMD)
EIEE. *See* Early infantile epileptic encephalopathy (EIEE)
Electromyography
    in dystonia, 976

Emery-Dreifuss muscular dystrophy (EDMD), 1014–1015
Epilepsy, **891–913**
    causes of
       genetic, 893–898
       structural/metabolic, 898–903
       syndromes with onset in childhood and adolescence, 897–898
       syndromes with onset in neonatal period and infancy, 893–897
    classification of, 892
    clinical findings in, 893–903
    defined, 891
    evaluation of, 903–906
    future directions in, 906–907
    genetics of, **891–913**
       introduction, 891–892
       primary, 893–898
       recent advances in, **891–913**
    management of, 906
    prevalence of, 891

F

Facioscapulohumeral muscular dystrophy (FSHD), 1011–1012
Fragile X–associated tremor/ataxia syndrome (FXTAS), **1073–1084**
    clinical course of, 1073–1074
    clinical findings in, 1075
    defined, 1073
    diagnosis of, 1075–1076
       future directions in, 1080
    evaluation of, 1079
    future directions in, 1080
    genetics of, 1076–1079
    imaging of, 1075–1076
    introduction, 1073–1076
    management of, 1079–1080
    models of, 1078–1079
    molecular pathogenesis of, 1078
    nature of, 1074–1075
    pathology of, 1076
    symptoms of, 1073–1074
Friedreich ataxia, **1095–1120**
    clinical course of, 1096
    clinical findings in, 1097–1098
    defined, 1095
    epidemiology of, 1096–1097
    evaluation of, 1105–1106
    future directions in, 1107–1114
    genetics of, 1100–1193
    genomics of, 1103–1105
    introduction, 1095
    management of, 1106–1107
    molecular pathogenesis of, 1101–1103

pathology of, 1098–1100
    symptoms of, 1096
FSHD. *See* Facioscapulohumeral muscular dystrophy (FSHD)
FXTAS. *See* Fragile X–associated tremor/ataxia syndrome (FXTAS)

G

GEFS+, 893
Genetic testing
    in ASDs, 957–962
Genetics
    of ASDs, 954–955
    of autosomal dominant SCAs, 988–993
    of dystonia, 979–980
    of epilepsy
        recent advances in, **891–913**. *See also* Epilepsy
    of Friedreich ataxia, 1100–1193
    of FXTAS, 1076–1079
    of HD, 1087–1089
    of neuropathic LSDs, 1061–1066
    of stroke, 918

H

HD. *See* Huntington disease (HD)
Huntington disease (HD), **1085–1094**
    clinical findings in, 1086–1087
    evaluation of, 1089–1091
    genetics of, 1087–1089
    introduction, 1085–1086
    management of, 1091–1092
        future directions in, 1092
    pathology of, 1087–1089

I

ICH. *See* Intracerebral hemorrhage (ICH)
Impulsion(s)
    obsessions and compulsions *vs.,* 1124–1125
Intracerebral hemorrhage (ICH)
    genetic architecture of, 921–922
Irritability
    inherited neurodegenerative diseases and, 1125
Ischemic stroke
    genetic architecture of, 920–921

L

LGMD. *See* Limb-girdle muscular dystrophy (LGMD)
Limb-girdle muscular dystrophy (LGMD), 1013–1014
Lithium toxicity
    inherited neurodegenerative disease management and, 1136

Lou Gehrig disease, **929–950**. *See also* Amyotrophic lateral sclerosis (ALS)
LSDs. *See* Lysosomal storage disorders (LSDs)
Lysosomal storage disorders (LSDs)
    neuropathic, **1051–1071**
        clinical course of, 1052
        clinical findings in, 1052, 1059–1060
        defined, 1051–1052
        diagnosis of
          future directions in, 1067
        evaluation of, 1066
        future directions in, 1067
        genetics of, 1061–1066
        introduction, 1051–1052
        management of, 1066–1067
        models of, 1065–1066
        molecular pathogenesis of, 1062–1065
        nature of, 1052
        symptoms of, 1052
        types of, 1053–1058

M

Mania
    inherited neurodegenerative diseases and, 1124
Metabolic disorders
    neurologic presentations of, **1031–1050**
        defects of amino acid metabolism, 1032–1041. *See also* Amino acid metabolism, defects of
        small molecular disorders, 1032, 1041–1048
Metabolic myopathies, 1018–1022
Monogenic stroke disorders, 918
Motor neuron disease, **929–950**. *See also* Amyotrophic lateral sclerosis (ALS)
Muscle channelopathies, 1022
Muscular dystrophy(ies), **1009–1029**. *See also specific types*
    autophagic vacuolar myopathies, 1022
    BMD, 1010–1011
    CMDs, 1017
    congenital myasthenic syndromes, 1017
    congenital myopathies, 1017
    diagnostic approach to, 1022–1025
    distal myopathies, 1015, 1016
    DMD, 1010–1011
    EDMD, 1014–1015
    FSHD, 1011–1012
    introduction, 1009–1010
    LGMD, 1013–1014
    metabolic myopathies, 1018–1022
    muscle channelopathies, 1022
    myotonic dystrophy, 1012–1013
    OPMD, 1015, 1017
    periodic paralysis, 1022

Myoclonic epilepsy of Doose, 897
Myopathy(ies)
    autophagic vacuolar, 1022
    congenital, 1017
    distal, 1015, 1016
    metabolic, 1018–1022
Myotonic dystrophy, 1012–1013

N

Neurodegenerative diseases
    inherited, **1121–1144**
        ADHD and, 1124
        aggression and, 1125
        anxiety *vs.* akathisia and, 1125
        apathy and, 1124
        behavioral management of, **1121–1144**
        bipolar affective disorder and, 1124
        clinical case, 1121–1122
        clinical findings in, 1122–1129
        evaluation of, 1126
        introduction, 1121–1122
        irritability and, 1125
        major depression in, 1122–1113
        management of, 1126–1129
            adverse effects related to, 1129–1137
                antidepressant-induced sexual dysfunction, 1131–1136
                AWS, 1131
                dopamine dysregulation syndrome, 1136–1137
                lithium toxicity, 1136
                serotonin syndrome, 1130
        mania and, 1124
        obsessions and compulsions *vs.* impulsions and, 1124–1125
        obsessions *vs.* perseveration and, 1125
        suicidality and, 1126
Neuropathic lysosomal storage disorders (LSDs), **1051–1071**. *See also* Lysosomal storage disorders (LSDs), neuropathic

O

Obsession(s)
    impulsions *vs.*, 1124–1125
    inherited neurodegenerative diseases and, 1124–1125
    perseveration *vs.*, 1125
Oculopharyngeal muscular dystrophies (OPMD), 1015, 1017
OPMD. *See* Oculopharyngeal muscular dystrophies (OPMD)
Organic acidemias, 1035–1039

P

Periodic paralysis, 1022
Perseveration

Perseveration (*continued*)
  obsessions *vs.*, 1125
Polysomnography
  in dystonia, 976
Psychiatric disorders
  ASDs and, 953

S

SCAs. *See also* Spinocerebellar ataxias (SCAs)
Sensory discrimination testing
  in dystonia, 978
Serotonin syndrome
  inherited neurodegenerative disease management and, 1130
Sexual dysfunction
  antidepressant-induced
    inherited neurodegenerative disease management and, 1131–1136
Small molecular disorders, 1032
Spinocerebellar ataxias (SCAs). *See also* Autosomal dominant spinocerebellar ataxias (SCAs)
  autosomal dominant, **987–1007**. *See also* Autosomal dominant spinocerebellar ataxias (SCAs)
  defined, 987
Stroke, **915–928**
  future research and clinical implications in, 923
  genetic disorders associated with, 918
  genetics of
    complex, 918–923
      genetic architecture of cerebrovascular disorders, 920–923
      overview of concepts and methodology, 918–920
  heritability of, 918
  introduction, 915–916
  ischemic
    genetic architecture of, 920–921
  as phenotype, 916–917
  phenotypes of
    intermediate cerebrovascular, 917
  subtypes of, 916–917
Suicidality
  inherited neurodegenerative diseases and, 1126

T

Transcranial magnetic stimulation
  in dystonia, 976

U

Urea cycle defects, 1041

W

White matter hyperintensity (WMH)
   genetic architecture of, 922–923
WMH. *See* White matter hyperintensity (WMH)

United States Postal Service

Statement of Ownership, Management, and Circulation
(All Periodicals Publications Except Requester Publications)

1. Publication Title
Neurologic Clinics

2. Publication Number
0 0 0 - 7 1 2

3. Filing Date
9/14/13

4. Issue Frequency
Feb, May, Aug, Nov

5. Number of Issues Published Annually
4

6. Annual Subscription Price
$285.00

7. Complete Mailing Address of Known Office of Publication (Not printer) (Street, city, county, state, and ZIP+4®)

Elsevier Inc.
360 Park Avenue South
New York, NY 10010-1710

Contact Person
Stephen R. Bushing

Telephone (Include area code)
215-239-3688

8. Complete Mailing Address of Headquarters or General Business Office of Publisher (Not printer)

Elsevier Inc., 360 Park Avenue South, New York, NY 10010-1710

9. Full Names and Complete Mailing Addresses of Publisher, Editor, and Managing Editor (Do not leave blank)

Publisher (Name and complete mailing address)

Linda Belfus, Elsevier, Inc., 1600 John F. Kennedy Blvd. Suite 1800, Philadelphia, PA 19103-2899

Editor (Name and complete mailing address)

Donald Mumford, Elsevier, Inc., 1600 John F. Kennedy Blvd. Suite 1800, Philadelphia, PA 19103-2899

Managing Editor (Name and complete mailing address)

Adrianne Brigido, Elsevier, Inc., 1600 John F. Kennedy Blvd. Suite 1800, Philadelphia, PA 19103-2899

10. Owner (Do not leave blank. If the publication is owned by a corporation, give the name and address of the corporation immediately followed by the names and addresses of all stockholders owning or holding 1 percent or more of the total amount of stock. If not owned by a corporation, give the names and addresses of the individual owners. If owned by a partnership or other unincorporated firm, give its name and address as well as those of each individual owner. If the publication is published by a nonprofit organization, give its name and address.)

Full Name	Complete Mailing Address
Wholly owned subsidiary of	1600 John F. Kennedy Blvd, Ste. 1800
Reed/Elsevier, US holdings	Philadelphia, PA 19103-2899

11. Known Bondholders, Mortgagees, and Other Security Holders Owning or Holding 1 Percent or More of Total Amount of Bonds, Mortgages, or Other Securities. If none, check box. ☐ None

Full Name	Complete Mailing Address
N/A	

12. Tax Status (For completion by nonprofit organizations authorized to mail at nonprofit rates) (Check one)
The purpose, function, and nonprofit status of this organization and the exempt status for federal income tax purposes:
☐ Has Not Changed During Preceding 12 Months
☐ Has Changed During Preceding 12 Months (Publisher must submit explanation of change with this statement)

13. Publication Title
Neurologic Clinics

14. Issue Date for Circulation Data Below
August 2013

15. Extent and Nature of Circulation

		Average No. Copies Each Issue During Preceding 12 Months	No. Copies of Single Issue Published Nearest to Filing Date
a. Total Number of Copies (Net press run)		913	880
b. Paid Circulation (By Mail and Outside the Mail)	(1) Mailed Outside-County Paid Subscriptions Stated on PS Form 3541. (Include paid distribution above nominal rate, advertiser's proof copies, and exchange copies)	439	390
	(2) Mailed In-County Paid Subscriptions Stated on PS Form 3541 (Include paid distribution above nominal rate, advertiser's proof copies, and exchange copies)		
	(3) Paid Distribution Outside the Mails Including Sales Through Dealers and Carriers, Street Vendors, Counter Sales, and Other Paid Distribution Outside USPS®	199	195
	(4) Paid Distribution by Other Classes Mailed Through the USPS (e.g. First-Class Mail®)		
c. Total Paid Distribution (Sum of 15b (1), (2), (3), and (4))	▶	638	585
d. Free or Nominal Rate Distribution (By Mail and Outside the Mail)	(1) Free or Nominal Rate Outside-County Copies Included on PS Form 3541	84	110
	(2) Free or Nominal Rate In-County Copies Included on PS Form 3541		
	(3) Free or Nominal Rate Copies Mailed at Other Classes Through the USPS (e.g. First-Class Mail)		
	(4) Free or Nominal Rate Distribution Outside the Mail (Carriers or other means)		
e. Total Free or Nominal Rate Distribution (Sum of 15d (1), (2), (3) and (4))	▶	84	110
f. Total Distribution (Sum of 15c and 15e)	▶	722	695
g. Copies not Distributed (See instructions to publishers #4 (page 83))	▶	191	185
h. Total (Sum of 15f and g)	▶	913	880
i. Percent Paid (15c divided by 15f times 100)		88.37%	84.17%

16. Publication of Statement of Ownership
☐ If the publication is a general publication, publication of this statement is required. Will be printed in the November 2013 issue of this publication.   ☐ Publication not required

17. Signature and Title of Editor, Publisher, Business Manager, or Owner

Stephen R. Bushing – Inventory Distribution Coordinator

Date: September 14, 2013

I certify that all information furnished on this form is true and complete. I understand that anyone who furnishes false or misleading information on this form or who omits material or information requested on the form may be subject to criminal sanctions (including fines and imprisonment) and/or civil sanctions (including civil penalties).

PS Form 3526, September 2007 (Page 1 of 3 (Instructions Page 3)) PSN 7530-01-000-9931 PRIVACY NOTICE: See our Privacy policy in www.usps.com

PS Form 3526, September 2007 (Page 2 of 3)

Printed and bound by CPI Group (UK) Ltd, Croydon, CR0 4YY

03/10/2024

01040492-0009

Moving?

Make sure your subscription moves with you!

To notify us of your new address, find your **Clinics Account Number** (located on your mailing label above your name), and contact customer service at:

Email: journalscustomerservice-usa@elsevier.com

800-654-2452 (subscribers in the U.S. & Canada)
314-447-8871 (subscribers outside of the U.S. & Canada)

Fax number: 314-447-8029

Elsevier Health Sciences Division
Subscription Customer Service
3251 Riverport Lane
Maryland Heights, MO 63043

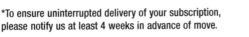